Middle Range Theory for Nursing

Second Edition

Mary Jane Smith, PhD, RN, earned her bachelor's and master's degrees from the University of Pittsburgh and her doctorate from New York University. She has held faculty positions at the following nursing schools: University of Pittsburgh, Duquesne University, Cornell University-New York Hospital, and The Ohio State University; and she is currently professor and associate dean for graduate academic affairs at West Virginia University School of Nursing. She has been teaching theory to nursing students for over 3 decades.

Patricia R. Liehr, PhD, RN, graduated from Ohio Valley Hospital, School of Nursing in Pittsburgh, Pennsylvania. She completed her baccalaureate degree in nursing at Villa Maria College, her master's in family health nursing at Duquesne University, and her doctorate at the University of Maryland–Baltimore, School of Nursing, with an emphasis on psychophysiology. She did postdoctoral education at the University of Pennsylvania as a Robert Wood Johnson scholar. Dr. Liehr is currently the associate dean for nursing research and scholarship at the Christine E. Lynn College of Nursing at Florida Atlantic University. She has taught nursing theory to master's and doctoral students for nearly 2 decades.

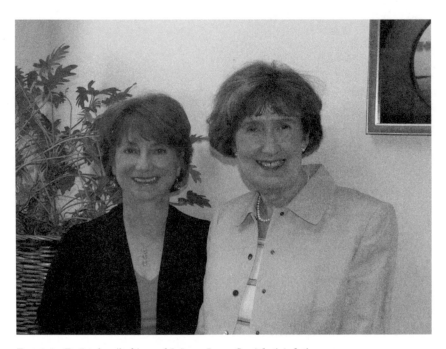

Patricia R. Liehr (left) and Mary Jane Smith (right).

Middle Range Theory for Nursing

Second Edition

Mary Jane Smith, PhD, RN
and
Patricia R. Liehr, PhD, RN
Editors

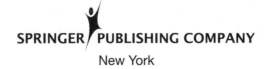

SPRINGER PUBLISHING COMPANY
New York

Springer Publishing Company, LLC
11 West 42nd Street
New York, NY 10036
www.springerpub.com

Acquisitions Editor: Allan Graubard
Production Editor: Julia Rosen
Cover design: Joanne E. Honigman
Composition: Apex CoVantage

08   09   10   11/   5   4   3   2   1

Library of Congress Cataloging-in-Publication Data

Middle range theory for nursing / Mary Jane Smith, Patricia R. Liehr, [editors]. — 2nd ed.
    p. ; cm.
  Includes bibliographical references and index.
  ISBN 978-0-8261-1916-2 (alk. paper)
   1. Nursing--Philosophy.   2. Nursing models.   3. Information science.   I. Smith, Mary Jane, 1938-   II. Liehr, Patricia R.
   [DNLM: 1. Nursing Theory.   2. Nursing Research.   WY 86 M627 2008]

RT84.5.M537 2008
610.7301—dc22   2008000940

Printed in the United States of America by Bang Printing.

Contents

Contributors

Bradley Aouizerat, PhD
Assistant Professor
University of California, San
Francisco
San Francisco, CA

**Virginia Carrieri-Kohlman,
DNSc, RN, FAAN**
Professor
School of Nursing
University of California, San
Francisco
San Francisco, CA

Heeseung Choi, DSN, RN
Assistant Professor
College of Nursing
University of Illinois at
Chicago
Chicago, IL

**Margaret F. Clayton, PhD,
RN, FNP**
Assistant Professor
School of Nursing
University of Utah
Salt Lake City, UT

**DorAnne Donesky-Cuenco,
PhD, RN**
Assistant Adjunct Professor
School of Nursing
University of California, San
Francisco
San Francisco, CA

Julia Faucett, PhD, RN, FAAN
Professor and Chair
School of Nursing
University of California, San
Francisco
San Francisco, CA

**Joyce J. Fitzpatrick, PhD, MBA,
RN, FAAN**
Elizabeth Brooks Ford Professor
of Nursing
Frances Payne Bolton School of
Nursing
Case Western Reserve University
Cleveland, OH

**Eugenie Hildebrandt, PhD,
RN, ANP**
Associate Professor
University of Wisconsin-
Milwaukee
School of Nursing
Milwaukee, WI

Janice Humphreys, PhD, RN,
   PNP, FAAN
Associate Professor
School of Nursing
University of California, San
   Francisco
San Francisco, CA

Susan Janson, DNSc, RN,
   ANP, FAAN
Professor and Harms/Alumnae
   Chair
School of Nursing
University of California, San
   Francisco
San Francisco, CA

Kathryn A. Lee, PhD, RN, FAAN
Professor and Livingston
   Chair
School of Nursing
University of California, San
   Francisco
San Francisco, CA

Elizabeth R. Lenz, PhD,
   RN, FAAN
Dean and Professor
The Ohio State University
School of Nursing
Columbus, OH

Geri LoBiondo-Wood, PhD,
   RN, FAAN
Associate Professor
University of Texas Health
   Sciences Center-Houston
School of Nursing
Houston, TX

Merle H. Mishel, PhD, RN, FAAN
Kenan Professor of Nursing
School of Nursing
The University of North Carolina
   at Chapel Hill
Chapel Hill, NC

Alvita Nathaniel, PhD, RN, APRN
Assistant Professor
West Virginia University School
   of Nursing
Charleston, WV

Cynthia Armstrong Persily, PhD,
   RN, FAAN
Professor and Associate Dean,
   Academic Affairs, Southern
   Region
West Virginia University School
   of Nursing
Charleston, WV

Linda C. Pugh, PhD, RNC
Professor
York College of Pennsylvania
School of Nursing
York, PA

Kathleen Puntillo, DNSc,
   RN, FAAN
Professor
School of Nursing
University of California, San
   Francisco
San Francisco, CA

Pamela G. Reed, PhD, RN,
   FAAN
Professor and Associate Dean
The University of Arizona College
   of Nursing
Tucson, AZ

Barbara Resnick, PhD, RN, FAAN
Professor
Sonya Ziporkin Gershowitz
    Chair in Gerontology
University of Maryland
School of Nursing
Baltimore, MD

Marlaine C. Smith, PhD,
    RN, FAAN
Helen K. Persson Eminent
    Scholar
Christine E. Lynn College of
    Nursing
Florida Atlantic University
Boca Raton, FL

Patricia L. Starck, DSN,
    RN, FAAN
Dean and Professor
University of Texas Health
    Sciences Center-Houston
School of Nursing
Houston, TX

Loretta A. Williams, PhD,
    RN, CNS, OCN
Department of Symptom
    Research
The University of Texas M.D.
    Anderson Cancer Center
Houston, TX

Foreword

This second edition of *Middle Range Theories for Nursing* extends the disciplinary boundaries of nursing and at the same time, deepens our understandings of core nursing content relevant to research and professional nursing practice. The importance of this contribution cannot be overestimated.

At the time of the publication of the first edition of the book, Smith and Liehr were pioneers in addressing middle range theories. Importantly, in that first edition the editors brought together eight middle range theories for nursing that had never been presented collectively. Since that time, doctoral education in nursing has vastly expanded, and the demand for knowledge of middle range theories has increased. While it is always important to introduce a movement, it is even more important to sustain a movement, especially for a developing discipline such as nursing.

In this new edition, there are 12 middle range nursing theories presented, evidence that the discipline has moved forward in the development of theoretical knowledge. Of the four new theories added, one, the theory of symptom management, serves as an umbrella for a considerable program of research in nursing. As such it has undergone much testing and provides strong support for application to professional nursing practice. The other new chapters, focused on theories of cultural marginality, caregiving dynamics, and moral reasoning are in the early stages of their development. It is important to include these new ideas so that, through systematic evaluation, nurse scholars can assist the authors in the theory refinement.

There also are new chapters that add considerable depth to the book. These chapters provide substantive content that will be useful to both faculty and students. They place middle range theory development within the context of disciplinary knowledge, a contribution that is needed for nurse scholars at all levels, including those in academic and clinical environments. One of the most important contributions that Smith and Liehr have made is to refocus attention on the theory lens of nursing knowledge development, particularly significant at a time when the focus has drifted to empirical and practical knowledge.

As with the first edition, there are key dimensions of the work that make it especially useful to new students of nursing theory, at the graduate and undergraduate levels. First, the structured format that is used across all theory chapters makes for a consistent level of explanation and analysis, and is especially useful for those trying to understand the similarities and differences in the theories. With this structure it is not difficult to assess knowledge development content components, or to evaluate the internal and external validity of the theories. Second, the ladder of abstraction diagrams that are presented for each of the theories provides a useful tool for those learning about middle range theories and how they are embedded in both philosophical and empirical referents. These figures also will serve as a springboard for future theorists, those who are using the middle range theories provided here to crystallize their own thinking about phenomena of interest within the discipline of nursing. And, importantly, each of the chapters is grounded in theory use in research and professional practice.

As with the first edition, this book is a welcome addition to nursing science literature. The content focus of the nursing discipline can be considered more critical for expansion, as nurse scholars search for their unique contribution to the understandings of health and wellness among individuals, families, and communities. This contribution extends our understandings and presents new opportunities for expanding the science of nursing through research and theory.

Joyce J. Fitzpatrick, PhD, MBA, RN, FAAN
Frances Payne Bolton School of Nursing
Case Western Reserve University

Preface

The interest in middle range theory continues to grow as demonstrated by the increased number of published theories as well as the desire among nursing faculty and researchers to have theories at the mid-range level to guide practice and research. The book is based on the premise that students come to know and understand a theory as the meaning of concepts are made clear and as they experience the way a theory informs practice and research in the everyday world of nursing. Over the past years, we have heard from students and faculty telling us that the book is user-friendly and truly reflects what they need as a reference to move middle range theory to the forefront of research and practice.

Middle range theory can be defined as a set of related ideas that are focused on a limited dimension of the reality of nursing. These theories are composed of concepts and suggested relationships among the concepts that can be depicted in a model. Middle range theories are developed and grow at the intersection of practice and research to provide guidance for everyday practice and scholarly research rooted in the discipline of nursing. We use the ladder of abstraction to articulate the logic of middle range theory as related to a philosophical perspective and practice/research approaches congruent with theory conceptualization.

The middle range theories chosen for presentation in this book cover a broad spectrum—from theories that were proposed decades ago and have been used extensively to theories that are newly developed and just coming into use. Some of the theories were originated by the primary nurse–author who wrote the chapter, and some were originally created by persons outside of nursing. After much thought and discussion with colleagues and students, we have come to the conclusion that theories for nursing are those that apply to the unique perspective of the discipline, regardless of origin, as long as they are used by nurse scholars to guide practice or research and are consistent with one of the paradigms presented by Newman and colleagues (Newman, Sime, & Corcoran-Perry, 1991). These paradigms, which are recognized philosophical perspectives unique to the discipline, present an ontological grounding for the middle range theories in this book. By connecting each theory with a paradigmatic perspective, we offer a view of the middle range theory's place within the larger scope of nursing science. This view was included to create a context for considering theories other than those developed by nurses that have been used to guide nursing practice and research.

We have added two new chapters on understanding and using middle range theory. Marlaine Smith's "Disciplinary Perspectives Linked to Middle Range Theories" elaborates on the structure of the discipline of nursing as a context for the development and use of middle range theories. This context is an important historical dimension for theory development today. It creates the foundation for what is shared in the chapters that follow. The second new chapter is titled "Building Structures for Research." This chapter presents a systematic approach to guide students in conceptualizing their ideas for research. The approach can also be used by faculty who teach courses in which students are working to establish their ideas for thesis and dissertation research. Included in this chapter are two exemplars written by students demonstrating use of the process. We decided to include this chapter as we simultaneously added to this edition of the book the theories of three new authors who had been our students. These students, like many others with whom we have engaged, contributed to our understanding of how to build structures for research. While this structure-building effort shares some of the processes of concept development, it is distinguished by its consistent foundation in nursing practice stories and its culmination in a newly created model to be used in research.

Four new middle range theories have been added to this second edition, bringing the total of theories in this book to 12. The new theories include: Symptom Management, Cultural Marginality, Caregiving Dynamics, and Moral Reckoning. The theory of Symptom Management has been in the forefront of practice and research by Humphreys and colleagues for over a decade. Inclusion of this established theory brings an added dimension to this second edition by representing the work of a team of researchers focused on symptoms. The three chapters describing new theories address major societal priorities that impact health in today's world. Immigration and the growing diversity of the nation call for related theory to inform understanding of health issues that arise for ethnically diverse populations. Choi's theory of cultural marginality describes one of these issues, being on the edge of two distinct cultures while trying to transition. The second societal priority is the growing population of frail elderly and persons with chronic illness who need help from caregivers in managing everyday living. Williams' theory of caregiving dynamics offers a perspective for guiding research and practice focused on the energy necessary to persist with caregiving over time. The third societal priority is the moral–ethical impact engendered by escalating use of technology and the complex nature of technologically driven health care delivery systems. Nathaniel's chapter on moral reckoning offers guidance in coming to terms with moral–ethical situational binds that arise in complex circumstances.

Those theories published in the first edition and included in this second edition are: Uncertainty, Meaning, Self-Transcendence, Community Empowerment, Unpleasant Symptoms, Self-Efficacy, Story, and Family Stress and Adaptation. Each chapter addressing a middle range theory follows a standard format. This includes purpose of the theory and how it was developed, concepts of the theory, relationships among the concepts and a model, use of the theory in nursing research, use of the theory in nursing practice, and conclusion. We believe this standard format facilitates a complete understanding of the theory and enables a comparison of the theories presented in the book.

Each theory is depicted on a ladder of abstraction that offers a clear and formal way of presenting the theories. The ladders were created by the editors and represent the editors' view of the philosophical grounding of the theory rather than the chapter authors' view. We have found that a ladder of abstraction can provide a starting place to guide students' thinking when they are trying to make sense of a theory. In addition, moving ideas up and down the ladder of abstraction generates scholarly dialogue. This process of moving up and down the ladder of abstraction is critical to building structures for research described in Chapter 3. The more dialogue on theory dimensions, the more likely it will be that theory will be understood, valued, and used as a guide for nursing practice and research.

The reader will notice when reading this book and comparing the theory descriptions from one edition of the book to the next that some theories have had ongoing development and use while others have received less attention and use during the last 5 years. The vibrancy of the theory is dependent on its use by scholars who critique and apply it, testing its relevancy to real-world practice and research. Proliferation of middle range theory without ongoing critique, application, and development is a concern that requires ongoing attention.

It is interesting that there are beginning clusters of middle range theories around important ideas for the discipline, such as symptoms. It would be useful to evaluate theory clusters, noting the common ground of guidance emerging from the body of scholarly work documented in the theory-cluster. An advantage of this effort would be that the thinking of unique nurse scholars would come together. One might expect that essential dimensions of the discipline could be made explicit by distilling and synthesizing messages from a theory-cluster. Although the analysis of theory clusters is not undertaken in this book, the information about middle range theory provided here creates a foundation for considering theory-cluster analysis.

In conclusion, this second edition represents a broader range of middle range theories including those that address societal priorities impacting health. The added chapters on disciplinary perspectives linked to middle range theory and on building structures for research contribute essential foundations related to the historical underpinning for middle range theory and the development and direction for future scholarly endeavors. As with the previous edition, we have edited and written with the intention of clarifying the contribution of middle range theory. We believe this clarification serves established as well as beginning nurse scholars seeking a theoretical foundation for practice and research.

Mary Jane Smith, PhD, RN
Patricia R. Liehr, PhD, RN

REFERENCE

Newman, M. A., Sime, A. M., & Corcoran-Perry, S. A. (1991). The focus of the discipline of nursing. *Advances in Nursing Science, 14,* 1–6.

Acknowledgments

An endeavor like this book is always the work of many. We are grateful to our students, who have prodded us with thought-provoking questions; our colleagues, who have challenged our thinking and writing; our contributors, who gave willingly of their time and effort; our publishers, who believed that we had something to offer; and our families, who have provided a base of love and support that makes anything possible.

CHAPTER 1

Disciplinary Perspectives Linked to Middle Range Theory

Marlaine C. Smith

Each discipline has a unique focus for knowledge development that directs its inquiry and distinguishes it from other fields of study. The knowledge that constitutes the discipline has some organization. Understanding this organization or the structure of the discipline is important for those engaged in learning the theories of the discipline and for those developing knowledge expanding the discipline. Perhaps this need is more acute in nursing because the evolution of the professional practice based on tradition and knowledge from other fields preceded emergence of substantive knowledge of the discipline. Nursing knowledge is the inclusive total of the philosophies, theories, research, and practice wisdom of the discipline. As a professional discipline this knowledge is important for guiding practice. Theory-guided, evidence-based practice is the hallmark of any professional discipline. The purpose of this chapter is to elaborate the structure of the discipline of nursing as a context for understanding and developing middle range theories.

The disciplinary focus of nursing has been debated for decades, but now there seems to be some general agreement. In 1978, Donaldson and Crowley stated that a discipline offers "a unique perspective, a distinct way of viewing . . . phenomena, which ultimately defines the limits and nature of its inquiry" (p. 113). They specified three recurrent themes that delimit the discipline of nursing:

1. Concern with principles and laws that govern the life processes, well-being, and optimum functioning of human beings, sick or well;
2. Concern with the patterning of human behavior in interaction with the environment in critical life situations; and
3. Concern with the processes by which positive changes in health status are affected (p. 113).

Nursing is a professional discipline (Donaldson & Crowley, 1978). Professional disciplines such as nursing, psychology, and education are different from academic disciplines such as biology, anthropology, and economics, in that they have a professional practice associated with them. According to the authors, professional disciplines include the same knowledge, descriptive theories, and basic and applied research common to academic disciplines. In addition, prescriptive theories and clinical research are included. So the differences between academic and professional disciplines are the additional knowledge required for professional disciplines. This is important, because many refer to nursing as a practice discipline. This seems to imply that the knowledge is about the practice alone and not about the substantive phenomena of concern to the discipline.

> Failure to recognize the existence of the discipline as a body of knowledge that is separate from the activities of practitioners has contributed to the fact that nursing has been viewed as a vocation rather than a profession. In turn, this has led to confusion about whether a discipline of nursing exists. (Conway, 1985, p. 73)

While we have made significant progress in building the knowledge base of nursing, this confusion about nursing lingers with other professions and in the public sphere.

Fawcett's (1984) explication of the nursing metaparadigm was another model for delineating the focus of nursing. According to Fawcett, the discipline of nursing is the study of the interrelationships among human beings, environment, health, and nursing. While the metaparadigm is widely accepted, the inclusion of nursing as a major concept of the nursing discipline seems tautological (Conway, 1985). Others have defined nursing as the study of the life process of unitary human beings (Rogers, 1970), caring (Boykin & Schoenhofer, 2001; Leininger, 1978; Watson, 1985), human–universe–health interrelationships (Parse, 1981), and "the health or wholeness of human beings as they interact with their environment" (Donaldson & Crowley, 1978, p. 113). Newman, Sime, and Corcoran-Perry (1991) created a parsimonious definition of the focus of nursing that synthesizes the unitary nature of human beings with caring: "Nursing is the study of caring in the human health experience" (p. 3).

My own definition uses similar concepts but shifts the direct object in the sentence: "Nursing is the study of human health and healing through caring" (Smith, 1994, p. 50). This definition can be stated even more parsimoniously: Nursing is the study of healing through caring. Healing comes from the same etymological origin as "health," haelen, meaning whole (Quinn, 1990, p. 553). Healing captures the dynamic meaning that health often lacks; healing implies a process of changing and evolving. Caring is the path to healing. In its deepest meaning it encompasses one's connectedness to all that is, a person-environment relatedness. Nursing knowledge focuses on the wholeness of human life and experience and the processes that support relationship, integration, and transformation. This is the focus of knowledge development in the discipline of nursing.

Defining nursing as a professional discipline does not negate or demean the practice of nursing. Knowledge generated from and applied in practice is contained within this description. The focus of practice comes from the definition of the discipline. Nursing has been defined as both science and art, with science encompassing the theories and research related to the phenomena of concern (disciplinary focus) and art as the creative application of that knowledge. Newman (1990) and others, perhaps influenced by critical/postmodern scholars, have used the term praxis to connote the unity of theory–research–practice lived in the patient–nurse encounter. Praxis breaks down the boundaries between theory and practice, researcher and practitioner, art and science. Praxis recognizes that the practitioner's values, philosophy, and theoretical perspective are embodied in the practice. Chinn refers to it as "doing what we know and knowing what we do" (Wheeler & Chinn, 1991, xii). Praxis reflects the embodied knowing that comes from the integration of values and actions and blurs the distinctions between roles of practitioner, researcher, and theoretician.

Middle range theories are part of the structure of the discipline. They address the substantive knowledge of the discipline by explicating and expanding on specific phenomena that are related to the caring-healing process. For example, the theory of self-transcendence explains how aging or vulnerability propels humans beyond self-boundaries to focus intrapersonally on life's meaning, interpersonally on connections with others and the environment, temporally to integrate past, present, and future, and transpersonally to connect with dimensions beyond the physical reality. Self-transcendence is related to well-being or healing, one of the identified foci of the discipline of nursing. This theory has been examined in research and used to guide nursing practice. With the expansion of middle range theories the skeletal outline of the discipline of nursing is enriched.

Several nursing scholars have organized the knowledge of the discipline into paradigms (Fawcett, 1995; Newman et al., 1991; Parse, 1987). The concept of *paradigm* originated in Kuhn's (1970) treatise on the development of knowledge within scientific fields. He asserted that the sciences evolve rather predictably from a preparadigm state to one in which there are competing paradigms around which the activity of science, normal science, is conducted. The activity of science to which he is referring is the inquiry examining the emerging questions and hypotheses surfacing from scientific theories and new findings. Paradigms are schools of shared assumptions, values and views about the phenomena addressed in particular sciences. It is common for mature disciplines to house multiple paradigms. If one paradigm becomes dominant and discoveries within it challenge the logic of other paradigms a scientific revolution may occur.

Parse (1987) modeled nursing with two paradigms: the totality and simultaneity. For her, the theories in the totality paradigm assert the view that humans are bio-psycho-social-spiritual beings responding or adapting to the environment, and health is a fluctuating point on a continuum. The simultaneity paradigm portends a unitary perspective. Unitary refers to the distinctive conceptualization of Rogers (1970, 1992) that humans are essentially whole and cannot be known by conceptually reducing them to parts. Also, the term unitary refers to the lack of separation between human and environment. Health is subjectively defined by the person (group or community) and reflects the process of evolving toward greater complexity and human becoming. Parse locates only two nursing conceptual systems/theories: the Science of Unitary Human Beings (Rogers, 1970, 1992) and the Theory of Human Becoming (Parse, 1981, 1987) in the simultaneity paradigm. For Parse, all nursing knowledge is related to the extant grand theories or conceptual models in the discipline. While she agrees that theories expand through research and conceptual development, she disagrees with the inclusion of middle range theories within the disciplinary structure if they are not grounded in the more abstract theoretical structure of an existing grand theory or conceptual model explicitly created by a nurse scholar.

Newman and colleagues (1991) identified three paradigms. These paradigms are conceptualized as evolving; the more complex paradigms encompass but extend the knowledge in a previous paradigm. The three paradigms are: particulate–deterministic, interactive–integrative, and unitary–transformative. From the perspective of the theories within the particulate–deterministic paradigm, human health and caring are understood through their component parts or activities; there is an underlying order and predictable antecedents and consequences, and knowledge development progresses to uncover these causal relationships. Reduction and causal inferences are characteristics of this paradigm. The interactive–integrative paradigm acknowledges contextual, subjective, and multidimensional relationships among the phenomena central to the discipline. The interrelationships among parts and the probabilistic nature of change are assumptions that guide the way phenomena are conceptualized and studied. The third paradigm is the unitary–transformative. Here, the person–environment unity is a patterned, self-organizing field within larger patterned self-organizing fields. Change is characterized by fluctuating rhythms of organization, disorganization, toward more complex organization. Subjective experience is primary and reflects the whole pattern (Newman et al., 1991, p. 4).

Fawcett (1995, 2000) joined the paradigm dialogue with her version of three paradigms. She named them: reaction, reciprocal interaction, and simultaneous action. This model was synthesized from the analysis of views of mechanism versus organism, persistence versus change, and the Parse and Newman and colleagues' nursing paradigm structure. In the reaction worldview, humans are the sum of the biological, psychological, sociological, and spiritual parts of their nature. Reactions are causal and stability is valued; change is a mechanism for survival. In the reciprocal interaction worldview, the parts are seen within the context of the whole, human–environment relationships are reciprocal; and change is probabilistic based on a number of factors. In the simultaneous action worldview, human beings are characterized by pattern and are in a mutual rhythmic open process with the environment. Change is continuous, unpredictable, and toward greater complexity and organization (Fawcett, 2000, p. 11–12).

Each middle range theory has its foundations in one paradigmatic perspective. The philosophies guiding the abstract views of human beings, human–environment interaction, and health and caring are reflected in each of the paradigms. This influences the meaning of the middle range theory, and for this reason it is important that the theory has a philosophical link to the paradigm clearly identified.

Figure 1.1 illustrates the structure of the discipline of nursing. This is adapted from an earlier version (Smith, 1994). The figure depicts the structure as clusters of inquiry and praxis surrounding a philosophic paradigmatic nexus. The levels of theory within the discipline based on the breadth and depth of focus and level of abstraction are represented. Theory comes from the Greek word, theoria, meaning "to see." A theory provides a particular way of seeing phenomena of concern to the discipline. Theories are patterns of ideas that provide a way of viewing a phenomenon in an organized way. Walker and Avant (1995) describe these levels of theory as metatheory, grand theory, middle range theory, and practice theory.

The figure depicts five levels of abstraction. The top oval includes the nursing metaparadigm and focus of the discipline of nursing. This is the knowledge beyond or at a more abstract level than theory per se. Grand theories are at the next level of the figure and include the abstract conceptual systems and theories that focus on the central phenomena of the discipline such as persons as adaptive systems, self-care deficits, unitary human beings, or human becoming. These grand theories are frameworks consisting of concepts and relational statements that explicate abstract phenomena. In the figure the grand theories cluster under the paradigms. Middle range theories are more circumscribed, elaborating more concrete concepts and relationships such as uncertainty, self-efficacy, meaning, and the others in this text. The number of middle range theories is growing. Middle range theory can be specifically derived from a grand theory or can be related directly to a paradigm. At the bottom level of the figure are the research and practice traditions related to the grand and middle range theories. Walker and Avant (1995) refer to this most specific level of theory as practice theory. Practice theories specify guidelines for nursing practice; in fact, the authors state that the word "theory" may be dropped to think of this level as "nursing practices" (p. 12) or what can be considered practice traditions. Both grand theories and middle range theories have practice traditions associated with them.

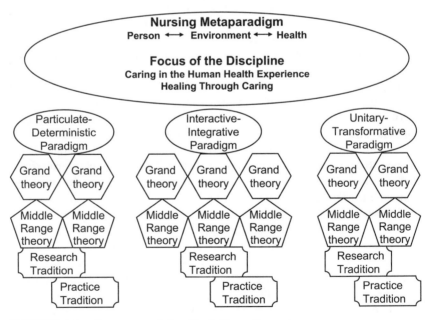

FIGURE 1.1   Structure of the discipline of nursing.

A practice tradition contains the activities, protocols, guidance, and practice wisdom that emerge from these theories. Models such as the LIGHT model (Andersen & Smereck, 1989) or the attendant nurse caring model (Watson & Foster, 2003) are examples. Smith and Liehr (2003) refer to these as micro-range theories, those that closely reflect practice events or are more readily operational and accessible to application in the nursing practice environment. Research traditions are the associated methods, procedures, and empirical indicators that guide inquiry related to the theory.

Some differentiate between grand theories and conceptual models. Fawcett (2000) differentiates them by how they address the metaparadigm concepts as she has defined them. Those that address the metaparadigm of human beings, environment, health, and nursing are labeled conceptual models, while those that do not are considered grand theories. Using her criteria, human caring theory (Watson, 1985) and Health as Expanding Consciousness (Newman, 1986) are considered grand theories. Walker and Avant (1995) include conceptual models under the classification of grand theories, and it seems more logical to define conceptual models by scope and level of abstraction instead of their explicit metaparadigm focus. In this chapter, the grand theories will be referred to as theories rather than conceptual frameworks.

The grand theories developed as nursing's distinctive focus became more clearly specified in the 1970s and 1980s. Prior to this time nursing scholars contributed to theoretical thinking without formalizing their ideas into theories. Nightingale's (1860/1969) assertions in *Notes on Nursing* about caring for those who are ill through attention to the environment are often labeled theoretical. Several grand theories share the same paradigmatic perspective. For example, the theories of Person as Adaptive System (Roy, 1989), Behavioral Systems (Johnson, 1980), and the Neuman (1989) System theory would share common views of the phenomena central to nursing that might locate them within the interactive–integrative paradigm. Others, such as the Science of Unitary Human Beings (Rogers, 1970), Health as Expanding Consciousness (Newman, 1986), and Human Becoming (Parse, 1998), cluster in the unitary–transformative paradigm.

There may be an explicit relationship between some grand theories and middle range theories. For example, Reed's (1991) middle range theory of self-transcendence and Barrett's (1988) theory of power are directly linked to Rogers's Science of Unitary Human Beings. Other middle range theories may not have such direct links to grand theories. In these instances, the philosophical assumptions underpinning the middle range theory may be located at the level of the paradigm rather than of the grand theory. Nevertheless, this linkage is important to establish the theory's validity as a nursing theory. Theoretical work is located in the discipline of nursing when it addresses the focus of the discipline and shares the philosophical assumptions of the nursing paradigms or one of the grand theories.

Some grand theories in nursing have developed research and/or practice traditions. Laudan (1977) asserts that sciences develop research traditions or schools of thought such as "Darwinism" or "quantum theory"; but in addition, Lauden's view includes the "legitimate methods of inquiry" open to the researcher from a given theoretical system (p. 79). Research traditions include the appropriate designs, methods, and instruments for data generation and analysis and emerging research questions and issues that are at the frontiers of knowledge development. They reflect the logical and consistent linkages between ontology, epistemology, and methodology. Ontology refers to the philosophical foundations of a given theory and is the essence or foundational meaning of the theory. Epistemology is about how one comes to know the theory and incorporates ways of understanding and studying the theory. Methodology is a systematic approach for knowledge generation and includes the processes of gathering, analyzing, synthesizing, and interpreting information. There is a correspondence between ontology (meaning), epistemology (coming to know), and methodology (approach to study) in order to give breadth and depth to the theory.

Examples of the connection between ontology, epistemology, and methodology are evident in several grand theories. For instance, the research-as-praxis method was developed by Newman (1990) for the study of phenomena from the Health as Expanding Consciousness (HEC) perspective, and a research method was developed from the theory of Human Becoming (Parse, 1998). Tools have been developed to measure theoretical constructs such as self-care agency (Denyes, 1982) or functional status within an adaptive systems perspective (Tulman et al., 1991), and debates on the appropriate epistemology and methodology in a unitary ontology (Cowling, 2007; Smith & Reeder, 1998) characterize the research traditions of some extant theories. These examples reflect the necessary relationship between theory, knowledge development, and research methods.

The practice traditions are the principles and processes that guide the use of a theory in practice. The practice tradition might include a classification or labeling system for nursing diagnoses or it might explicitly eschew this type of labeling. It might include the processes of living the theory in practice such as Barrett's (1988) deliberative mutual patterning or the developing practice traditions around Watson's theory such as ritualizing hand washing and creating quiet time on nursing units (Watson & Foster, 2003). The practice traditions are the ways that nurses live the theory and make it explicit and visible in their practice.

Middle range theories have direct linkages to research and practice. They may be developed inductively through qualitative research and practice observations or deductively through logical analysis and synthesis. They may evolve through retroductive processes of rhythmic induction–deduction. As scholarly work extends middle range theories we can expect research and practice traditions to continue developing. For example, scholars advancing uncertainty theory will continue to test hypotheses derived from the theory with different populations. Nurses in practice can take middle range theories and develop practice guidelines based on them. For example, oncology nurses whose worldviews are situated in the interactive–integrative paradigm may develop protocols to care for patients receiving chemotherapy using the theory of unpleasant symptoms. The use of this protocol in practice will feed back to the middle range theory, extending the evidence for practice and contributing to ongoing theory development. The use of middle range theories to structure research and practice builds the substance, organization, and integration of the discipline.

The growth of the discipline of nursing is dependent on the systematic and continuing application of nursing knowledge in practice and development of new knowledge. Few grand theories have been added to the discipline since the 1980s. Some suggest that there is no longer a need to differentiate knowledge and establish disciplinary boundaries because interdisciplinary teams will conduct research around common problems, eliminating the urge to establish disciplinary boundaries. Even the National Institutes of Health Roadmap rewards interdisciplinary research enterprises. This emphasis can enrich perspectives through interdisciplinary collaboration, but it is critical to approach interdisciplinary collaboration with a clear view of nursing knowledge to enable meaningful weaving of disciplinary perspectives.

Nursing remains on the margin of the professional disciplines and is in danger of being consumed or ignored if sufficient attention is not given to the uniqueness of nursing's field of inquiry and practice. There are hopeful indicators that nursing knowledge is growing. The blossoming of middle range theories signifies a growth of knowledge development in nursing. Middle range theories offer valuable organizing frameworks to phenomena being researched by interdisciplinary teams. These theories are useful to nurses and persons from other disciplines in framing phenomena of shared concern. Hospitals seeking magnet status are now required to articulate some nursing theoretic perspective that guides nursing practice in the facility. The quality of the practice environment is important for the quality of care and the retention of nurses. Theory-guided practice elevates the work of nurses leading to fulfillment and satisfaction and providing a satisfying professional model of practice.

The new role of the doctor of nursing practice has the potential to enrich the current level of advanced practice by moving it toward true nursing practice guided by nursing theory. The movement toward translational research and enhanced absorption of research findings into the front lines of care will demand practice models that bring coherence and sense to research findings. Isolated, rapid cycling of findings can result in confusion and chaos if not sensibly synthesized into a model of care that is guided not only by evidence but also by a guiding compass of values and a framework that synthesizes research into a meaningful whole. This is the role of theory. With this continuing shift to theory-guided practice and research, productive scientist–practitioner partnerships will emerge committed to the application of knowledge to change care and improve quality of life for patients, families, and communities.

REFERENCES

Andersen, M. D., & Smereck, G. A. D. (1989). Personalized nursing LIGHT model. *Nursing Science Quarterly, 2,* 120–130.

Barrett, E. A. M. (1988). Using Roger's Science of Unitary Human Beings in nursing practice. *Nursing Science Quarterly, 1*(2), 50–51.

Boykin, A., & Schoenhofer, S. O. (2001). *Nursing as caring.* Sudbury, MA: Jones & Bartlett.

Conway, M. E. (1985). Toward greater specificity of nursing's metaparadigm. *Advances in Nursing Science, 7*(4), 73–81.

Cowling, W. R. (2007). A unitary participatory vision of nursing knowledge. *Advances in Nursing Science, 30*(1), 71–80.

Denyes, M. J. (1982). Measurement of self-care agency in adolescents (Abstract). *Nursing Research, 31,* 63.

Donaldson, S. K., & Crowley, D. M. (1978). The discipline of nursing. *Nursing Outlook, 26,* 113–120.

Fawcett, J. (1984). The metaparadigm of nursing: Current status and future refinements. *Image: Journal of Nursing Scholarship, 16,* 84–87.

Fawcett, J. (1995). *Analysis and evaluation of conceptual models of nursing* (3rd ed.). Philadelphia: F.A. Davis.

Fawcett, J. (2000). *Analysis and evaluation of contemporary nursing knowledge: Nursing models and theories.* Philadelphia: F. A. Davis.

Johnson, D. E. (1980). The behavioral system model for nursing. In J. P. Riehl & C. Roy (Eds.), *Conceptual models for nursing practice* (2nd ed., pp. 207–216). New York: Appleton-Century-Crofts.

Kuhn, T. S. (1970). *The structure of scientific revolutions* (2nd ed.). Chicago: University of Chicago Press.

Laudan, L. (1977). *Progress and its problems: Toward a theory of scientific growth.* Berkeley: University of California Press.

Leininger, M. (1978). *Transcultural nursing: Concepts, theories and practices.* New York: Wiley.

Neuman, B. (1989). *The Neuman systems model* (2nd ed.). Norwalk, CT: Appleton & Lange.

Newman, M. A. (1986). *Health as expanding consciousness.* St. Louis: Mosby.

Newman, M. A. (1990). Newman's theory of health as praxis. *Nursing Science Quarterly,* *3*(1), 37–41.

Newman, M. A., Sime, A. M., & Corcoran-Perry, S. A. (1991). Focus of the discipline of nursing. *Advances in Nursing Science, 14*(1), 1–6.

Nightingale, F. (1860/1969). *Notes on nursing: What it is and what it is not.* London: reprinted by Lippincott, Philadelphia, 1946.

Parse, R. R. (1981). *Man-living-health: A theory of nursing.* New York: Wiley.

Parse, R. R. (Ed.). (1987). *Nursing science. Major paradigms, theories and critiques.* Philadelphia: Saunders.

Parse, R. R. (1998). *The human becoming school of thought: A perspective for nurses and other health professionals.* Thousand Oaks, CA: Sage.

Quinn, J. A. (1990). On healing, wholeness and the haelen effect. *Nursing and Health Care, 10*(10), 553–556.

Reed, P. G. (1991). Toward a nursing theory of self-transcendence: Deductive reformulation using developmental theories. *Advances in Nursing Science, 13*(4), 64–77.

Rogers, M. E. (1970). *An introduction to the theoretical basis of nursing.* New York: F. A. Davis.

Rogers, M. E. (1992). Nursing science and the space age. *Nursing Science Quarterly, 5,* 27–34.

Roy, C. (1989). The Roy adaptation model. In J. P. Riehl & C. Roy (Eds.), *Conceptual models for nursing practice* (2nd ed., pp. 179–188). New York: Appleton & Lange.

Smith, M. C. (1994). Arriving at a philosophy of nursing. In J. F. Kikuchi & H. Simmons (Eds.), *Developing a philosophy of nursing* (pp. 43–60). Thousand Oaks, CA: Sage.

Smith, M. C., & Reeder, F. (1998). Clinical outcomes research and Rogerian science: Strange or emergent bedfellows. *Visions: Journal of Rogerian Nursing Science, 6,* 27–38.

Smith, M. J., & Liehr, P. R. (2003). *Middle range theory for nursing.* New York: Springer Publishing.

Tulman, L., Higgins, K., Fawcett, J., Nunno, C., Vansickel, C., Haas, M. B., et al. (1991). The inventory of functional status-antepartum period: Development and testing. *Journal of Nurse-Midwifery, 36*(2), 117–123.

Walker, L., & Avant, K. (1995). *Strategies for theory construction in nursing.* Norwalk, CT: Appleton & Lange.

Watson, J. (1985). *Nursing: The philosophy and science of caring.* Boulder, CO: Associated University Press.

Watson, J., & Foster, R. (2003). The Attending Nurse Caring Model: Integrating theory, evidence and advanced caring-healing therapeutics for transforming professional practice. *Journal of Clinical Nursing, 12,* 360–365.

Wheeler, C. E., & Chinn, P. L. (1991). *Peace and power: A handbook of feminist process* (3rd ed.). New York: NLN.

CHAPTER 2

Understanding Middle Range Theory by Moving Up and Down the Ladder of Abstraction

Mary Jane Smith and Patricia R. Liehr

Every discipline has a process of reasoning that is rooted in the philosophy, theories, and empirical generalizations that define it. The reasoning process is logical when all levels come together and make sense in an orderly and coherent manner. The ladder of abstraction is a logical system for locating and relating three different and distinct levels of discourse: the philosophical, theoretical, and empirical. The purpose of this chapter is to describe the ladder of abstraction as central to understanding and using middle range theory in research and practice. The philosophical, theoretical, and empirical dimensions of the middle range theories presented in this book will be considered relative to the ladder of abstraction. The ladder of abstraction is a structure that maps the connection between levels of discourse (see Figure 2.1).

If one pictures a ladder with three rungs, the highest is the philosophical, the middle the theoretical, and the lowest the empirical. These rungs represent levels of discourse, or differing ways of describing ideas. The philosophical is the highest level, representing beliefs and assumptions that are accepted as true and fundamental to the theory. The philosophical level of abstraction represents belief systems essential to the reasoning found in the theoretical and empirical expression of middle range theories.

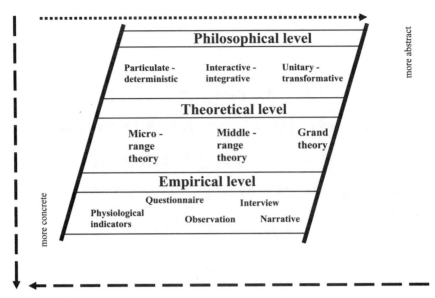

FIGURE 2.1   Ladder of abstraction.

The theoretical is in the realm of the abstract, consisting of symbols, ideas, and concepts. Many of the theories in this book are known by a central abstraction. For instance: uncertainty, meaning, and self-transcendence are some of the theoretically abstract ideas that will be discussed in this book. Implicit in abstraction is an outer shadow of vagueness that enables the ongoing development of the idea. This bit of vagueness can throw a person off guard and engender confusion about the meaning of an idea. However, the abstract nature of theory is not intended to be confusing or abstruse. In deciphering the abstract and differentiating ideas according to the philosophical, theoretical, and empirical, one figures out meaning and comes to know what is explicit about an abstract idea.

The empirical is the lowest rung on the ladder, at a concrete level of discourse. For instance, if ideas are expressed as practice stories, they are low on the ladder. The empirical represents what can be observed through the senses and moves beyond to include perceptions, symbolic meanings, self-reports, observable behavior, biological indicators, and personal stories (Ford-Gilboe, Campbell, & Berman, 1995; Reed, 1995).

Ideas are languaged to explain and describe their essence. Ideas at the theoretical level are concepts specific to a theory. Concepts characterize properties that describe and explain the theory at a middle range level of discourse. Levels of discourse are differing ways of expressing, defining, and specifying an idea. If one idea is more abstract than another, then it is more encompassing, enveloping a broader scope. On the other hand, if an idea is less abstract it is more concrete. This notion of the relationship between levels of abstraction is key to understanding and making sense of the theoretical. Levels of abstraction apply to each rung of the ladder in relation to the other rungs. That is to say, the philosophical is at a higher level than the theoretical. When one is grappling with understanding the theoretical or middle level on the ladder, the process is to move the idea up to evaluate the philosophical premise and move down to empirical indicators, where the theory connects to the world of practice and research. The concepts defining the structure of theory are learned by thinking through meaning in the context of nursing practice and research. To have a complete understanding one moves the theoretical idea back and forth, along the rungs of the ladder and within the rungs of the ladder. For example, if you were trying to understand a theory, a start at the middle rung of the ladder would lead to the question: How is the theory defined conceptually? What are the concepts, and what do the concepts mean? Then given the answers to the first set of questions, you would move to a lower ladder rung and ask: What does this mean to me and how does it connect with what I already know, namely my experience? Then one might look at how personal experience fits with the description of the theory. One might also question what values and beliefs are included in the assumptions of the theory, thus moving the theory up the ladder of abstraction. The point is that in coming to know the realm of the theoretical, one thinks through the theory by moving up and down the rungs of the ladder. The theory becomes understandable through discourse with self and with others through reading, thinking, and dialogue. Such discourse is always both tacit and explicit. This means that a person can begin to describe in words the meaning of an abstract idea and at the same time hold more knowledge about the idea than can be made explicit. Each time the idea is described through talking, writing, and discussion, a greater grasp is achieved.

It should be pointed out that staying on one rung deters understanding and limits ability to use the theory in practice or research. Persons may choose to stay on the rung that is most comfortable. For example, theorists may stay at the theoretical, and researchers may stay at the empirical, while meta-theorists may be more comfortable at the philosophical. It is a premise of this work on middle range theory that in order to move nursing science to the front lines of practice and research, nurses must be skilled in moving up and down and back and forth on the ladder of abstraction when studying, practicing, and researching the science of nursing.

When all levels of an idea can be mapped on the ladder of abstraction and the levels cohere with each other, the theoretical is guided by a logical process that provides clarity and facilitates understanding and use of the theory in research and practice. To understand a theory at all levels of abstraction requires a process of reasoning. By moving from the lower rung of the ladder to the middle and then the upper rung, one is making sense of phenomena through inductive reasoning. And conversely, movement from the upper philosophical rung to the theoretical and then to the empirical is deductive reasoning. The substantive knowledge of the discipline structured by logic guides thinking through nursing research and advanced nursing practice. This point flies in the face of the notion that theory is bewildering logic, abstruse and rather incomprehensible. There is logic to the abstract that can be reasoned through with the ladder of abstraction. Each level of the ladder will be discussed in the context of the middle range theories presented in this book.

PHILOSOPHICAL LEVEL

The philosophical level includes assumptions, beliefs, paradigmatic perspectives, and points of view. Reasoning through a nursing situation for practice and for research is based on assumptions. Assumptions are beliefs accepted as true about what constitutes reality. Assumptions about how individuals change are at the backbone of a theory. A paradigm is a worldview that includes disciplinary values and perspectives that are at the philosophical level.

Multiple paradigmatic schemas have been developed in nursing, and several of these are discussed in the first chapter. The schema used to guide discussion in this book is the one developed by Newman, Sime, and Corcoran-Perry (1991), who identified caring in the human health experience as the focus of the discipline of nursing. Then they identified three paradigms that guide the discipline: the particulate–deterministic, interactive–integrative, and unitary–transformative. Each paradigm incorporates unique values about health and caring and how change comes about. In the particulate–deterministic paradigm, the person is viewed as an isolated entity, change as primarily linear and causal, and the knowledge base is grounded in the perspective of the biophysical sciences. The interactive–integrative paradigm describes persons as reciprocal interacting entities, change as probabilistic and related to multiple factors, and grounding in the perspective of the social sciences. In the unitary–transformative paradigm, the person is viewed as unitary, evolving in a mutual and simultaneous process where change is creative and unpredictable, and the knowledge base is grounded in the human sciences.

One can clearly see that the three paradigms are at differing levels of philosophical abstraction because all three hold assumptions, values, and a point of view at differing levels of abstraction. The most abstract is the unitary–transformative, next is the interactive–integrative, and lowest in level of abstraction is the particulate–deterministic. This is an example of levels of abstraction within the philosophical rung of the ladder. Although theorists may not explicate their assumptions or paradigmatic perspective, a careful reading of the theory will lead to understanding about where the theorist stands in relation to a point of view and what makes up the philosophical underpinnings of the proposed theory.

The ladder of abstraction (Figure 2.1) depicts the highest level of abstraction as the philosophical level, including the particulate–deterministic, interactive–integrative, and unitary–transformative paradigms. The middle range theories presented in this book have been placed by the editors in one of these paradigms on the philosophical rung of the ladder. This was a judgment reflecting the view of two people that occurred through scholarly discourse. It is important for the reader to understand that different judgments may be made by different people who have a different understanding of the theory and the paradigms. There isn't a "right" way to link a theory with a paradigm, but there are always substantiated reasons for the linking decisions that are based on logical coherence. The editors made the decision about the theory–paradigm link based on the knowledge roots of the middle range theories.

The middle range theories of Uncertainty, Community Empowerment, Unpleasant Symptoms, Self-Efficacy, Family Stress and Adaptation, Symptom Management, Cultural Marginality, Caregiving Dynamics, and Moral Reckoning are rooted primarily in the social sciences and relate to a multidimensional and contextual reality. These nine theories have substantiated links to the interactive–integrative paradigm. The middle range theories of Story, Meaning, and Self-Transcendence are primarily rooted in the human sciences and relate to reality as a process of mutual and creative unfolding. These three theories describe values consistent with the unitary–transformative paradigm. There is value in understanding the paradigmatic perspective of a theory because it helps one lay out a starting point for a theory by establishing its philosophical foundation, where there is meaning for the theory's content, structure, and use in practice and research.

THEORETICAL LEVEL

The reader will note that the middle range theories found in this book are presented in the historical order of publication. This ordering decision was made based on the year the author introduced ideas relevant to the theory in a peer-reviewed publication. All theories in the book comply with the focus of nursing as presented by Newman and colleagues (1991), who say that nursing "is the study of caring in the human health experience" (p. 3). They go on to say "A body of knowledge that does not include caring and human health experience is not nursing knowledge" (p. 3). Caring is described as a moral imperative having a service identity. All 12 middle range theories described in this work have a focus of caring in the human health experience. Application of any one of these theories in practice or in research aims at facilitating change in the human health experience.

The human health experience is explicit in each of the theories as experiencing: uncertainty, suffering, vulnerability, community power, symptoms, decisions to make behavioral change, a complicating health challenge, family stress, living at the margin of cultures, giving care to another, and situation binds that demand moral reckoning. It is noteworthy that two of the middle range theories, Unpleasant Symptoms and Symptom Management, share the common human experience of symptoms. There is also common ground for the theories of Meaning and Self-Transcendence through their respective focus on suffering and vulnerability, which are intricately connected human health experiences.

Caring in the human health experience requires consideration of how the nurse lives relationships with people regarding their health. Based on these theories, some of the ways that caring transpires in the context of nursing are through promoting structure and order, inviting and engaging in dialogue, supporting inner resources, involving the community in creating health programs, understanding symptom experience and offering relief, tailoring information, responding to struggle, counseling caregivers, and discussing situational binds.

The middle range theories in this book add to the body of knowledge about nursing regardless of their discipline of origin. All of the theories have been applied in nursing practice and research to enhance caring in the human health experience. Theories belong to many disciplines. What is important to nursing science is that the research and practice based on a theory can be grounded in the focus and paradigmatic perspective of the discipline of nursing.

The theoretical rung on the ladder of abstraction includes concepts, frameworks, and theories. A theoretical concept is different from an everyday concept because it is a mental image of an aspect of reality that is put into words to describe and explain the meaning of a phenomenon significant to the discipline of nursing. A theoretical framework is a structure of interrelating concepts that describe and explain the meaning of a phenomenon. What then is a theory? Theory is described in the literature at all levels of abstraction. The accepted definition of a theory rests in the eye of the beholder. Chinn and Kramer (1999, p. 258) define theory as "a creative and rigorous structuring of ideas that project a tentative, purposeful and systematic view of phenomena." Im and Meleis (1999, p. 11) define theory as "an organized, coherent and systematic articulation of a set of statements related to significant questions in a discipline that are communicated in a meaningful whole to describe or explain a phenomena or set of phenomena." McKay (1969), on the other hand, describes theory as a logically interrelated set of confirmed hypotheses. Chinn and Kramer's definition of theory is at the highest level of abstraction, next is Im and Meleis, and at the lowest level is McKay. Given this array of theory definitions it is easy to understand why one could argue several ways about whether a particular theory is indeed a theory: it all depends on the way theory is defined.

Furthermore, there are levels of theory within the theoretical rung of the ladder. At the most abstract level, there are the grand theories. These are theories that have a very broad scope. The conceptual focus of some of these grand theories includes goal attainment (King, 1996), self-care (Orem, 1971), adaptation (Roy & Andrews, 1991), becoming (Parse, 1992), and unitary human field processes (Rogers, 1994). Each of these grand theories shares the common ground of offering a structure that enables description and explanation of essential conceptualizations of nursing. However, even on the common ground of grand theory, some are more abstract than others. For instance, becoming is more abstract than goal attainment.

Middle range theories, the subject of this book, are described by Merton (1968, p. 9) as those "that lie between the minor but necessary working hypotheses that evolve in abundance during day-to-day research and the all-inclusive systematic efforts to develop unified theory." He goes on to say that the principal ideas of middle range theories are relatively simple. Simple, here, means rudimentary straightforward ideas that stem from the focus of the discipline. Thus, middle range theory is a basic, usable structure of ideas, less abstract than grand theory and more abstract than empirical generalizations or micro range theory.

Micro range theories, described as situation-specific by Im and Meleis (1999, p. 13), are theories that focus on "specific nursing phenomena that reflect clinical practice and that are limited to specific populations or to particular fields of practice." These theories "offer a blue print that is more readily operational and/or has more accessible utility in clinical situations" (p. 19). It can be seen that this level of theory is lower on the ladder of abstraction than middle range theory. Examples of situation-specific theories are menopausal transition of Korean immigrant women, learned response to chronic illness of patients with rheumatoid arthritis, and women's responses when dealing with their multiple roles (Im & Meleis, 1999). The Ladder of Abstraction depicts micro range theory, middle range theory, and grand theory on ascending levels of discourse (Figure 2.1). The ladders for each theory presented here show a description of the philosophical, conceptual, and empirical connections. Each chapter's author has specifically identified theory concepts, so the inclusion of concepts on the ladder was a straightforward process. This may not always be true; sometimes the authors of published articles on middle range theory do not clearly identify concepts. In that instance, the reader is left to decipher what the concepts of the theory are and how they are defined. For some middle range theories it may be necessary to differentiate concepts by a very careful reading of the manuscript and examination of the model. When this interpretative process is needed, there is always a risk that the concepts identified by the reader are not exactly what the author of the theory intended.

EMPIRICAL LEVEL

The empirical level represents discourse that brings a theory to research and practice. Empirics include physiologic indicators, what can be learned from questionnaires, observation, and interview and narrative (Figure 2.1). Like other rungs on the ladder, the empirical level of discourse moves from the most concrete (physiologic indicators) to the most abstract (narrative). Even at this lowest level of discourse there is a range of abstraction.

Whether doing practice or research, the nurse connects with the empirical level. The advanced practice nurse may use physiologic indicators, interview, and observation while applying theory to caring in the human health experience. The nurse researcher may use observation and narrative in a single study while applying theory to examine caring in the human health experience. Decisions about empirics are guided by philosophy and theory. It is important that the nurse choose empirics that fit with philosophic and theoretical perspectives.

MIDDLE RANGE THEORIES ON THE
LADDER OF ABSTRACTION

There are 12 middle range theories in the book, presented in chronological order according to when the chapter author introduced the idea in a refereed publication. For instance, although the Theory of Meaning was first presented by Starck as a theory in 2003, she began using Viktor Frankl's ideas in her dissertation research, where she studied perception of meaning and purpose in life for people who had suffered spinal cord injury. The first date noted in her chapter citing this work is 1979 in *Dissertation Abstracts*. In 1985, she published an article on logotherapy, which we identified as the first related work published in a refereed journal. Starck's place in the order of authors reflects the 1985 citation. This approach to ordering the chapters places explicit emphasis on the continued work necessary to grow ideas over time; implicit emphasis suggests that nursing scholars must be willing to persist with the sometimes tedious work of theory building, and this work occurs with spurts and stalls usually over decades.

The first middle range theory encompasses the Uncertainty in Illness and Reconceptualized Uncertainty in Illness middle range theories. Mishel and Clayton address both of these theories in Chapter 4. The original uncertainty theory pertains to acute illness while the reconceptualized theory pertains to the continual uncertainty experienced in chronic illness. On the ladder, the reconceptualization is represented in bold print at the philosophical and theoretical level. The theories are consistent with beliefs associated with the interactive–integrative paradigm.

Persons experience uncertainty during diagnosis and treatment and when illness has a downward trajectory, and persons experience continual uncertainty in ongoing chronic illness and also with the possibility of recurrence of an illness. Concepts at the theoretical level in both theories are antecedents of uncertainty, appraisal of uncertainty, and coping with uncertainty. Concepts added in the reconceptualized theory include self-organization and probabilistic thinking. Moving to the empirical level with practice is offering information and explanation, providing structure and order, and focusing on choices and alternatives. An instrument has been developed that is directly related to the theory, the uncertainty in illness scale (see Figure 2.2).

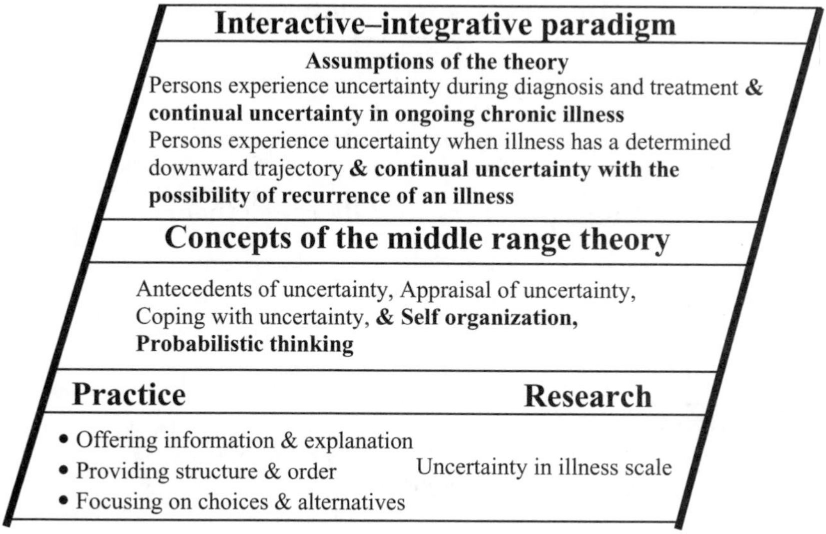

Interactive–integrative paradigm

Assumptions of the theory
Persons experience uncertainty during diagnosis and treatment **&
continual uncertainty in ongoing chronic illness**
Persons experience uncertainty when illness has a determined
downward trajectory **& continual uncertainty with the
possibility of recurrence of an illness**

Concepts of the middle range theory

Antecedents of uncertainty, Appraisal of uncertainty,
Coping with uncertainty, **& Self organization,
Probabilistic thinking**

Practice   **Research**

• Offering information & explanation
• Providing structure & order   Uncertainty in illness scale
• Focusing on choices & alternatives

FIGURE 2.2 Ladder of abstraction: Uncertainty in illness.

The second middle range theory presented is Starck's Theory of Meaning, based on the work of Viktor Frankl. This theory is grounded in the unitary–transformative paradigm. It is assumed that through a transformative process, persons find meaning. When confronted with a hopeless situation, meaning can be freely and responsibly realized in every moment. Concepts at the theoretical level include life purpose, freedom to choose, and suffering. Practice approaches at the empirical level include dereflection, paradoxical intention, and Socratic dialogue. Empirical indicators for research include questionnaires, interview, and other narrative approaches (see Figure 2.3).

The third middle range theory, Self-Transcendence developed by Reed, is grounded in assumptions of the unitary–transformative paradigm. Self-transcendence is a unitary process. The theory assumes that persons are integral and coextensive with their environment and capable of an awareness that extends beyond physical and temporal dimensions. Concepts at the theoretical level of discourse include vulnerability, self-transcendence, and well-being. Taking the theory to the empirical level with practice includes integrative spiritual care, support of inner resources, and expansion of intrapersonal, interpersonal, temporal, and transpersonal boundaries. Like the theory of uncertainty, a research instrument has been developed that is directly related to the theory, the self-transcendence scale (see Figure 2.4).

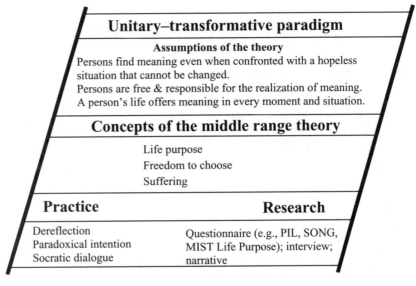

FIGURE 2.3   Ladder of abstraction: Meaning.

The fourth middle range theory, Community Empowerment, is presented by Persily and Hildebrandt. This theory is grounded in the beliefs of the interactive–integrative paradigm, in which change is an interactive process related to multiple factors in the community. Communities are empowered through an interactive–integrative reciprocal process. Specific assumptions for this theory are that communities are complex, experience can be generalized, and answers to health problems lie in and with the community. Theoretical concepts are involvement, lay workers, and reciprocal health. Reciprocal health is the outcome of community involvement with lay workers. Practice and research at the empirical level includes lay workers at the interface with traditional health care providers in the community (see Figure 2.5).

The fifth theory presented in the book is Symptom Management Theory by Humphreys, Lee, Carrieri-Kohlman, Puntillo, Faucett, Janson, Aouizerat, and Donesky-Cuenco. This theory is grounded in assumptions of the interactive–integrative paradigm, in which persons manage their symptoms in interaction with the environment. The specific assumptions of the theory include that health and illness affect symptom management, that improvement in symptoms extends beyond personal health, and that symptoms are subjective and experienced in clusters. There are three concepts at the middle range level of discourse. The concepts are symptom experience, symptom management strategies, and symptom status outcomes. At the empirical level, practice application occurs with patient–provider

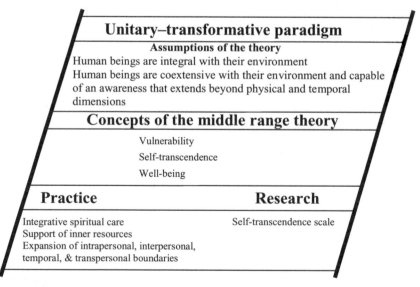

Unitary–transformative paradigm

Assumptions of the theory
Human beings are integral with their environment
Human beings are coextensive with their environment and capable of an awareness that extends beyond physical and temporal dimensions

Concepts of the middle range theory

Vulnerability

Self-transcendence

Well-being

Practice   **Research**

Integrative spiritual care   Self-transcendence scale
Support of inner resources
Expansion of intrapersonal, interpersonal,
temporal, & transpersonal boundaries

FIGURE 2.4   Ladder of abstraction: Self-transcendence.

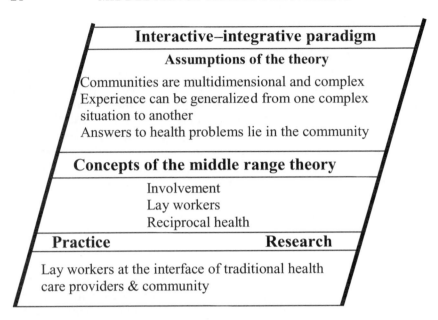

FIGURE 2.5   Ladder of abstraction: Community empowerment.

communication marked by an understanding of the symptom experience and the implementation of effective strategies. Research application includes measurement of symptom-specific outcomes and contextual factors related to the symptom under study (see Figure 2.6).

The sixth middle range theory is Unpleasant Symptoms by Lenz and Pugh. The theory is grounded in the beliefs and assumptions associated with the interactive–integrative paradigm. Specific beliefs of the theory are that there are commonalities across different symptoms experienced by persons in varied situations, and symptoms are subjective phenomena occurring in family and community contexts. Concepts at the theoretical level include symptoms, influencing factors, and performance. Practice application at the empirical level includes assessment of the symptom, symptom management, and relief intervention. Empirical measurements are gathered through scales and observations that capture the symptom experience (see Figure 2.7).

The seventh middle range theory is Self-Efficacy by Resnick, grounded in the assumptions of the interactive–integrative paradigm. Persons change in a reciprocal interactive process when they exercise influence over what they do and decide how to behave. Concepts at the theoretical level include self-efficacy expectations and self-efficacy outcomes. Examples of practice applications at the empirical level include learning about exercise, addressing unpleasant sensations, and cueing to exercise. Research based on this middle range theory uses self-efficacy scales (see Figure 2.8).

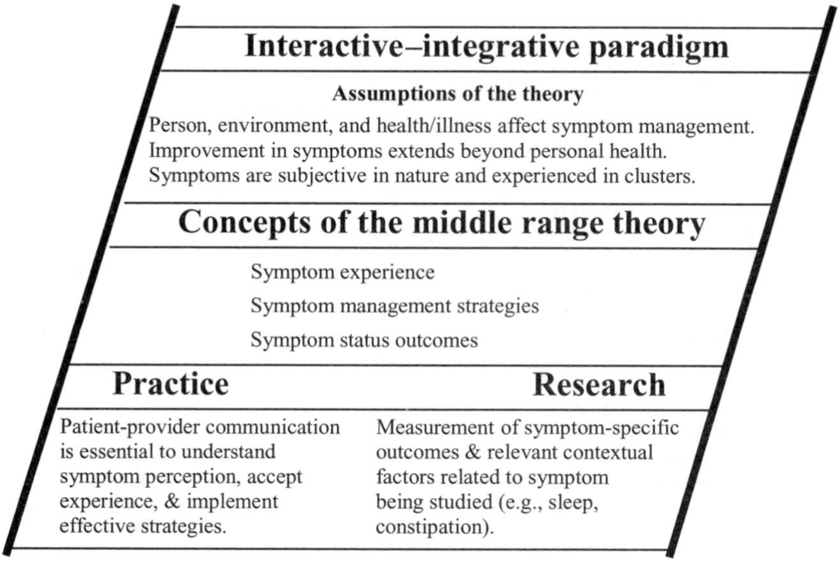

FIGURE 2.6   Ladder of abstraction: Symptom management.

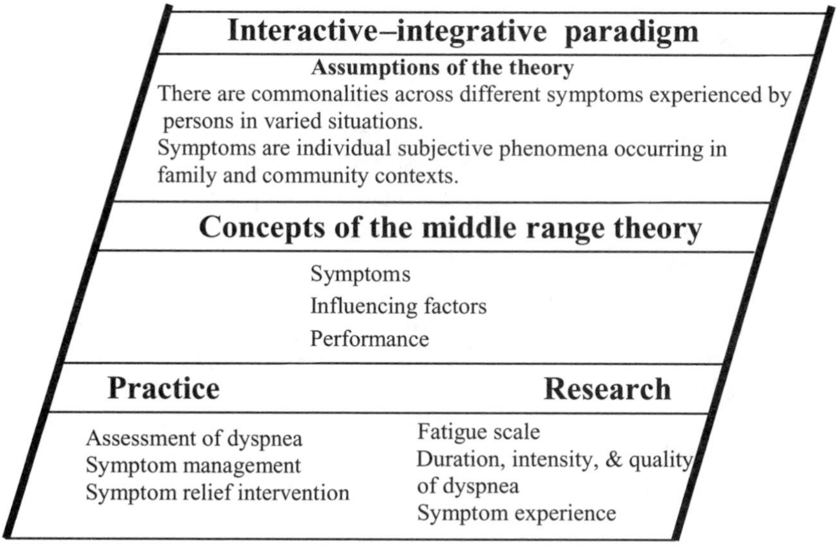

FIGURE 2.7   Ladder of abstraction: Unpleasant symptoms.

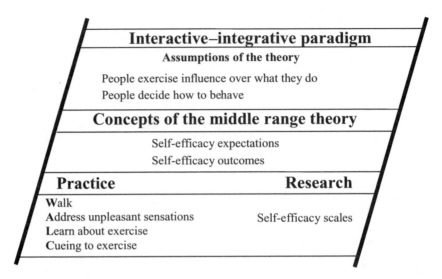

FIGURE 2.8   Ladder of abstraction: Self-efficacy.

The eighth middle range theory presented is Liehr and Smith's Story Theory, which is grounded in the assumptions of the unitary–transformative paradigm where change is viewed as creative and unpredictable. The name of this theory has changed over the last several years from "attentively embracing story" to Story Theory. Story is a narrative happening that enables transformative experience in the unitary nurse–person process. The specific assumptions of the theory include that persons change in interrelationship with their world as they live an expanded present and experience meaning. There are three concepts at the theoretical level: intentional dialogue, connecting with self-in-relation, and creating ease. At the empirical level the health story is the basis for both practice and research. Examples of empirical approaches in practice include creation of a story path and family tree. Health story data may be analyzed using phenomenological, linguistic, case study, or story inquiry methods (see Figure 2.9).

The ninth middle range theory, Family Stress and Adaptation by LoBiondo-Wood, is grounded in the interactive–integrative paradigm. Families change through reciprocal interactive processes that are related to multiple factors. Beliefs about family stress and adaptation are that hardship is natural and predictable; basic competencies foster family growth; families give to and take from a relationship network; and families facing crisis work together. Concepts of this theory include stressor, existing resources, perception of the stressor, crisis, pile-up, existing and new resources, perception, coping, and adaptation. Empirics related to this theory include practice interventions based on illness trajectories and research measures of stress and adaptation (see Figure 2.10).

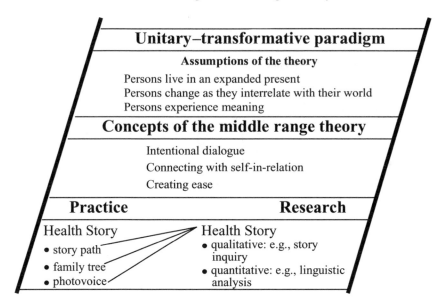

FIGURE 2.9   Ladder of abstraction: Story.

The 10th theory presented in this book is the Theory of Cultural Marginality developed by Choi. This theory is embedded in the interactive–integrative paradigm and it describes the experience of people who are caught between two cultures. Assumptions specific to the theory include across-cultural conflict recognition, marginal living, and easing cultural tension. Examples of practice applications include promoting parent–child engagement through cross-cultural understanding and being sensitive to the struggle of immigration. Research activities are aimed at developing an instrument to measure cultural marginality and studying mental health outcomes of persons living through across-culture conflict (see Figure 2.11).

The 11th theory found in the book is the Theory of Caregiving Dynamics by Williams. This theory is in keeping with the assumptions of the interactive–integrative paradigm and holds that the interactive caregiving relationship extends over time. Specific assumptions include recognition of the coexistence of negative and positive aspects of caregiving, distinction between informal and formal caregiving, and the emerging nature of the caregiving relationship over time. Concepts descriptive of the theory are commitment, expectation management, and role negotiation. Application of the theory in practice consists of caregiver classes with tailored information, attention to exercise and nutrition, and counseling. Research based on the theory focuses on the care recipient's view and testing interventions that enhance the caregiving relationship (see Figure 2.12).

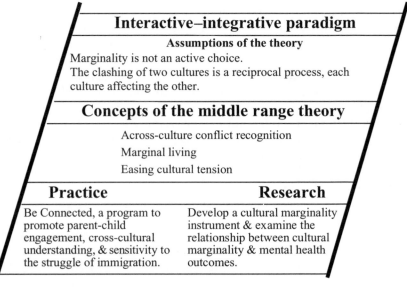

Interactive–integrative paradigm	
Assumptions of the theory	
Hardship is a natural & predictable aspect of family life	
Families develop basic competencies, patterns, & capabilities that foster growth, protect, & enable recovery	
Families draw from & contribute to a relationship network	
Families faced with crisis work to restore order	
Concepts of the middle range theory	
Stressor	Pile-up
Existing resources	Existing & new resources
Perception of the stressor	Family perception of the stressor
Crisis	Coping
	Adaptation
Practice	**Research**
Understanding family response to illness trajectory enables intervention	Measures such as FILE, FIRM, CHIP, FCCI, FAD

FIGURE 2.10   Ladder of abstraction: Family stress and adaptation.

Interactive–integrative paradigm	
Assumptions of the theory	
Marginality is not an active choice.	
The clashing of two cultures is a reciprocal process, each culture affecting the other.	
Concepts of the middle range theory	
Across-culture conflict recognition	
Marginal living	
Easing cultural tension	
Practice	**Research**
Be Connected, a program to promote parent-child engagement, cross-cultural understanding, & sensitivity to the struggle of immigration.	Develop a cultural marginality instrument & examine the relationship between cultural marginality & mental health outcomes.

FIGURE 2.11   Ladder of abstraction: Cultural marginality.

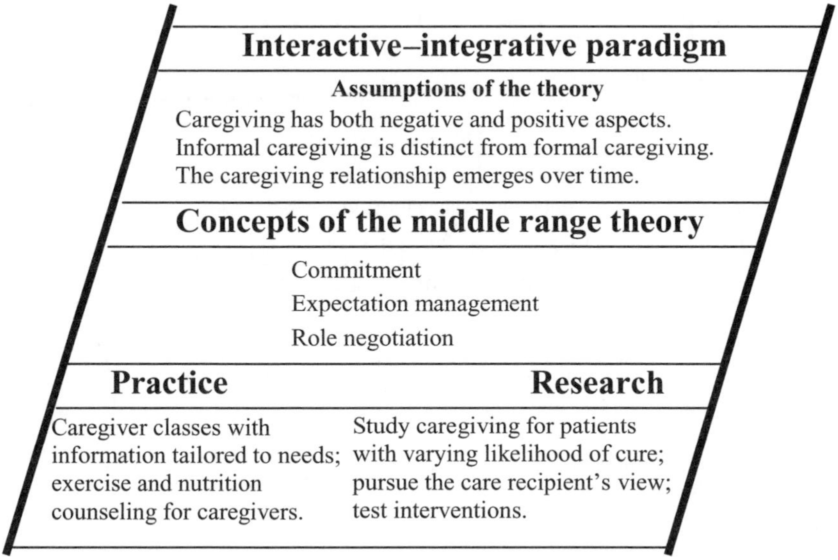

FIGURE 2.12   Ladder of abstraction: Caregiving dynamics.

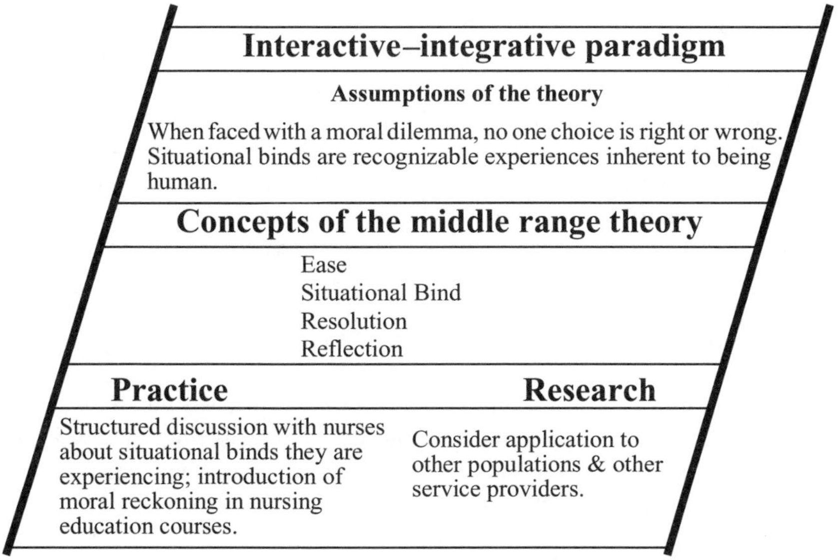

FIGURE 2.13   Ladder of abstraction: Moral reckoning.

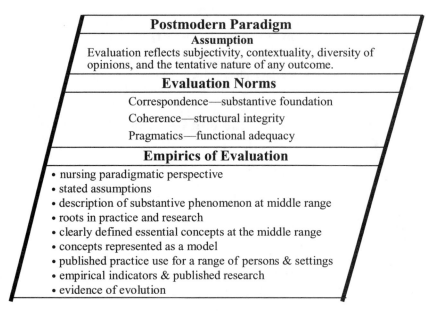

FIGURE 2.14   Ladder of abstraction: Evaluation.

The 12th theory is Nathaniel's Theory of Moral Reckoning, grounded in the interactive–integrative paradigm. According to this theory persons engage in a social process of deliberating when faced with a moral dilemma. Assumptions supporting the theory include facing a moral dilemma where no one choice is right or wrong and experiencing situational binds that are inherent to being human. Concepts in the theory are ease, situational bind, resolution, and reflection. Practice based on the theory includes providing structured discussion with nurses about situational binds and introduction of moral reckoning in nursing education courses. Research guided by the theory includes study of moral reckoning with nurses. Because moral reckoning is a human experience that is increasingly common in this day and age, it warrants consideration for guiding nursing practice and structuring study for people who are in a moral bind (see Figure 2.13 on previous page).

There is one final ladder of abstraction in this book in the evaluation chapter by Smith. In this chapter, Smith offers a process for understanding and evaluating middle range theories based on postmodern beliefs (see Figure 2.14). Overall, the ladders of abstraction provide a structure to guide the student in deciphering theory so that it can be used productively in advanced nursing practice and research. So, we urge you to begin climbing the ladders . . . stay long enough on each rung to get comfortable and spend enough time on all three rungs to get the whole picture of any theory. Also, expect to be uncomfortable when a rung is new to you. Discomfort is a space for growing and connecting what you know with what you are learning.

REFERENCES

Chinn, P., & Kramer, M. K. (1999). *Theory and nursing: Integrated knowledge development.* St. Louis: Mosby.

Ford-Gilboe, M., Campbell, J., & Berman, H. (1995). Stories and numbers: Coexistence without compromise. *Advances in Nursing Science, 18*(1), 14–26.

Im, E., & Meleis, A. I. (1999). Situation-specific theories: Philosophical roots, properties, and approach. *Advances in Nursing Science, 22*(2), 11–24.

King, I. (1996). The theory of goal attainment in research and practice. *Nursing Science Quarterly, 9,* 61–66.

McKay, R. P. (1969). Theories, models, and systems for nursing. *Nursing Research, 18,* 393–399.

Merton, R. K. (1968). *Social theory and social structure.* New York: Free Press.

Newman, M., Sime, A. M., & Corcoran-Perry, S. A. (1991). The focus of the discipline of nursing. *Advances in Nursing Science, 14*(1), 1–6.

Orem, D. (1971). *Nursing: Concepts of practice.* New York: McGraw-Hill.

Parse, R. R. (1992). Human becoming: Parse's theory of nursing. *Nursing Science Quarterly, 5*(1), 35–42.

Reed, P. (1995). A treatise on nursing knowledge development for the 21st century: Beyond postmodernism. *Advances in Nursing Science, 17,* 70–84.

Rogers, M. E. (1994). The science of unitary human beings: Current perspectives. *Nursing Science Quarterly, 7,* 33–35.

Roy, C., & Andrews, H. A. (1991). *The Roy adaptation model: The definitive statement.* Norwalk, CT: Appleton & Lange.

CHAPTER 3

Building Structures
for Research

Patricia R. Liehr and Mary Jane Smith

In this book, there are three middle range theories that grew out of the authors' work with doctoral students. These students started the process of inquiry by identifying a concept and clarifying the meaning of the concept through an established method of concept analysis found in the work of Rodgers and Knafl (2000). Even though we used the established concept analysis methods, we began to adjust our approach using the ladder of abstraction, moving down the ladder for stories and up the ladder for theories. Paley (1996) states, "The meaning of a term is made specific when it becomes part of a specific theory" (p. 577). He advocates locating concepts within a theoretical niche so that the meaning of a concept is specified by the overall structure of the theory. From this perspective, students are guided to develop a solid understanding of a theory and select congruent methodologies for researching the theory acknowledging the niche for their phenomenon of interest.

In our present work with doctoral students, we have developed a logical process that has helped students think through their ideas for research with peer–student input guided by a teacher–mentor. In this chapter, we will describe the process of building structures for research, offering guidance to graduate students and to faculty teaching courses where students are working to establish ideas for research. The chapter may also be helpful to practitioners and junior nursing faculty who are actively engaged in developing a focus for research. The systematic approach to be described in this chapter includes a 10-phase process. The phases include (1) a story that captures the phenomenon as lived in an actual practice situation, (2) naming the phenomenon of interest,

(3) identifying the theoretical lens for viewing the phenomenon, (4) exploring the literature related to the phenomenon, (5) gathering and reconstructing a story from a person who has experienced the phenomenon, (6) writing a mini-saga that captures the reconstructed story, (7) determining the core qualities of the phenomenon, (8) formulating a definition that integrates the core qualities, (9) drawing a model that depicts relationships between the core qualities, and (10) creating a mini-synthesis that integrates all phases of the structure building process. The process is not meant to be linear, where the student completes one phase and then goes on to the next. Rather, the process begins and then touches back to previous phases, always creating a work in progress with care to maintain correspondence between the phases and ongoing clarification of the defining core qualities.

PRACTICE STORY

The first phase begins with evidence from a practice story. The practice story addresses a critical incident in nursing practice related to caring in the human health experience that stirs the students' interest and is tied to the area they want to study. Prior to writing the story, students are engaged in a discussion about their research interest and then requested to think about a practice situation. Writing the story can take place in class or as an assignment. Students are invited to bring the practice situation into focus, place themselves in a quiet place where they can stay with their focus, and begin writing. They are instructed to begin by describing their first encounter and writing the story event by event, ending with how the situation came to a close. The practice story has a beginning, middle, and end and is centered on a nurse–person situation. Students are told not to worry about grammar or spelling but just to write the story as it comes to them. They then set the story aside and attend to details about the situation that come to them in their everyday coming and going. After a few days, they can edit their story for sentence mechanics and add detail.

PHENOMENON OF INTEREST

The phenomenon of interest is a human health experience conceptualized as the central idea for research. The phenomenon begins to emerge as the practice story is evaluated in relation to a student's area of interest. This evaluation can be a group endeavor led by a faculty mentor where all participants in a seminar receive a copy of the practice story to establish a foundation for dialogue, or it can occur through an Internet discussion board. Once the phenomenon is articulated, it must be named.

Naming the phenomenon requires considerable scrutiny and deliberation. It is an arduous process aimed at addressing a substantive area for study about which the student is passionate. Keeping the name at the middle range level of abstraction will enable development of a meaningful structure to guide research. If the name of the phenomenon is at a too-high level of abstraction then going to the empirical may be difficult; if at a too-low level the ensuing research will be narrow in scope. Maximum flexibility is attained when the phenomenon is named at a middle range level of abstraction. A common mistake when beginners name a phenomenon is that they name a population like congestive heart failure patients instead of a human health experience. In this situation, they are called to name the human health experience of persistent tiredness instead of the population.

THEORETICAL LENS

The theoretical lens is a perspective for viewing the phenomenon of interest. This perspective can emerge directly from a paradigm, from a grand theory, or from a middle range theory. The perspective shapes the meaning of the phenomenon for study. For instance, persistent tiredness will be described differently if one is looking through the lens of the particulate–deterministic paradigm (Newman, Sime, & Corcoran-Perry, 1991), as compared to Human Becoming theory (Parse, 1992), as compared to the theory of Unpleasant Symptoms (Lenz & Pugh, 2003). If viewing persistent tiredness through the lens of the particulate–deterministic paradigm, the meaning of the phenomenon will be imbued with cause–effect values. If viewing through Human Becoming grand theory, the meaning of the phenomenon might reflect multidimensional moving to possibilities in the person–universe process. If viewing through the middle range theory of Unpleasant Symptoms, the meaning of the phenomenon could include physiological, psychological, and situational factors influencing persistent tiredness and symptoms that interact and accentuate tiredness.

For phenomena named at a middle range level of abstraction, middle range theories create contextual niches that enable meaningful guidance for research. The logical connection between a phenomenon and a middle range theory is more explicit than if using a paradigmatic perspective or a grand theory. A stronger logical connection enhances clarity of meaning for the phenomenon and logical coherence between the ontology, epistemology, and methodology.

In the appendix of this book, there is a list of middle range theories published over the last 2 decades. Theories in this table were identified through a Cumulative Index of Nursing and Health Literature (CINAHL) search using the search terms "middle range theory," "mid-range theory," and "midrange theory." Students could use this table to identify a theoretical lens associated with their phenomenon of interest.

RELATED LITERATURE

The related literature is the existing body of knowledge associated with the phenomenon of interest. The question guiding the literature review is: What are the core qualities related to the phenomenon of interest? This is usually not accessed directly from the name of the phenomenon. Therefore, several steps for beginning exploration of related literature will be provided. It is best to begin with the lens for viewing the phenomenon by exploring the foundational literature supporting the theoretical perspective. One way to do this is to look at the reference list in a published source about the selected theory serving as a lens and identify relevant papers to ground understanding.

The second step requires identifying a population of interest and exploring the phenomenon as it relates to a population of interest. It is important in this step to address what matters about this phenomenon to the population. For instance, if studying persistent tiredness in persons with congestive heart failure, the student would pursue understanding of how tiredness permeates their lives. This step often takes the student to the literature of other disciplines; however, if it does not, then it is important to consider the phenomenon through the writings of scholars from diverse disciplines.

The third step is to explore the literature associated with the phenomenon name. For instance, if the phenomenon is persistent tiredness, then tiredness would be a search term that would be explored. If the phenomenon is more abstract, such as cultural belonging, then exploring the literature on social support to identify descriptions of belonging would be helpful. Even literature about gangs might provide insight about the meaning of the phenomenon of belonging.

At the completion of this phase, students will have a rudimentary list of core qualities of their phenomenon of interest that is rooted in the literature. Core qualities are the defining properties of the phenomenon.

RECONSTRUCTED STORY

The reconstructed story combines the phenomenon, population, and theoretical perspective. It is gathered from someone who has lived the phenomenon. The organizing structure for story gathering will include attention to the core qualities that have been identified in the previous phase. Sometimes the person sharing the story will describe different core qualities than originally identified and sometimes it may be necessary to gather a story from two or three people to affirm/disaffirm the significance of the identified core qualities. In writing the reconstructed story, the student creates a beginning, middle, and end that highlight the core qualities situated in the storytellers' experience.

MINI-SAGA

The mini-saga is a short story that synthesizes the reconstructed story. According to Pink (2005), "Mini-sagas are *extremely* short stories—just fifty words long . . . no more, no less" (p. 117). Like the reconstructed story, there is a beginning, middle, and end. The mini-saga captures the core meaning of the storyteller, so that anyone hearing it has a sense of the importance of the phenomenon. The purpose of the mini-saga is to crystallize the essence of the phenomenon of interest so that it can be readily shared with others. Writing the mini-saga is hard work and requires dialogue with peers and mentors that can be structured through either face-to-face seminars or Internet discussion boards.

CORE QUALITIES

The core qualities are the defining properties of the phenomenon. The student has been formulating the core qualities throughout the phases of this process, and at this phase of the structure-building process there is enhanced clarity about the nature of the qualities. The student is asked to stay with the identified core qualities at each phase of the continuing process.

DEFINITION

The definition is a sentence that begins with the name of the phenomenon followed by "is" (e.g., "Persistent tiredness is . . ."). The rest of the sentence arranges the core qualities as related to each other to describe the phenomenon. Although this seems straightforward, it is often difficult to create this defining sentence, which is the original contribution of the researcher at this point in the structure-building process. Regardless of difficulty, the researcher is called to take a stand and make a unique contribution.

MODEL

The model is a structural representation of the definition, depicting the relationships between the core qualities of the phenomenon. It is expected that there is congruence between the definition and the model. That is, the core qualities that appear in the definition will appear in the model. It is understood that the model is situated in a theory niche, and the student will be able to discuss the link between the theoretical perspective, phenomenon definition, and the model.

MINI-SYNTHESIS

The mini-synthesis is a 50-word three-sentence creation that pulls together the structure-building process thus far. The first sentence addresses the significance of the phenomenon in the context of a particular population. The second sentence identifies the phenomenon by name, linking it to the core qualities. The third sentence suggests an approach for moving toward a research question.

EXEMPLARS

Two exemplars written by students at the completion of the first year in their doctoral program are offered to facilitate understanding of the structure-building process. The exemplars are snapshots of their idea development after a year of doctoral study. However, the reader will notice that these students have moved a long way in conceptualizing their ideas for dissertation research.

REFERENCES

Lenz, E. R., & Pugh, L. C. (2003). The theory of unpleasant symptoms. In M. J. Smith & P. R. Liehr, *Middle range theory for nursing*. New York: Springer Publishing.

Newman, M., Sime, A. M., & Corcoran-Perry, S. A. (1991). The focus of the discipline of nursing. *Advances in Nursing Science, 14*(1), 1–6.

Paley, J. (1996). How not to clarify concepts in nursing. *Journal of Advanced Nursing, 24,* 572–578.

Parse, R. R. (1992). Human becoming: Parse's theory of nursing. *Nursing Science Quarterly, 5*(1), 35–42.

Pink, D. H. (2005). *A whole new mind: Moving from the information age to the conceptual age.* New York: Penguin Group.

Rodgers, B. L., & Knafl, K. A. (2000). *Concept development in nursing: Foundations, techniques, and applications.* Philadelphia: W. B. Saunders.

Exemplar #1: Yearning to Be Recognized

Anthony R. Ramsey

PRACTICE STORY

Nursing practice in an emergency setting offers the opportunity to care for patients experiencing many different illnesses or trauma. I have cared for police officers killed in the line of duty, children lethargic from fever, and women engaged in a battle with migraine headache. Women with migraine utilize health care resources and the emergency room more frequently than women without migraine (Elston Lafata et al., 2004). Based on my observations, the headache experience for these women is a powerful force that invokes physical pain as well as emotional turmoil. Most of the women say that the emergency room is the last place they want to visit, especially on a day off from work or when another responsibility is being neglected such as providing care for their child. These women are sometimes labeled "frequent flyers" or "drug seekers" by the emergency room staff. Furthermore, these women are often viewed by staff as "the migraine in room 3," a dehumanizing approach to patient care. The story of one particular woman had a profound impact on my nursing practice.

The first time I met Stacy was in the triage room. She was shielding her eyes from the bright fluorescent lights while holding a damp cloth to her mouth. I went through the normal procedure of obtaining vital signs and gathering the history of the present illness. Stacy explained that she had a history of migraine, but the headache usually resolved with abortive therapies prescribed by her physician. Along with her husband, we proceeded to a room that was relatively private and I dimmed the lights. The ER physician examined her and ordered the intramuscular administration of pain medication accompanied by an antiemetic. After receiving the medication, Stacy's pain decreased from 10 on a 10-point scale to 2. The nausea and photophobia had subsided, but Stacy was obviously sleepy from the medication. She was discharged with orders to follow up with her primary care physician.

Stacy periodically arrived to the ER with a migraine in the years following our initial encounter. I came to know Stacy and her husband very well during this period. I learned that together they both were working long hours and raising a rebellious 13-year-old daughter. I became interested in migraine and started reading everything I could about the illness. Whenever Stacy arrived, I tried to share with her and her husband information regarding migraine prevention and the importance of family counseling during and after crisis. They were receptive and stated over and again they wanted any information that would help keep Stacy out of the ER and at home living a productive life. Stacy eventually told me that the fact that I "believed her" provided both her and her husband with comfort. Stacy wanted her suffering to be acknowledged and she deeply appreciated my acceptance of her as a person experiencing pain.

In time I left the ER for an academic position without fully realizing that I might never see Stacy again. On the other hand, I live in a small, close-knit community and should have expected the possibility of a chance meeting. I almost didn't recognize Stacy when we first met in our local grocery store because of her significant weight gain. She explained that she had enrolled in a migraine study at a major university. She did not know the medications she was taking, but she did know two things for sure. First, she gained a significant amount of weight after entering the study. Second and most importantly, she had experienced only two migraines since enrollment, neither requiring emergency care. Our chance meeting ended with her once again thanking me for believing that she had pain and embracing her situation. Again, I was able to evaluate my practice and incorporate a new understanding of living in pain and the fear that frequently accompanies the experience.

PHENOMENON OF INTEREST

The phenomenon of interest related to Stacy's story is the migraine patient's outward cry for physical and emotional affirmation and relief, best described as "yearning to be recognized." "Yearning to be recognized" was synthesized as the result of work completed for classes leading to a PhD in a nursing theory course where a group of nine students, with the mentoring of an experienced nurse educator, engaged in ferreting out areas of focus for doctoral study. Following a systematic approach, each student presented the practice problem of interest and received feedback from the group and mentor as ideas were discussed and developed.

"Yearning to be recognized" was first labeled as "making valid." However, I, along with my mentor and group members, never fully accepted this name, yet the literature seemed to be pointing toward the nurse's validation of suffering through actively listening to the patient. Later in the year, after classes had concluded, I continued to work with my mentor regarding this idea. We determined that women who experience migraine headaches are in fact yearning for the physical and emotional pain to be recognized as real.

THEORETICAL LENS

The foundation supporting the nursing phenomenon is directly linked to a middle range nursing theory and a metaparadigm. Newman and colleagues' (1991) unitary–transformative metaparadigm serves as the philosophical umbrella for the phenomenon of yearning to be recognized. This metaparadigm holds that each patient's situation is unique and dynamic. It is through the understanding of past and current health events that persons create meaning and discover their true healing potential. The nurse's role is to provide a healing environment, understand the contextual nature of the patient situation, and aid in the discovery of the patient's healing potential. The phenomenon of yearning to be recognized is facilitating relief and validating suffering to promote healing, providing a direct link to Newman's metaparadigm.

The phenomenon of yearning to be recognized is directly linked to the theory of attentively embracing story (Smith & Liehr, 2003). This theory centers on the nurse's presence with another to validate suffering through story. In the context of true presence there is intentional focus on dialogue to summon a story. The migraine experience of pain is the complicating health challenge that initiates the sharing of a story. The nurse is charged with remaining free from distraction while embracing the reality of another through sharing of her migraine story. In true presence the nurse withholds judgment while listening, allowing for the identification of story patterns that facilitate understanding of the meaning of suffering with migraine headaches. Humans experience suffering in many different forms, and any form of suffering is considered a complicating health challenge. Finally, relief, another attribute of yearning to be recognized, involves the understanding of another. This understanding enables ease that Smith and Liehr describe, creating the potential for an optimal outcome for those who are suffering.

RELATED LITERATURE

The work of coming to know this idea required a significant literature review to identify essential qualities of the phenomenon. Frustration mounted as I searched unsuccessfully for terms related to nurses hearing and acknowledging the unique patient experience. Many different search strategies were used, including searches on migraine, women, care, validation, pain and suffering. However, "yearning to be recognized" with these exact words is not found in the nursing or medical literature. Instead, this idea is informed through related concepts. Suffering, threat to integrity, attentive presence, help-seeking, and release of pressure were concepts defined in various studies. Although they are developed in the literature, these concepts will be connected to yearning to be recognized through the use of key sources.

Suffering

The literature clearly identifies the need for establishing a therapeutic relationship between the practicing nurse and a patient who is experiencing suffering in any form. The current body of literature offers many definitions of suffering, often including the concepts of physical and emotional pain. However, suffering was best described at the theoretical level by Kahn and Steeves (1986), who stated that "suffering is experienced when some crucial aspect of one's own self, being or existence is threatened" (p. 626). This suffering is not only articulated words but also bodily expressions of the experience of deep pain. It is through attending to this voice that the nurse is called to explore with patients what is going on in their unique situation. This voice as an expression of suffering connects past and future all in the present moment, thus creating meaning and providing relief (Fredriksson & Eriksson, 2001). To alleviate suffering, a consoling dialogue that allows the patient to examine wounds leads to an understanding of the suffering experienced (Norberg, Bergsten, & Lundman, 2001). Suffering is defined as a threat against a person's integrity, identity, or connectedness (Norberg et al., 2001).

Attentive Presence

Smith and Liehr's (2003) middle range theory of attentively embracing story identifies attentive presence as a key concept of the theory. Here, the nurse is truly present with another to validate what matters most to the patient and gather the story. As the story unfolds, the nurse aids the patient to clarify and connect the everyday thoughts and feelings about living with the health challenge. Additional research verified the importance of active provider engagement to create an avenue for the sharing of health challenges and concerns (Fredriksson & Eriksson, 2001; Sundin, Axelsson, Jansson, & Norberg, 2000).

Release of Pressure

Persons experience suffering in many different forms, and any form of suffering is considered a complicating health challenge. Migraine headache often invokes fear of pain, fear of missed work and leisure activities as well as a fear of submitting to the disease and ultimately disappointing loved ones (Moloney, Strickland, DeRossett, Melby, & Dietrich, 2006). These fears, combined with physical pain, create an internal pressure that may become unbearable. When another acknowledges the physical and emotional aspects of the migraine, an avenue for the release of pressure has been created through belief and affirmation. In the end, the woman with a migraine is able to create meaning, which serves as framework for a new approach to illness management. The release of the pressure often created by suffering is defined throughout the literature as the development of understanding and ease through validation of suffering (Fredriksson & Eriksson, 2001; Sundin et al., 2000; Wikberg, Jansson, & Lithner, 2000). Smith and Liehr (2003) hold that this release of pressure may occur with the aid of a nurse, when everyday thoughts and feelings are connected to the current health challenge.

RECONSTRUCTED STORY

The reconstructed story is an actual story gathered from a woman who has lived yearning to be recognized. The intention of this story-gathering is to take a grass-roots approach and hear about the phenomenon from someone who has experienced it. This story was obtained from a 31-year-old woman who was recently divorced and had no children. She had suffered from severe migraine headaches since the age of 14. The nurse has been the primary care provider for 1 year. The nurse began by asking Joan what happens when she goes to the emergency room with a migraine headache.

She said that she gets really scared when she gets a headache and is afraid that she will have to go to the hospital. She indicated that a previous experience in the hospital with abdominal pain was horrible. Her words were

> I was in the ER crying in pain and the woman doctor told me that she wouldn't treat me unless I stopped crying, but I couldn't help it. She told me that I was bothering everybody else in the ER. And then when she did the pelvic, I swear it was like she balled her whole fist up and pushed it up to do the exam. I was horrified. And she just said I had appendicitis and would have to wait for surgery.

Joan told me she knows hospital people are busy yet she is in so much pain that she can't help herself. When seeking care for her migraine headache she found that the experience was the same as when she was in the emergency room with severe abdominal pain. Her words were

They said you have to stop crying yet I was throwing up and so upset. The doctor told me I was bothering everybody and had to stop. I couldn't speak, but Charlie [ex-husband] told them to just give me a shot like they always do. The doctor told him that he had nothing to do with this and that I needed to stop crying. Then when I returned a couple of months later, they were just like "Oh, it's you again."

When asked to talk more about care in the hospital emergency room, she described the process as

You don't see the nurses that much. I mean, you see them for the first time in that little room before they take you back. Then, when they take you back, another nurse asks you the same questions. After a long wait, a doctor comes in and asks the same questions once more. The mood of the nurses seems to change after they talk to the doctor. When they first see me they are all about helping me and then after talking to him they change. When they come back they are quiet and won't look you in the eye.

MINI-SAGA

Crying with pain in the emergency room, she was told to stop crying if she wanted help. She couldn't stop. The doctor told her she was bothering all the patients and the ensuing medical approach was aggressive, escalating her pain. From then on, the label "drug seeker" superseded her personhood.

SYNTHESIZED DEFINITION

Webster's Ninth New Collegiate Dictionary defines yearning as "longing persistently, wistfully or sadly." Recognize is defined as "to acknowledge formally; to admit as being one entitled to be heard" (Merriam-Webster, 1988). Based on the supporting literature and the real-world stories of women with migraines, the phenomenon of yearning to be recognized is defined as attending to the voice of suffering that calls for relief. The attributes of the phenomenon are attending, voice of suffering, and relief. Attending is defined as being truly present with another through story to validate what matters most to the person. The second attribute, the voice of suffering, is defined as the bodily expression of deep pain. For a person with migraine headache, deep pain is a profound, all-consuming state of unrelenting pressure. Relief is defined as the release of emotional and physical pressure.

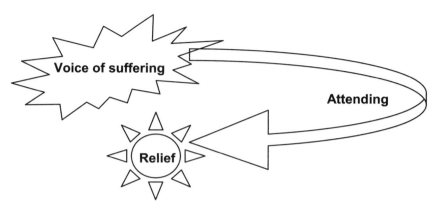

FIGURE 3.1   Yearning to be recognized.

MODEL

The model is presented in Figure 3.1.

MINI-SYNTHESIS

In the emergency room, women suffering migraine headaches are disaffirmed when labeled "drug seekers" in the midst of their excruciating pain. Yearning to be recognized, they call for attention to their suffering to enable relief. The truly present nurse hears the voice of suffering and takes action to reduce pain.

REFERENCES

Elston Lafata, J., Moon, C., Leotta, C., Kolodner, K., Poisson, L., & Lipton, R. B. (2004). The medical care utilization and costs associated with migraine headache. *Journal of General Internal Medicine, 19*(10), 1005–1012.

Fredriksson, L., & Eriksson, K. (2001). The patient's narrative of suffering: A path to health? An interpretive research synthesis on narrative understanding. *Scandinavian Journal of Caring Sciences, 15,* 3–11.

Kahn, D. L., & Steeves, R. H. (1986). The experience of suffering: Conceptual clarification and theoretical definition. *Journal of Advanced Nursing, 11,* 623–631.

Merriam-Webster. (1988). *Webster's ninth new collegiate dictionary* (9th ed.). Springfield, MA: Author.

Moloney, M. F., Strickland, O. L., DeRossett, S. E., Melby, M. K., & Dietrich, A. S. (2006). The experiences of midlife women with migraines. *Journal of Nursing Scholarship, 38*(3), 278–285.

Newman, M., Sime, A. M., & Corcoran-Perry, S. A. (1991). The focus of the discipline of nursing. *Advances in Nursing Science, 14*(1), 1–6.

Norberg, A., Bergsten, M., & Lundman, B. (2001). A model of consolidation. *Nursing Ethics, 8*(6), 544–553.

Smith, M. J., & Liehr, P. R. (2003). *Middle range theory for nursing.* New York: Springer Publishing.

Sundin, K., Axelsson, K., Jansson, L., & Norberg, A. (2000). Suffering from care as expressed in the narratives of former patients in somatic wards. *Scandinavian Journal of Caring Sciences, 14*(1), 16–22.

Wikberg, A., Jansson, L., & Lithner, F. (2000). Women's experience of suffering repeated severe attacks of acute intermittent porphyria. *Journal of Advanced Nursing, 32*(6), 1348–1355.

Exemplar #2: Catastrophic Cultural Immersion

Lisa Marie Wands

PRACTICE STORY

During my time as a volunteer in Mississippi after Hurricane Katrina, I heard many heartbreaking stories of loss and struggle as people labored long days to clean up the remains of their property and possessions and move on with their lives, but I did not witness hopelessness or defeat. Instead, Katrina's survivors faced their tasks with fortitude and purpose, and witnessing this admirable determination made me question how people can pick themselves up after a catastrophe and forge ahead into the unknown future. The following story of Marcie and Dave exemplifies the spirit I witnessed. They shared their story with me as we talked about how they were getting through these days.

Marcie and Dave had rented a backhoe to remove the mountain of rubble that had once been their dream home in a little town in Mississippi that had been flooded by Hurricane Katrina's tidal surge. The house that had been a source of pride and joy was reduced to a pile of busted boards and broken windows. Like most of their neighbors and friends, Marcie and Dave went about the task of clearing the land in preparation for rebuilding. They would have to furnish a new home with replacements for every household item from the bedspread to the toaster.

One day, Marcie noticed something glint in the sun in the dirt that Dave was about to scoop up with the backhoe. She yelled to him to stop so she could see what it was, and much to their amazement, what Marcie pulled from the ground was a completely intact china plate from her grandmother's antique collection. There were no scratches or chips on the plate; it was as if someone had purposefully placed the plate there under just a light layer of soil. Marcie and Dave reveled at finding the plate, and their friends and neighbors celebrated with them as they started spreading the news.

I marveled to see the joy that they found in finding a solitary plate as their house lay in ruins. My presence in that moment was that of an outsider as my role was that of a volunteer and not of a local who had endured the same hardship, and I wondered if that was why I could not appreciate what the plate represented. Did it epitomize hope that "not all was lost"? Did they recognize that a piece of their past had survived the wreckage, therefore making it easier to recognize themselves in this present world of "hurricane survivors"?

PHENOMENON OF INTEREST

When people experience a catastrophe, such as a hurricane, they find themselves immersed in a culture that was unknown prior to the event. For example, Marcie and Dave's previous identities were not wiped out by the storm; however, their lives were changed by an event, Hurricane Katrina, which drastically altered their physical environment. A week prior to the storm, Marcie and Dave were leading normal lives: working, enjoying their new home, and planning for the future. After the storm passed, this normalcy was gone, their jobs were on hold, and their house was destroyed. They now belonged to a group of people known as survivors and had to seek a new normalcy in a new culture.

My first attempt at labeling the phenomenon I witnessed was to name it "cultural immersion." The term "cultural immersion" is commonly used in regard to voluntary expeditions into unfamiliar societies by people who wish to learn something about that group. Nursing students learn cultural competence by traveling to a foreign place and participating in providing health care to that area's people. Students of languages travel to live with families in countries where a language is spoken so that they may learn to speak fluently in a real-world setting. Some people immerse themselves in a foreign culture simply to become more educated about that culture's population. All of these experiences are done with purpose and by choice. Further development of the concept name required that I include a sense of the culture in which a person becomes immersed or the traumatic process by which the immersion occurs. This further development required continued dialogue about the idea.

For a while, I considered whether I wanted to study nurses working in catastrophe circumstances or whether I wanted to study the survivors of catastrophe. In looking at these two groups through my perspective as a nurse, I realized that I was more curious about the process that the survivors of the storm were experiencing. Online discussions with my doctoral classmates validated my decision to concentrate on survivors of catastrophe, especially given that nurses need to try to understand what the population experiences if we are to be of service to them. In order to fully identify the population, I added the word "catastrophic" to the phrase "cultural immersion" to capture the essence of trauma for those who had survived Katrina's flood waters; these people had experienced a catastrophe that had immersed them in a culture of survivorship that they did not know prior to the storm. The immersion was abrupt, and those affected were required to step back and take inventory of where they were and who they were in the context of the new culture.

In further refining catastrophic cultural immersion, a class exercise required viewing the concept at different levels of abstraction. I found the story of Marcie and Dave to be at a lower level of abstraction in its quality of hands-on practice and individuality. As I defined the concept at a higher level of abstraction and separated the concept from the population that initiated my thoughts, I realized that the concept could be applied across a wide range of situations and populations. For example, a diagnosis of cancer is a catastrophic cultural immersion for the individual that suddenly belongs to the culture of cancer patients. During this time, I was transcribing interviews for a faculty member who had gathered stories of veterans of World War II who had survived the bombing at Pearl Harbor, and I realized that these veterans had experienced catastrophic cultural immersion when they lived through the surprise attack. Catastrophic cultural immersion could be applied to survivors of storm, cancer, or war, and there were numerous other possibilities.

THEORETICAL LENS

Development of the concept of catastrophic cultural immersion was guided by Starck's (2003) theory of meaning, which is based on Viktor Frankl's work on the human experience of suffering. While a prisoner of a concentration camp, Frankl made observations about how people have the ability to make choices while in the midst of dreadful circumstances. He believed that there are three dimensions that affect how we as human beings move through a traumatic experience: the physical, the mental, and the spiritual. Disruption in one element can manifest in a different element, but the spiritual can transcend both the physical and mental facets enabling people to rise above the challenge at hand.

Starck (2003) used Frankl's work as a foundation to create a middle range theory for nursing, the Theory of Meaning. In addition to defining the human dimensions, Starck provides descriptions of the concepts, or "building blocks" (p. 128), of the theory, which are life purpose, freedom to choose, and human suffering. The first theoretical concept of finding purpose in life is equated with finding meaning in life, and meaning is considered to be a completely individual discovery. No person can dictate what another person's meaning is or will be. Frankl explained three ways in which a person can find meaning: transcending oneself to reach out to others; having an experience through relationships with others; and choosing one's attitude "in spite of difficult circumstances" (Starck, 2003, p. 131). In the concept of freedom to choose, persons retain the ability to choose their attitude and maintain dignity while immersed in a catastrophic event. In the face of great adversity, any person may present with a wide variety of reactions, ranging from indifference to courage. Starck (2003) refers to this as "spiritual freedom or independence of mind" (p. 132). Frankl wrote "the way in which [a person] accepts, the way in which he bears his cross, what courage he manifests in suffering, what dignity he displays in doom and disaster, is the measure of his human fulfillment" (Starck, 2003, p. 132). The main idea of the third theoretical concept of suffering is that it is individually defined. Only a person in the midst of an experience knows how it is to live that experience. As with finding meaning in life, an outsider can neither explain nor dictate what suffering means to a person. In their description of how our individual experiences are shaped by multiple factors, Sharpe and Curran (2006) state that patients view illness based not only on present factors but also in terms of prior experiences, beliefs, and knowledge as well as personal hopes and dreams for the future.

The theory of meaning as offered by Starck (2003) and based on Frankl's work can be used to inform understanding of the concept of catastrophic cultural immersion and explore the process as individuals experience it. Experiencing a catastrophe displaces one from a known culture into an unknown culture. The meaning a person ascribes to the experience is completely individual because the meaning that existed prior to the catastrophe was specific to the individual and has become a part of personal history. Re-evaluating self in the context of the new culture may be part of finding meaning in new surroundings (Sharpe & Curran, 2006). At all times in this migration from one culture to another a person retains the ability to choose which path to take. The choices may later be judged to be negative, positive, or even neutral, but judgment can only be made by the individual making the choices.

RELATED LITERATURE

Catastrophic events can create effects at the individual, family, or national level. While the impact of any event is ultimately individual and personal, catastrophes are generally thought of as being of the natural, man-made, or personal kind. Unfortunately, we are all too familiar with examples of large-scale catastrophes in our recent history. While Hurricane Katrina is an example of a natural catastrophe, the argument could be made that the inadequate maintenance of the levees and insufficient response of rescue aid are attributable to human error, therefore creating a man-made catastrophic situation. The tragedies of September 11, 2001, are a vivid example of a man-made catastrophe. Individuals' responses to these kinds of events could be counted as personal catastrophes; other examples of personal catastrophes include being diagnosed with cancer, experiencing a stroke, or becoming disabled as a result of an automobile accident.

Natural and man-made catastrophes have the capacity to impact entire communities (Tremblay, Blanchard, Pelletier, & Vallerand, 2006). Hurricane Katrina caused widespread havoc for hundreds of thousands of people living along the coast of the Gulf of Mexico and ultimately caused $81 billion in property damage (Habib, 2007). The events of September 11 not only directly impacted people at the sites of the terrorist attacks but also created psychological distress across the nation; "seventeen percent of the U.S. population outside of New York City" reported having symptoms of stress associated with September 11 (Silver, Holman, McIntosh, Poulin, & Gil-Rivas, 2002). Tremblay et al. (2006) studied the effects of a 1998 ice storm that lasted for 11 days, interrupting life-as-usual in southeastern Canada and northeastern United States by causing widespread power outages and forcing people to evacuate their homes. In their literature review, which included natural disasters such as eruption of a volcano, earthquakes, and floods, Tremblay et al. (2006) found that "responses to natural disasters cover a wide range of psychological, behavioral, and physical disturbances" (p. 1503).

While large-scale catastrophes can impact entire communities, each individual of that community is uniquely affected by the event. In addition, individuals can experience wholly personal catastrophe, such as being diagnosed with cancer or enduring a stroke. Backe, Larsson, and Fridlund (1996) conducted interviews with six people who had recently suffered from a stroke and discovered feelings of confusion and disassociation with self amidst loss of functional independence. Mathieson and Stam (1995) found that people who had been diagnosed with cancer expressed feelings of uselessness, questioned self-identities, and believed that their bodies had betrayed them. Though some commonalities can be found, the impact of a catastrophe no matter how large or small is unique to the individual.

Similarly, the process by which an individual moves through the experience of a catastrophe is unique, though common threads can be found among varying experiences. One of the first steps in dealing with a catastrophic event is to take stock of new surroundings. Mathieson and Stam (1995) address the experience of recapturing a sense of self-identity in the midst of illness by stating that one's entire life is an ongoing story in which meaning and hopes for the future continually add to a person's identity. Backe et al. (1996) describe how "a person suffering from a stroke suddenly finds him/herself in a new life situation" (p. 286) and discovers the need to "deal with [his/her] situation both emotionally and intellectually" (p. 289).

Once a person takes stock of the new environment, personal choice about how to overcome effects of the catastrophe are considered. Finding meaning and purpose in life is the essential driving force guiding choices. Mathieson and Stam (1995) assert that finding meaning in a new life situation with cancer "is imperative because the former meanings upon which the non-ill person based her life may no longer be available to her" (p. 296). Plans for the future also must be modified in the person's new life story. Backe et al.'s (1996) interviews with people who had experienced a stroke led to the discovery that once acceptance of the new life situation was achieved it was possible to begin "look[ing] for new opportunities to attain the best possible life" (p. 290).

"Culture" is one more dimension of the phenomenon name that must be considered in the "related literature" phase of this process. Traditionally, culture is viewed as a static set of traits, including value judgments and belief systems, and we think of culture largely related to ethnic or racial groups. The concept of catastrophic cultural immersion, however, assumes a much broader meaning. Chiu and Hong's (2005) description of culture as a "network of knowledge and practices that is produced, distributed, and reproduced among a collection of interconnected people" (p. 490) is a much better fit for the emerging idea. As people become immersed in the new culture, they can use their extant personal knowledge to negotiate it and gain insight about it, enabling creation of their new normal.

RECONSTRUCTED STORY

The idea of catastrophic cultural immersion began in the context of natural disaster, but my interest was growing in the area of war survivors, so I composed a reconstructed story from a World War II Pearl Harbor survivor for this phase of concept development.

Oscar was 19 years old and aboard the U.S.S. Phoenix when Japanese aircraft started dropping bombs on the U.S. Naval fleet. At first, he and his shipmates thought that the Air Force was running an unannounced mock attack until they saw nearby battleships burst into flames. The harbor became a scene of death and destruction full of burning, sinking ships. Once the chaos started to subside, Oscar and a few others were recruited to help retrieve the bodies of those who hadn't survived. He continued to serve in the Navy until the war was over and feels fortunate to have emerged relatively unscathed from the various battles in which he fought. Looking back at his experience almost 65 years later, Oscar identifies two main ideas about why he feels he was not as affected by the Pearl Harbor tragedy as others. The first is that he was too young to really grasp what was happening all around him, and the second is recognition that combat is different for soldiers depending on their proximity to the enemy. Shooting at an airplane with a gun mounted on a battleship deck is worlds apart from being face-to-face with a guy and shooting him with a handheld rifle.

Oscar's ship traveled to Pearl Harbor twice during the war, but he never felt the need to return again because "he didn't leave anything there." When he returned home, Oscar went right to work. He never told the story of his experience to his family. He doesn't feel that his Pearl Harbor experience has affected his health at all. As he looks toward the future, he hopes to live out his remaining days as independently as possible and would like to see today's youth, including his grandkids, become more self-reliant and more patriotic toward their country. In the meantime, he's enjoying good health, being able to do the things he wants, and appreciates the occasional "thank you" he gets from people when they see the "Pearl Harbor Survivor" license plate on his car.

MINI-SAGA

One of the final pieces of this concept development process was to create an exactly 50-word mini-saga that represents the reconstructed story with a beginning, middle, and end.

All his buddies thought it was a mock drill when the bombs started falling from the sky. He never told his family how that day changed his life forever. Watching the flag flutter in the wind brings tears to his eyes, and he hopes kids will come to understand someday.

SYNTHESIZED DEFINITION

Catastrophic cultural immersion is the abrupt displacement of persons into sudden unfamiliarity from which they struggle to transcend.

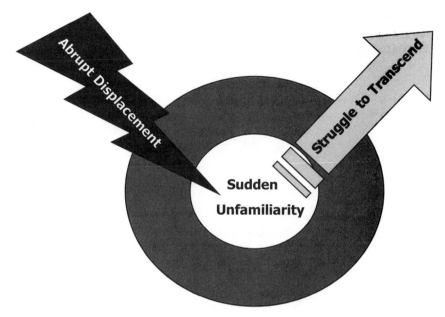

FIGURE 3.2   Concept: Catastrophic cultural immersion.

MODEL

The model is presented in Figure 3.2.

MINI-SYNTHESIS

The mini-synthesis locates the phenomenon of interest within the context of a particular population. For me, the context was veterans returning from the war in Iraq.

When coming home from war, American soldiers are faced with the challenge of reintegrating into everyday living. This is a catastrophic cultural immersion characterized by struggle to find meaning in a once familiar and now unfamiliar environment. Understanding their challenge creates a foundation for helping them move on with living.

REFERENCES

Backe, M., Larsson, K., & Fridlund, B. (1996). Patients' conceptions of their life situation within the first week after a stroke event: A qualitative analysis. *Intensive and Critical Care Nursing, 12,* 285–294.

Chiu, C.-Y., & Hong, Y-Y. (2005). Cultural competence: Dynamic processes. In A. J. Elliot & C. S. Dweck (Eds.), *Handbook of competence and motivation* (pp. 489–505). New York: Guilford.

Habib, L. (2007, August 28). Katrina's statistics tell story of its wrath. Retrieved October 4, 2007, from The Weather Channel's website at http://www.weather.com/news center/topstories/060829katrinastats.html?from=hurricane_tracker

Mathieson, C. M., & Stam H. J. (1995). Renegotiating identity: Cancer narratives. *Sociology of Health & Illness, 17*(3), 283–306.

Sharpe, L., & Curran, L. (2006). Understanding the process of adjustment to illness. *Social Science & Medicine, 62,* 1153–1166.

Silver, R. C., Holman, A., McIntosh, D. N., Poulin, M., & Gil-Rivas, V. (2002). Nationwide longitudinal study of psychological responses to September 11. *JAMA, 288,* 1235–1244.

Starck, P. L. (2003). The theory of meaning. In M. J. Smith & P. R. Liehr (Eds.), *Middle range theory for nursing* (pp. 125–144). New York: Springer Publishing.

Tremblay, M. A., Blanchard, C. M., Pelletier, L. G., & Vallerand, R. J. (2006). A dual route in explaining health outcomes in natural disaster. *Journal of Applied Social Psychology, 36*(6), 1502–1522.

CHAPTER 4

Theories of Uncertainty in Illness

Merle H. Mishel and Margaret F. Clayton

In this chapter, two theories of uncertainty in illness will be described. The original uncertainty in illness theory was developed to address uncertainty during the diagnostic and treatment phases of an illness or an illness with a determined downward trajectory. This theory will be referred to by the acronym UIT (Mishel, 1988). The reconceptualized uncertainty in illness theory was developed to address the experience of living with continuous uncertainty in either a chronic illness requiring ongoing management or an illness with the possibility of recurrence. This reconceptualized theory will be referred to by the acronym RUIT (Mishel, 1990). The acronyms will be used to discuss each theory in the remainder of the chapter.

The uncertainty in illness theory (UIT) proposes that uncertainty exists in illness situations that are ambiguous, complex, unpredictable, and when information is unavailable or inconsistent. Uncertainty is defined as the inability to determine the meaning of illness-related events. It is a cognitive state created when the individual cannot adequately structure or categorize an illness event because of insufficient cues (Mishel, 1988). The theory explains how patients cognitively structure a schema for the subjective interpretation of uncertainty in illness, treatment, and outcome. The theory is composed of three major themes: (1) antecedents of uncertainty, (2) appraisal of uncertainty, and (3) coping with uncertainty. Uncertainty and cognitive schema are the major concepts of the theory.

The reconceptualized theory of uncertainty (RUIT) retains the definition of uncertainty and major themes as in the UIT. The two concepts of self-organization and probabilistic thinking are added. The RUIT addresses the process that occurs when a person lives with unremitting uncertainty found in chronic illness or in illness with a potential for recurrence. The desired outcome from the RUIT is growth to a new value system, whereas the outcome of the UIT is a return to the previous level of adaptation or functioning (Mishel, 1990).

PURPOSE OF THE THEORIES AND
HOW THEY WERE DEVELOPED

The purpose of the theories is to describe and explain uncertainty as a basis for practice and research. The UIT applies to the pre-diagnostic, diagnostic, and treatment phases of acute and chronic illness, and the RUIT applies to enduring uncertainty in chronic illness or illness with the possibility of recurrence and where self-management is the primary focus for treatment. The theories focus on the individual in the context of illness or a treatable condition, and to the family or parent of an ill individual. Use with groups or communities is not consistent with the conceptualization of either theory.

The finding that uncertainty was reported to be a common experience of people experiencing illness or receiving medical treatment led to the creation of the UIT (Mishel, 1988). Although the concept was cited in the literature, there was no substantive exploration of how uncertainty developed or was resolved by ill individuals. It was a personal experience with my (M. M.) ill father that catalyzed the concept for me. He was dying from colon cancer, and his body was swollen in some places and emaciated in others. He didn't understand what was happening to him to cause these diverse physiological responses, so he focused on whatever he could control to provide some degree of predictability for himself. The effort he spent on achieving some understanding brought the significance of uncertainty home to me. Although I explored the work on the concept of uncertainty, it was not until I entered doctoral study in psychology that I focused on the concept in earnest.

Developing the UIT included a synthesis of the research on uncertainty, cognitive processing, and managing threatening events, as well as clinical data and discussion with colleagues. The UIT was revised from the original measurement model published in 1981 to the theory published in 1988. During my doctoral study, I focused my dissertation on the development and testing of a measure of uncertainty. At that time, I was influenced by the literature on stress and coping that discussed uncertainty as one type of stressful event (Lazarus, 1974). As I began to explore the literature, I discovered the work of Norton (1975), who identified eight dimensions of uncertainty. His work, along with that of

Moos and Tsu (1977), formed the framework for interviews leading to the development of the Mishel Uncertainty in Illness Scale.

My early ideas were further influenced by Bower (1978) and Shalit (1977), who described uncertainty as a complex cognitive stressor, along with Budner (1962), who considered ambiguous stimuli that are novel or complex as a source for uncertainty. These cognitive psychologists did not apply their work to a specific context; however, their ideas about uncertainty influenced me to view uncertainty as a cognitive state instead of an emotional response. This was an important distinction that directed ongoing theory development. Uncertainty as a stressor or threat was reinforced by the work of both Shalit (1977) and Lazarus (1974). Coping resulting from primary appraisal of the uncertainty and secondary appraisal of the response to uncertainty was adapted from the work of Lazarus (1974). The measurement model of uncertainty (Mishel, 1981) incorporated the work of these primary sources to conceptualize uncertainty in illness and to develop the Uncertainty in Illness Scale.

When the Uncertainty in Illness Scale was published, a body of findings on uncertainty quickly emerged in the nursing literature (Mishel, 1983, 1984; Mishel & Braden, 1987, 1988; Mishel, Hostetter, King, & Graham, 1984; Mishel & Murdaugh, 1987). The findings on uncertainty flushed out the antecedents of uncertainty presented in the measurement model. The stimuli frame variable, composed of familiarity of events and congruence of events, was formed from a combination of research on uncertainty in illness and research in cognitive psychology. The third component of stimuli frame, which is symptom pattern, was developed from qualitative studies (Mishel & Murdaugh, 1987) describing the importance of consistency and predictability of symptoms to form a symptom pattern. Following this mode for theory development, the antecedent of cognitive capacities was based on cognitive psychology (Mandler, 1979) and practice knowledge about instructing patients when cognitive processing abilities are compromised. The final antecedent of structure providers was developed from research on uncertainty in illness.

The appraisal section of the theory was developed using sources from the 1981 model and was expanded based on clinical data and discussions with colleagues. Colleagues identified the need to consider personality variables in the evaluation of uncertainty, and clinical data indicated that uncertainty could be a preferred state under specific circumstances. This led to include inference and illusion as two phases of appraisal and to support and define these phases using research from nursing and psychology (Mishel & Braden, 1987; Mishel & Murdaugh, 1987).

The RUIT was developed through discussion with colleagues, qualitative data from chronically ill individuals, and an awareness of the limitations of the UIT theory. There was the need to rethink the theory for application with the chronically ill. The UIT explained uncertainty in the acute and treatment phases of illness but did not address life changes expressed by persons with chronic illness. Furthermore, the UIT was linear and did not incorporate change over time. Qualitative interviews with chronically ill individuals revealed that many acknowledged continuous uncertainty and a new view of life that incorporated uncertainty. Furthermore, questions emerged from an examination of the role of uncertainty in Western society. From the perspective of critical social theory (Allen, 1985), the patient's desire for certainty may reflect the goals of control and predictability that form the socio-historic values of Western society (Mishel, 1990). Clinical data revealed that those who chose to incorporate uncertainty into their lives were living a value system on the edge of mainstream ideas. In order to explain the clinical data, a framework that conceptualized uncertainty as a preferred state was needed. Using the process of theory derivation described by Walker and Avant (1989), chaos theory was chosen as the parent theory to reconceptualize the uncertainty theory. The reconceptualization was compatible with the parent theory and advanced the understanding of uncertainty in a new light. Chaos theory emphasizes disorder, instability, diversity, disequilibrium, and restructuring as the healthy variability of a system. The reconceptualized theory included ideas of disorganization and reformulation of a new stability to explain how a person with enduring uncertainty emerges with a new view of life.

Drawing from the concepts in chaos theory (Prigogine & Stengers, 1984), uncertainty is viewed as a force that spreads from illness to other areas of a person's life and competes with the person's previous mode of functioning. As uncertain areas of life increase, they can disrupt ongoing life patterns. Pattern disruption occurs as uncertainty feeds back on itself and generates more uncertainty such as questions about the ability to meet desired goals and to maintain desired relationships. When uncertainty persists, the concentration of uncertainty increases and exceeds a person's level of tolerance. There is a sense of disorganization that promotes personal instability. With a high level of disorganization comes a loss of a sense of coherence (Antonovsky, 1987). A system in disorganization begins to reorganize at an imperceptible level. This reorganization represents a gradual transition from a perspective of life oriented to predictability and control to a new view of life in which multiple contingencies are preferable.

CONCEPTS OF THE THEORIES

The UIT theory is organized around three major themes: antecedents of uncertainty, appraisal of uncertainty, and coping with uncertainty.

Uncertainty is the central concept in the theory and is defined as the inability to determine the meaning of illness-related events occurring when the decision maker is unable to assign definite value to objects or events and/or is unable to accurately predict outcomes. Another concept central to the uncertainty theory is cognitive schema, which is defined as the person's subjective interpretation of illness-related events (see Figure 4.1).

The ideas included in the antecedent theme of the theory include stimuli frame, cognitive capacity, and structure providers. Stimuli frame is defined as the form, composition, and structure of the stimuli that the person perceives. The stimuli frame has three components: symptom pattern, event familiarity, and event congruence. Symptom pattern refers to the degree to which symptoms are present with sufficient consistency to be perceived as having a pattern or configuration. Event familiarity is the degree to which the situation is habitual, repetitive, or contains recognized cues. Event congruence refers to the consistency between the expected and the experienced illness-related events. Cognitive capacity and structure providers influence the three components of the stimuli frame. Cognitive capacity is the information-processing ability of the individual.

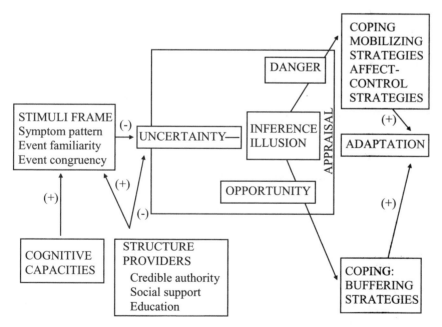

FIGURE 4.1   Perceived uncertainty in illness.

Note: Reprinted with permission from: Mishel, M. H. (1988). Uncertainty in illness. *Image: The Journal of Nursing Scholarship, 20*(4), 225–232.

Structure providers are the resources available to assist the person in the interpretation of the stimuli frame. Structure providers include education, social support, and credible authority.

The second major theme in the UIT is appraisal of uncertainty, which is defined as the process of placing a value on the uncertain event or situation. There are two components of appraisal: inference or illusion. Inference refers to the evaluation of uncertainty using related examples and is built on personality dispositions, general experience, knowledge, and contextual cures. Illusion refers to the construction of beliefs formed from uncertainty that have a positive outlook. The result of appraisal is the valuing of uncertainty as a danger or an opportunity.

The third theme in the UIT is coping with uncertainty, and the concepts include danger, opportunity, coping, and adaptation. Danger is the possibility of a harmful outcome. Opportunity is the possibility of a positive outcome. Coping with a danger appraisal is defined as activities directed toward reducing uncertainty and managing the emotion generated by a danger appraisal. Coping with an opportunity appraisal is defined as activities directed toward maintaining uncertainty. Adaptation is defined as biopsychosocial behavior occurring within the person's individually defined range of usual behavior.

The RUIT includes the antecedent theme in the UIT and adds the two concepts of self-organization and probabilistic thinking. Self-organization is the reformulation of a new sense of order, resulting from the integration of continuous uncertainty into one's self-structure in which uncertainty is accepted as the natural rhythm of life. Probabilistic thinking is a belief in a conditional world in which the expectation of certainty and predictability is abandoned. The RUIT proposes four factors that influence the formation of a new life perspective. These are prior life experience, physiological status, social resources, and health care providers. In the process of reorganization, the person re-evaluates uncertainty by gradual approximations, from an aversive experience to one of opportunity. Thus uncertainty becomes the foundation for a new sense of order and is accepted as the natural rhythm of life. There is a new ability to focus on multiple alternatives, choices, and possibilities; re-evaluate what is important in life; consider variation in personal investment; and appreciate the impermanence and fragility of life. The theory identifies conditions under which the new ability is maintained or is blocked.

The concepts of both theories tie clearly to nursing by describing and explaining human responses to illness situations. Uncertainty crosses all phases of illness from pre-diagnosis symptomatology to diagnosis, treatment, treatment residuals, recovery, potential recurrence, and exacerbation. Thus the theories are pertinent to the health experience for all age groups. Uncertainty is experienced by ill persons, caregivers, and parents of ill children.

The theories incorporate a consideration of the health care environment as a component of the stimuli frame as well as the broader support network. Nursing care is represented under the concept of structure providers. Since an important part of nursing involves explaining and providing information, it follows that nursing actions are interventions to help patients manage uncertainty. The outcomes of both theories are directly related to health. The health outcome is either to regain personal control, as in adaptation in the UIT, or consciousness expansion, as in the RUIT.

RELATIONSHIPS AMONG THE CONCEPTS: THE MODELS

As seen in Figure 4.1, the UIT is displayed as a linear model with no feedback loops. According to the model, uncertainty is the result of antecedents. The major path to uncertainty is through the stimuli frame variables. Cognitive capacities influence stimuli frame variables. If the person has a compromised cognitive capacity due to fever, infection, pain, or mind-altering medication, the clarity and definition of the stimuli frame variables are likely to be reduced, resulting in uncertainty. In such a situation, it is assumed that stimuli frame variables are clear, patterned, and distinct, and only become less so because of limitations in cognitive capacity. However, when cognitive capacity is adequate, stimuli frame variables may still lack a symptom pattern or be unfamiliar and incongruent due to lack of information, complex information, information overload, or conflicting information. The structure provider variables then come into play to alter the stimuli frame variables by interpreting, providing meaning, and explaining. These actions serve to structure the stimuli frame, thereby reducing or preventing uncertainty. Structure providers may also directly impact uncertainty. The health care provider can offer explanations or use other approaches that directly reduce uncertainty. Similarly, uncertainty can be reduced by one's level of education and resultant knowledge. Social support networks also influence the stimuli frame by providing information from similar others, providing examples, and offering supportive information.

Uncertainty is viewed as a neutral state and is not associated with emotions until evaluated. During the evaluation of uncertainty, inference and illusion come into play. Inference and illusion are based on beliefs and personality dispositions that influence whether uncertainty is appraised as a danger or as an opportunity. Because uncertainty renders a situation amorphous and ill defined, positively oriented illusions can be generated

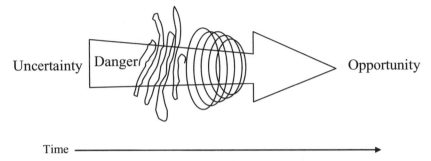

FIGURE 4.2   Uncertainty in chronic illness.

Note: Reprinted with permission from: Bailey, D. E., & Stewart, J. L. (2001). Mishel's theory of uncertainty in illness. In A. M. Mariner-Tomey & M. R. Alligood (Eds.), *Nursing theorists and their work* (5th ed., pp. 560–583). St. Louis, MO: Mosby.

from uncertainty, leading to an appraisal of uncertainty as an opportunity. Uncertainty appraised as an opportunity implies a positive outcome and buffering coping strategies are used to maintain it. In contrast, beliefs and personality dispositions can result in uncertainty appraised as danger. Uncertainty evaluated as danger implies harm. Problem-focused coping strategies are employed to reduce it. If problem-focused coping cannot be used, then emotional coping strategies are used to respond to the uncertainty. If the coping strategies are effective, adaptation occurs. Difficulty in adapting indicates inability to manipulate uncertainty in the desired direction.

The RUIT (Figure 4.2) represents the process of moving from uncertainty appraised as danger to uncertainty appraised as an opportunity and resource for a new view of life. As noted earlier in this chapter, the reconceptualized theory builds on the original theory at the appraisal portion. The RUIT describes enduring uncertainty that is initially viewed as danger due to its invasion into broader areas of life resulting in instability. The jagged line within the arrow represents both the invasion of uncertainty and the growing instability. The patterned circular portion of the line represents the repatterning and reorganization resulting in a revised view of uncertainty. The bottom arrow indicates that this is a process that evolves over time.

USE OF THE THEORIES IN
NURSING RESEARCH

Beginning with the publication of the Uncertainty in Illness Scale (Mishel, 1981), there has been extensive research into uncertainty in both acute and chronic illnesses. The research on uncertainty is voluminous and includes studies in nursing and other disciplines. Several comprehensive reviews of research have summarized and critiqued the current state of the knowledge on uncertainty in illness (Bailey & Stewart, 2001; Barron, 2000; Mast, 1995; McCormick, 2001; Mishel, 1997a, 1999; Neville, 2003; Stewart & Mishel, 2000). Other authors have attempted to develop an expanded definition of uncertainty (Penrod, 2001) or have critiqued the current work based upon a misunderstanding of the reconceptualized uncertainty theory (Parry, 2003). In this chapter, the research review will be limited to studies that directly address components of the UIT and the RUIT and will not include studies that use the uncertainty scales but do not consider aspects of the theories in study design, literature review, or discussion of findings.

While some studies focus on components of the UIT or RUIT, in the past few years more studies have used uncertainty as the conceptual framework for the study and directly tested major sections of the UIT, elaborated upon the UIT, or elaborated upon selected antecedents and outcomes adding richness to the theory (Jurgens, 2006; Kang, 2005, 2006; Kang, Daly, & Kim, 2004; McCormick, Naimark, & Tate, 2006; Sammarco, 2001; Santacroce, 2003; Wonghongkul, Dechaprom, Phumivichuvate, & Losawatkul, 2006). The theory has also been used as the basis for revising the Parent's Perception of Uncertainty Scale (Santacroce, 2001). In the study by Kang and colleagues (2004) the researchers operationalized and tested the antecedents of social support and education as structure providers along with the stimuli frame variable of symptom pattern on uncertainty in patients with atrial fibrillation. Findings were generally supportive of the theory, with symptom severity as the strongest predictor of uncertainty, while the structure provider variables of education and social support reduced uncertainty. An unusual study using grounded theory explored children's perception of uncertainty during treatment for cancer, citing the uncertainty theory as the sensitizing theory (Stewart, 2003). The uncertainty theory grown through research studies is the area of credible authority and social support from investigators in nursing and in health communication (Brashers et al., 2003; Brashers, Neidig, & Goldsmith, 2004; Clayton, Mishel, & Belyea, 2006).

Many studies have focused on the antecedents of stimuli frame and structure providers. Three aspects of illness have been found to cause uncertainty: (1) severity of illness, (2) erratic nature of symptoms, and (3) ambiguity of symptoms. Severity of illness and ambiguity of symptoms correspond to the stimuli frame component of symptom pattern, while the erratic nature of symptoms corresponds to the stimuli component of event congruence.

Studies that focus on severity of illness and uncertainty are classified as those that address the theoretical link between symptom pattern and uncertainty. Severity of illness refers to symptoms with such intensity that they do not clearly reflect a discernable, understandable pattern. Several studies have shown that severity of illness is a predictor of uncertainty, although the indicators of severity of illness have varied across studies (Mishel, 1997a). Among patients in the acute or treatment phase of illnesses such as cardiovascular disease (Christman et al., 1988), cancer (Galloway & Graydon, 1996; Hilton, 1994), chronic illness such as pain in fibromyalgia (Johnson, Zautra, & Davis, 2006), and parenting of critically ill children and children recently diagnosed with cancer (Santacroce, 2002; Tomlinson, Kirschbaum, Harbaugh, & Anderson, 1996), severity of illness was positively associated with uncertainty. According to the UIT, the nature of the severity presents difficulty delineating a symptom pattern about the extent of the disease, resulting in uncertainty.

Stimuli Frame: Symptom Pattern

Studies that address the process of identifying symptoms of a disease or condition and reaching a diagnosis are classified as addressing symptom pattern. The process of receiving a diagnosis requires that a symptom pattern exist and can be labeled as an illness or condition. In the UIT, absence of the symptom pattern is associated with uncertainty. Uncertainty levels have been reported to be highest in those without a diagnosis and undergoing diagnostic examinations (Hilton, 1993; Mishel, 1981). In studies where patients' symptoms are not clearly distinguishable from those of other comorbid conditions or where symptoms of recurrence can be confused with signs of aging or other natural processes and not recognizable as signs of disease, such as in lupus, survivors of breast cancer, and cardiac disease, these symptoms are associated with uncertainty (Hilton, 1988; Mishel & Murdaugh, 1987; Nelson, 1996; Winters, 1999). In a study of long-term breast cancer survivors, it was not the symptoms that elicited uncertainty but events that triggered thoughts of recurrence or the meaning of physical symptoms from long-term treatment side effects (Gil et al., 2004). High levels of symptoms such as pain are associated with uncertainty when one does not know how to manage them (Johnson et al., 2006). Similarly, research has demonstrated the association between uncertainty and experienced physical symptoms of breast cancer survivors, demonstrating that unpredictable physical symptoms that may come and go, such as fatigue and arm problems, can create uncertainty about breast cancer recurrence (Clayton, Mishel, & Belyea, 2006; Wonghongkul et al., 2006). Other research has focused on understanding the ambiguity of symptoms associated with pre-term labor (Weiss, Saks, & Harris, 2002). Even previous experience with pre-term labor did not reduce the ambiguity associated with this condition.

The erratic nature of symptom onset and disease progression is a major antecedent of uncertainty in chronic illness (Mishel, 1999). Symptoms that occur unpredictably fit the description of the stimuli frame component of event incongruence because there is no congruity between the cue and the outcome. The timing and nature of symptom onset, duration, intensity, and location are unforeseeable, characterized by periods of stability and erratic flares of exacerbation or unpredictable recurrence resulting in uncertainty (Brown & Powell-Cope, 1991; Mast, 1998; Mishel & Braden, 1988; Sexton, Calcasola, Bottomley, & Funk, 1999). Similarly, difficulty being aware of physical symptoms and determining their meaning in acute heart failure patients has also been found to be related to greater uncertainty (Jurgens, 2006). Among parents of ill children, unpredictable trajectories with few markers of illness are also positively associated with uncertainty (Cohen, 1993b). Determining the cause of an illness is another example of cue–outcome congruence. If a specific cause can be identified, the cause functions as the cue with illness as the outcome. Difficulty in determining cause of illness has been found to be associated with uncertainty (Cohen, 1993a; Sharkey, 1995; Turner, Tomlinson, & Harbaugh, 1990). Recent work on patients with endometriosis found that since no cure exists and treatment effectiveness varies, patients experience uncertainty surrounding the relationship of diagnosis to treatment outcomes (Lemaire, 2004). In young adults with asthma, uncertainty has been proposed to occur due to episode severity and/or frequency, which is not contingent upon the person's attempt to manage the illness (Mullins, Chaney, Balderson, & Hommel, 2000).

Stimuli Frame: Event Familiarity

Studies that focus on the health care or home environment for treatment of illness fit under the stimuli frame component of event familiarity. Although fewer studies have addressed this component of stimuli frame, the studies that have been conducted support that unfamiliarity with health care environment, organization, and expectations is associated with uncertainty. Health care environments characterized by novelty and confusion where the rules and routines are unknown and equipment and treatments are unfamiliar are associated with uncertainty (Horner, 1997; Stewart & Mishel, 2000; Turner, Tomlinson, & Harbaugh, 1990).

Structure Providers: Social Support

In the UIT, social support from friends, family, and those with similar experiences are proposed to reduce uncertainty directly and indirectly by influencing the stimuli frame. Those with similar experience have been found to influence the stimuli frame by providing information about illness-related events and symptom pattern (Van Riper & Selder, 1989; White & Frasure-Smith, 1995). There are a number of studies that support the role of social support in reducing uncertainty among parents of ill children, adult and adolescent patients, and their care providers (Bennett, 1993; Davis, 1990; Mishel & Braden, 1987; Neville, 1998; Tomlinson et al., 1996). However, when the illness is stigmatized, the questionable acceptance by others limits the use of social support to manage uncertainty (Brown & Powell-Cope, 1991; Weitz, 1989). Social interaction also may not always be supportive. Unsupportive interactions serve to heighten uncertainty (Wineman, 1990). The dual impact of social support has also been investigated in men with HIV or AIDS. Brashers, Neidig, and Goldsmith (2004) reported that other individuals help HIV patients manage uncertainty by providing instrumental support, facilitating skill development, giving acceptance or validation, allowing ventilation, and encouraging a perspective shift. They also report that there are problems associated with social support and uncertainty management including a lack of coordination in managing uncertainty, the addition of relational uncertainty, and the burden of caregiver uncertainty. Other investigators have found that family members experience high levels of uncertainty, which may impair their ability to provide support for the patient (Brown & Powell-Cope, 1991; Mishel & Murdaugh, 1987; Wineman, O'Brien, Nealon, & Kaskel, 1993). In a study of uncertainty in African American and White family members of men with localized prostate cancer, uncertainty was associated with family members feeling less positive about treatments and patient recovery, feeling more psychological distress, and engaging in less active problem solving (Germino et al., 1998). These findings bring into question the ability of family members to be supportive of the patient when family members are trying to deal with their own uncertainties. Among younger breast cancer survivors, both social support and uncertainty together explained 27% of the variance in quality of life, with higher levels of social support functioning to reduce uncertainty (Sammarco, 2001). Current research supports the theoretical relationship between social support and uncertainty and provides information on factors that influence effective social support.

Structure Providers: Credible Authority

Credible authority refers to health care providers who are seen as credible information givers by the patient or family member. As experts, health care providers have been proposed to reduce uncertainty by providing information and promoting confidence in their clinical judgment and performance. Trust and confidence in the health care provider's ability to make a diagnosis, to control the illness, and to provide adequate treatment has been reported to be related to less uncertainty across a variety of acute and chronic illnesses (Mishel & Braden, 1988; Santacroce, 2000). On the other hand, patients' lack of confidence in the provider's abilities increases uncertainty (Becker, Janson-Bjerklie, Benner, Slobin, & Ferdetich, 1993; Smeltzer, 1994). Uncertainty has also been found to increase when patients report that they are not receiving adequate information from health care providers (Galloway & Graydon, 1996; Hilton, 1988; Nyhlin, 1990; Small & Graydon, 1993; Weems & Patterson, 1989).

Recently there has been a resurgence of interest in the study of doctor–patient communication. Clayton, Mishel, and Belyea (2006) report the testing of a model based on the UIT with an emphasis on the role of doctor–patient communication in older breast cancer survivors. Findings did not support the role of doctor–patient communication in relation to uncertainty or to well-being. Various explanations for the lack of influence of doctor–patient interaction in the model may be that the need for information from the physician may decrease over time from diagnosis through recovery unless there is a recurrence. This idea is supported by the work of Brashers, Hsieh, Neidig, and Reynolds (2006), who found that patients with an enduring chronic illness such as HIV held beliefs and attitudes about health care providers in a variety of dimensions. Brashers and colleagues describe the criteria used by these patients to evaluate the provider and strategies for managing their relationship with the provider. This work clearly contributes to the theory; however, further research is needed to determine if the information is applicable to individuals with other diagnoses.

Appraisal of Uncertainty

According to the UIT, appraisal of uncertainty involves personality dispositions, attitudes, and beliefs, which influence whether uncertainty is appraised as a danger or an opportunity. There is support for the impact of uncertainty on reducing personality dispositions such as optimism, sense of coherence, and level of resourcefulness (Christman, 1990; Hilton, 1989; Mishel et al., 1984). Certain dispositions such as generalized negative outcome expectancies interact with uncertainty to predict psychological distress (Mullins et al., 1995). However, selected cognitive and personality factors have been reported to mediate the relationship between uncertainty and danger or opportunity. Mediators that decrease the impact of uncertainty on danger and adjustment include higher enabling skill, self-efficacy, mastery, hope, challenge, and existential well-being (Braden, Mishel, Longman, & Burns, 1998; Landis, 1996; Mishel, Padilla, Grant, &

Sorenson, 1991; Mishel & Sorenson, 1991; Wonghongkul et al., 2006; Wonghongkul, Moore, Musil, Schneider, & Deimling, 2000). Some studies where appraisals were found to be positive are of populations that are a number of years post-treatment. Others have reported that positive appraisals of uncertainty can be found along with negative appraisals, enabling both to exist simultaneously. This has been reported for patients awaiting coronary artery bypass surgery where uncertainty can be seen as a source for hope (McCormick et al., 2006). However, recent work by Kang (2006) with a sample of patients with atrial fibrillation reported that appraisal of uncertainty as an opportunity had a negative relationship with depression, and appraisal of uncertainty as a danger was positively associated with depression. As uncertainty increased, so did the danger appraisal, which was related to a decrease in mental health (Kang, 2005).

Coping With Uncertainty

Numerous investigators who have studied the management of uncertainty have found that higher uncertainty is associated with danger and resultant emotion-focused coping strategies such as wishful thinking, avoidance, and fatalism (Christman, 1990; Hilton, 1989; Mishel & Sorenson, 1991; Mishel et al., 1991; Redeker, 1992; Webster & Christman, 1988). Severe symptoms such as high levels of pain in interaction with uncertainty have been reported to reduce one's ability to cope with the symptom (Johnson et al., 2006). Others report more varied coping strategies for managing uncertainty including cognitive strategies such as downward comparison, constructing a personal scenario for the illness, use of faith or religion, and identifying markers and triggers (Baier, 1995; Mishel & Murdaugh, 1987; Wiener & Dodd, 1993). Mishel (1993) offered a review of major uncertainty management methods; however, there is little evidence for the use of any of these coping strategies mediating the relationship between uncertainty and emotional distress (Mast, 1998; Mishel & Sorenson, 1991; Mishel et al., 1991). While there has not been much study of the role of hopefulness in managing uncertainty, findings from a study of participation in a clinical drug trial revealed that uncertainty was related to a decrease in hope during time in the trial. Those with more uncertainty and less hopefulness reported more negative moods (Wineman, Schwetz, Zeller, & Cyphert, 2003). In the area of uncertainty in children, Stewart (2003) reported that children emphasized the routine and ordinariness of their lives despite their cancer diagnosis and treatment.

Uncertainty and Adjustment

According to the UIT, adjustment refers to returning to the individual's level of pre-illness functioning. However, most of the research has interpreted this as emotional stability or quality of life. Few studies have tested the complete outcome portion of the theory, including uncertainty, appraisal, coping strategies, and adjustment. Most studies examine the relationship between uncertainty and an outcome and relate these findings to the theory. The findings from these studies have consistently shown positive relationships between uncertainty and negative emotional outcomes (Bennett, 1993; Mast, 1998; Mishel, 1984; Mullins et al., 2001; Sanders-Dewey, Mullins, & Chaney, 2001; Small & Graydon, 1993; Taylor-Piliae & Molassiotis, 2001; Wineman, Schwetz, Goodkin, & Rudick, 1996). Further evidence for the significant effect of uncertainty on depression was reported by Mullins and colleagues (2000) in young adults with asthma. The effect of uncertainty on depression was at its maximum under conditions of increased illness severity. Uncertainty has also been related to poorer psychosocial adjustment in the areas of less life satisfaction (Hilton, 1994), negative attitudes toward health care, family relationships, recreation and employment (Mishel et al., 1984; Mishel & Braden, 1987), less satisfaction with health care services (Green & Murton, 1996), and poorer quality of life (Carroll, Hamilton, & McGovern, 1999; Padilla, Mishel, & Grant, 1992). Santacroce (2003) has identified the linkage between uncertainty and negative outcomes in her literature review on parental uncertainty and posttraumatic stress in serious childhood illness.

There has been extensive study of uncertainty in illness based on the UIT, and most of the research supports sections of the theory. Although some studies were not done to test the theory, the findings are consistent with the UIT. Overall, the theory has been very useful in guiding research, and sections of the theory are well-supported by published studies with a variety of clinical populations and caregivers.

Research on RUIT

Less attention has been given to study of the RUIT, possibly due to the difficulty in studying a process that evolves over time. Support for the RUIT has been found in qualitative studies that favor a transition through uncertainty to a new orientation toward life with acceptance of uncertainty as a part of life (Mishel, 1999). The samples for these studies included long-term diabetic patients (Nyhlin, 1990), chronically ill men (Charmaz, 1994), HIV patients (Brashers et al., 2003; Katz, 1996), persons with schizophrenia (Baier, 1995), spouses of heart transplant patients (Mishel & Murdaugh, 1987), family caregivers of AIDS patients (Brown & Powell-Cope, 1991), breast cancer survivors (Mishel et al., 2005; Nelson, 1996; Pelusi, 1997), adolescent survivors of childhood cancer (Parry, 2003), and women recovering from cardiac disease (Fleury, Kimbrell, & Kruszewski, 1995). Bailey, Wallace, and

Mishel (2007), using the RUIT as the organizing framework for the study, interviewed men who were undergoing watchful waiting as their treatment for prostate cancer. Although the findings were not totally supportive of the RUIT, men did express that they had generated options, created opportunities for themselves, and remained hopeful of a positive outcome. Parry's (2003) study of childhood cancer survivors suggests that uncertainty can be a catalyst for growth, for a greater appreciation for life, and for greater awareness of life purpose. However, in another study of survivors of childhood cancer, findings showed that uncertainty mediated the relationship between posttraumatic stress disorder and health promotion behaviors, indicating that uncertainty exists over time and reduces health promotion activities (Santacroce & Lee, 2006).

The findings supporting the RUIT seem to differ by subject population and methodology where more qualitative studies, as compared with quantitative studies, support the RUIT. The transition through uncertainty toward a new view of life was framed differently by each investigator and included themes such as a revised life perspective, new ways of being in the world, growth through uncertainty, new levels of self-organization, new goals for living, devaluating what is worthwhile, redefining what is normal, and building new dreams (Bailey & Stewart, 2001). All of the investigators described the gradual acceptance of uncertainty and the restructuring of reality as major components of the process, both of which are consistent with the RUIT.

An instrument to measure the change theoretically proposed in the RUIT was developed by Mishel and Fleury and is being tested for construct validity. The scale addresses growth through uncertainty toward a new view of life and was developed to address the discrepancy noted above between qualitative and quantitative approaches to study the RUIT. Initial use of the scale was reported by Mast (1998), and further testing of the scale is occurring before it is available for general use. The Growth Through Uncertainty Scale, GTUS, has been used in a few clinical investigations. In a recent intervention study involving both authors of this chapter, baseline analysis of the data included use of the GTUS. The analysis was to identify variables that would predict either negative mood state or personal growth (GTUS) in older African American and White long-term breast cancer survivors. Of the variables found to be significant predictors, negative cognitive state, which included uncertainty, was a significant predictor of both outcomes. The overall findings were supportive of the RUIT since cognitive reappraisal, defined as the tendency to address concerns from a positive point of view, predicted 40% of the variance in personal growth (GTUS) (Porter et al., 2006). Also, in the findings from this intervention study, at 10 months and 20 months post-intervention, older long-term African American breast cancer survivors in the treatment group maintained and increased scores on the GTUS over time while scores for subjects in the control group declined over time (Gil et al., 2006; Mishel et al., 2005).

Interventions to Manage Uncertainty

An uncertainty management intervention has been developed and tested in four clinical trials for breast cancer patients and patients with localized or advanced prostate cancer (Braden et al., 1998; Mishel, 1997b; Mishel et al., 2002; Mishel et al., 2003). The intervention was structured to follow the theory of the UIT and was delivered by weekly phone calls to cancer patients. All studies included equal numbers of White and minority samples. The intervention was effective in teaching patients skills to manage uncertainty including improvements in problem solving, cognitive reframing, treatment-related side effects, and patient–provider communication. Improvement was also found in ability to manage the uncertainty related to side effects from cancer treatment. Religious participation and education were found to be moderators of the treatment outcomes of cancer knowledge and patient–provider communication in the intervention trial for men with localized prostate cancer. Education was a covariate in the study of older women during treatment for breast cancer. Using the UIT and the RUIT as the framework for study of an intervention for older long-term African American and White breast cancer survivors, a self-delivered uncertainty management intervention with nurse assistance was tested and results indicated that the intervention at 10 months and 20 months follow-up produced significant differences in experimental and control groups in cognitive reframing, cancer knowledge, patient–provider communication, and a variety of coping skills. The most important results were the improvement in the treatment groups' pursuit of further information along with declines in uncertainty and stable effects in personal growth over time (Gil et al., 2006; Mishel et al., 2005).

Further intervention work based on the UIT and RUIT was conducted by Bailey, Mishel, Belyea, Stewart, and Mohler (2004) among men selecting watchful waiting in prostate cancer. The results from this clinical trial showed that men in the intervention improved on the GTUS on the subscale of living life in a new light and believing that their future would be improved. An intervention program for women with recurrent breast cancer and their family members was found to be well-received. This program was not developed on the uncertainty theory but did contain a core component on uncertainty reduction. This component offered women and families factual information about cancer recurrence and treatments, encouraged assertive approaches with health care providers, and focused on learning to live with uncertainty in preference to negative certainty (Northouse et al., 2002). An intervention trial for newly diagnosed breast cancer patients in Taiwan used the UIT framework and provided information to questions raised by patients. This continual supportive care was given at four points during treatment. The findings indicated that support was increased and uncertainty was decreased 1 month after surgery and 4 months after diagnosis (Liu, Li, Tang, Huang, & Chiou, 2006). Other intervention studies included uncertainty as a variable but did not use either the UIT or RUIT as the framework for the study or for the intervention (Kreulen & Braden, 2004; McCain et al., 2003; Taylor-Piliae & Chair, 2002). The number of intervention studies using the uncertainty theory or including intervention to address uncertainty is continually increasing in the literature.

USE OF THE THEORIES IN NURSING PRACTICE

Nurses are included in the UIT as part of the antecedent variable of structure providers. The clinical literature supports delivery of information as the major method to help patients manage uncertainty. Nurses provide information that helps patients develop meaning from the illness experience by providing structure to the stimuli frame. When considering the RUIT, nurses help patients manage chronic uncertainty by assisting with the patient's reappraisal of uncertainty from stressful to hopeful in addition to providing relevant information.

Understanding the sources of patient uncertainty can help nurses plan for effective information giving and may greatly assist nurses to help patients manage or reduce their uncertainty. In one of the few articles to address the environmental component of the stimuli frame, Sharkey (1995) discussed how family coping could be enhanced by home care nurses normalizing health care into the familiar routines of families caring for a terminally ill child at home. Among cardiac patients, White and Frasure-Smith (1995) suggested that nurses promote the use of patient-solicited social support to manage uncertainty in percutaneous transluminal coronary angioplasty (PTCA) patients. These researchers suggested that the benefit from the social support received by PTCA patients was due to direct requests tailored to specific needs versus unsolicited social support due to simply being ill. Additionally, information from nurses about the potential long-term success of this procedure might help reduce the higher uncertainty found in PTCA patients 3 months after surgery. Among breast cancer survivors, Gil and colleagues (2004, 2005) suggested that nurses can help women identify their personal triggers of uncertainty about recurrence, then teach coping skills such as breathing relaxation, pleasant imagery, calming self-talk, and distraction to help survivors manage their uncertainty.

The RUIT has also been used to inform clinical practice and help nurses understand sources of patient uncertainty. An example of how mental health nurses can assist patients by understanding sources of uncertainty is found in research by Brashers and colleagues (2003) describing the medical, social, and personal forms of uncertainty for persons living with HIV/AIDS. Further, this research suggests nurses should be aware that subgroups of this population such as women, drug users, gay men, and parents can experience different sources of uncertainty based on social stigma, role and/or identity confusion, and lack of familiarity with the medical system. Other research using the RUIT indicates that childhood cancer survivors often have late emerging side effects that impact quality of life and the experience of uncertainty similar to other long-term cancer survivors (Lee, 2006; Santacroce & Lee, 2006). These studies suggest that childhood cancer survivors who lack effective coping and uncertainty management skills may be unable to reappraise uncertainty and are at risk for the development of posttraumatic stress symptoms (PTSS) as a way of avoiding uncertainty when life demands become excessive (Lee, 2006). Health professionals who are aware of the increased risk of PTSS created by an inability to reappraise uncertainty can offer developmentally appropriate information, thereby clarifying the ambiguity of future survivorship and helping childhood cancer survivors manage the continual uncertainty in their lives (Santacroce & Lee, 2006).

Recognizing uncertainty and then providing contextual cues to reduce ambiguity and increase understanding explains how nurses communicate with patients. Contextual cues provide explanations of what patients will see, hear, and feel during procedures and tests, as well as what signs and symptoms they will experience at various points in their illness trajectory. Providing information and explanations about treatments and medications has been proposed to be the most important and frequent approach to reducing patient uncertainty (Mishel et al., 2002; Wineman et al., 1996). Galloway and Graydon (1996), who based their findings on recently discharged colon cancer patients, noted that nurses could provide information to alleviate the uncertainty of being discharged to the home environment. Correspondingly, Mitchell, Courtney, and Coyer (2003) found that nurses provide beneficial contextual cues and information to both families and patients upon transfer from the intensive care unit to a general hospital floor. Families of patients who received clear information were more able to make decisions for patients, reported less anxiety, and were better able to provide emotional and physical patient support. Other effective methods for reducing patient uncertainty can include encouraging communication with patients who have successfully managed their uncertainties. Weems and Patterson (1989) suggest sharing the uncertainties of waiting for a renal transplant with someone who has already received a transplant or sharing uncertainties of how to live with chronic obstructive pulmonary disease (COPD) with someone who is successfully managing this chronic disease (Small & Graydon, 1993). This type of communication provides information to patients for structuring the stimuli and also functions as a source of social support.

Offering comprehensive information allows the nurse to function as a credible authority, strengthening the stimuli frame by enhancing disease predictability and reducing symptom ambiguity. Righter (1995) used the UIT to describe the role of an enterostomal therapy (ET) nurse as a credible authority for the ostomy patient. She describes the ET nurse as providing structure and order to the experience of the new ostomy patient through clinical expertise and experience. The ET nurse reduces the ambiguity of the ostomy experience by providing information, counseling, and support. This facilitates ostomy patients' adaptation to their newly altered perception of themselves and helps them regain a sense of control and mastery by creating order and predictability. Other ideas on changing clinical practice to reduce patient uncertainty include educational interventions delivered in person, by telephone, or by individualized patient information packets delivered through the mail (Calvin & Lane, 1999; Mishel et al., 2002). Research by Bailey and colleagues (2004) found that nurses can clarify information about treatment options that create confusion for men who have selected watchful waiting as their treatment choice for prostate cancer. Nurses can answer patient questions about variations in prostate-specific antigen (PSA) values, thus reducing uncertainty about both disease progression and future events. Understanding the meaning of lab values helped men sort out the confusion associated with mixed messages given to them by family who promoted aggressive treatment and urologists who promoted watchful waiting. Mishel and colleagues (2002) found that prostate cancer patients immediately post-surgery or during radiation therapy felt reassured when their questions were answered by a nurse, resulting in reduced anxiety and uncertainty. These men also expressed appreciation for the concern of a health professional and subsequently reported feeling less alone in their battle with cancer.

When considering the predictability of illness trajectories, Sexton and colleagues (1999) found that advanced practice nurses helped patients manage a diagnosis of asthma by implementing nursing actions that helped patients predict and manage their asthma attacks. Similarly, among breast cancer survivors, unpredictable physical symptoms that may come and go such as fatigue and arm problems can create uncertainty about breast cancer recurrence (Clayton, Mishel, & Belyea, 2006; Wong-hongkul et al., 2006). Thus, providers, including advance practice nurses, should try to communicate in a manner that fully explains existing symptoms and their relationship or lack thereof to cancer recurrence (Clayton, Dudley, & Musters, 2006).

Clinical journals are increasingly identifying patient uncertainty as an important part of the illness experience and provide suggestions for nursing actions to reduce patient uncertainty or facilitate a new outlook by focusing on choices and alternatives. Suggestions for managing uncertainty in clinical practice include work by Crigger (1996), who suggests that nurses can help women adapt positively to multiple sclerosis by shifting the emphasis from the management of physical disability to the management of uncertainty, thereby helping women achieve mastery over their daily lives. Similarly, Calvin and Lane (1999) suggested incorporating preoperative psycho-educational interventions to reduce uncertainty as part of orthopedic preadmission visits. Other examples of using UIT to develop and implement nursing interventions to reduce uncertainty and regain control in clinical settings are suggested by Allan (1990) for HIV-positive men, Sterken (1996) for fathers of pediatric cancer patients, Northouse, Mood, Templin, Mellon, and George (2000) for patients with colon cancer, and Sharkey (1995) for homebound pediatric oncology patients. Ritz and colleagues (2000) report another nursing intervention to manage uncertainty in clinical practice. These clinicians investigated the effect of follow-up nursing care by the advanced practice nurse after discharge of newly treated breast cancer patients. Six months after diagnosis, uncertainty was reduced and quality of life was improved.

Based on the antecedent variables of UIT, Northouse and colleagues (2000) suggested that health professionals keep in mind individual characteristics of patients, social environments, and methods of illness appraisal when caring for patients with colon cancer. They suggested that nurses provide patients with a framework of expectations about the physical and emotional illness trajectory associated with the first year of managing this diagnosis. Thus, use of the UIT can help nurses recognize groups of patients and/or caregivers that may be at risk for increased uncertainty. For example, Sterken (1996) found that younger fathers did not understand the information given to them about their child's treatment and disease patterns as well as older fathers, illustrating how cognitive capacity influences uncertainty. Santacroce (2002) found that African American parents of children newly diagnosed with cancer experienced greater uncertainty than White parents. She posits that past experiences with the health care system can impact parental uncertainty. These studies illustrate the difficulty as well as the potential benefit in using demographic characteristics to identify persons at risk for heightened uncertainty.

Current investigators have explained how the theory can be applied to understanding a clinical situation, clinical diagnosis, or clinical practice. For example, it is important to realize when increased uncertainty can place patients at risk for additional illnesses, such as recognizing that uncertainty is a major factor contributing to depression in patients with hepatitis C (Saunders & Cookman, 2005). Some clinical areas such as women's health and cardiovascular disease have been studied in depth. In the area of women's health, Sorenson (1990) discusses the concepts of symptom pattern, event familiarity and congruency, cognitive capacity, structure providers, and credible authority, using examples from normal pregnancy to help nurses relate the theory to women who are experiencing difficulty adapting to the uncertainties of pregnancy. For women experiencing high-risk pregnancy, they preferred the coping strategy of avoidance as a means for managing uncertainty and preserving their sense of well-being (Giurgescu, Penckofer, Maurer, & Bryant, 2006). Suggestions are made about how perinatal nurses can help women accept impending motherhood and utilize more effective coping mechanisms to reduce uncertainty and improve psychological well-being. Lemaire and Lenz (1995) applied the UIT to the condition of menopause. The stimuli frame for menopause was defined as the symptoms that indicate approaching menopause, including mood swings, hot flashes, dry skin, and memory changes. If women received factual information from a source deemed credible, such as nurses and health care providers, it was thought that familiarity with the event of menopause would be increased and uncertainty about this normal life event would be decreased. Consistent with predictions of UIT, uncertainty declined after receipt of understandable information delivered by a credible source, allowing women to construct meaning from the ambiguity and unpredictability of their symptoms surrounding the normal process of menopause. Similarly, Lemaire (2004) suggests that nurses who understand the uncertainty associated with the symptoms of endometriosis are better able to care for women experiencing this condition. Nursing actions such as providing informational material, offering referrals to support groups, and sharing electronic resources can help women better understand and manage the ambiguity and unpredictability of symptoms such as cramping, non-menstrual pain, and fatigue. Other research has focused on understanding the ambiguity of symptoms associated with preterm labor (Weiss et al., 2002). Weiss and colleagues found that women lacked familiarity with the symptom pattern of preterm labor. They suggest that language used by women in describing preterm labor be incorporated into educational materials available to all pregnant women to help them recognize preterm labor as differentiated from term labor. They stress that every expectant woman needs education about the cues to use in recognizing preterm labor.

In patients diagnosed with atrial fibrillation, UIT can help nurses identify patients at risk for increased uncertainty (Kang et al., 2004). Focusing on the antecedents of uncertainty, findings showed that patients with more severe symptoms and those with less education experienced greater uncertainty, helping nurses to be more aware of which patients may be at risk. Other research has found that those patients who receive an implantable cardioverter defibrillator (ICD) experience great uncertainty, never knowing when their arrhythmias may reoccur and when the device may "fire" (Flemme et al., 2005). Further, hospital nurses may have little time to prepare these patients for discharge since there is no need for further hospitalization postimplantation of the device. Outpatient clinic and office nurses, therefore, can provide key information and support to these patients, recognizing that the high levels of uncertainty frequently experienced by these patients put them at risk for poorer quality of life. Similarly, Rydström and colleagues (2004) note the uncertainty that affects the whole family when a child has asthma, suggesting education for both parents and siblings about asthma as well as the impact of asthma on family dynamics. Further, these authors stress the importance of communicating to families that their nurse is approachable about both disease issues and family dynamics issues as part of holistic disease management.

Another approach to improving patient care is recognizing the importance of professional education on uncertainty to effect change in clinical practice. Wunderlich, Perry, Lavin, and Katz (1999) suggested that critical care nurses would benefit from staff development sessions on how to address the uncertainty that patients experience during the process of weaning from mechanical ventilation. Dombeck (1996) commented that health care professionals need to increase their own tolerance for ambiguity and uncertainty to effectively listen to clients who are experiencing ambiguity and uncertainty. Similarly Light (1979) noted that health care professionals have been socialized to minimize uncertainty; this socialization may make it difficult to effectively address patient uncertainty until health care workers learn more about it (Baier, 1995). Recognizing the importance of integrating UIT into a management strategy for asthma patients, the American Nurses Credentialing Center's Commission on Accreditation offered 3 credit hours for successful completion of a continuing education unit (CEU) quiz following the published article (Sexton et al., 1999) about coping with uncertainty. Other CEU offerings incorporating uncertainty theory have been offered following a case study on spiritual disequilibrium (Dombeck, 1996) and an article on weaning a patient from mechanical ventilation (Wunderlich et al., 1999).

CONCLUSION

The Uncertainty in Illness theories have been used in multiple ways to inform clinician understanding of patients, families, and illness situations. Clinical research guided by both the original UIT (1988) and the RUIT (1990) for those coping with both acute and chronic illnesses will continue to help identify appropriate nursing interventions for many types of illnesses and patients. Ultimately the recognition of the importance of uncertainty can change clinical practice, allowing the development of nursing interventions that facilitate a positive patient adaptation to the illness experience.

REFERENCES

Allan, J. D. (1990). Focusing on living, not dying: A naturalistic study of self-care among seropositive gay men. *Holistic Nursing Practice, 4*(2), 56–63.

Allen, D. G. (1985). Nursing research and social control: Alternative models of science that emphasize understanding and emancipation. *Image: Journal of Nursing Scholarship, 17,* 58–64.

Antonovsky, A. (1987). *Unraveling the mystery of health: How people manage stress and stay well.* San Francisco: Jossey-Bass.

Baier, M. (1995). Uncertainty of illness for persons with schizophrenia. *Issues in Mental Health Nursing, 16,* 201–212.

Bailey, D. E., Mishel, M. H., Belyea, M., Stewart, J. L., & Mohler, J. (2004). Uncertainty intervention for watchful waiting in prostate cancer. *Cancer Nursing, 27*(5), 339–346.

Bailey, D. E., & Stewart, J. L. (2001). Mishel's theory of uncertainty in illness. In A. M. Mariner-Tomey & M. R. Alligood (Eds.), *Nursing theorists and their work* (5th ed.). St. Louis, MO: Mosby. pp. 560–583.

Bailey, D. E., Wallace, M., & Mishel, M. H. (2007). Watching, waiting and uncertainty in prostate cancer. *Journal of Clinical Nursing, 16*(4), 734–741.

Barron, C. R. (2000). Stress, uncertainty, and health. In V. H. Rice (Ed.), *Handbook of stress, coping and health: Implications for nursing research, theory, and practice* (pp. 517–539). Thousand Oaks, CA: Sage.

Becker, G., Janson-Bjerklie, S., Benner, P., Slobin, K., & Ferdetich, S. (1993). The dilemma of seeking urgent care: Asthma episodes and emergency service use. *Social Science and Medicine, 37,* 305–313.

Bennett, S. J. (1993). Relationships among selected antecedent variables and coping effectiveness in postmyocardial infarction patients. *Research in Nursing and Health, 16,* 131–139.

Bower, G. H. (1978). *The psychology of learning and motivation: Advances in research and theory.* New York: Academic Press.

Braden, C. J., Mishel, M. H., Longman, A. J., & Burns, L. (1998). Self-help intervention project: Women receiving breast cancer treatment. *Cancer Practice, 6*(2), 87–98.

Brashers, D. E., Hsieh, E., Neidig, J. L., & Reynolds, N. R. (2006). Managing uncertainty about illness: Health care providers as credible authorities. In R. M. Dailey & B. A. Le Poire (Eds.), *Applied interpersonal communication matters.* New York: Peter Lang.

Brashers, D. E., Neidig, J. L., & Goldsmith, D. J. (2004). Social support and the management of uncertainty for people living with HIV. *Health Communication, 16,* 305–331.

Brashers, D. E., Neidig, J. L., Russell, J. A., Cardillo, L. W., Haas, S. M., Dobbs, L. K., et al. (2003). The medical, personal, and social causes of uncertainty in HIV illness. *Issues in Mental Health Nursing, 24*(5), 497–522.

Brown, M. A., & Powell-Cope, G. M. (1991). AIDS family caregiving: Transitions through uncertainty. *Nursing Research, 40,* 337–345.

Budner, S. (1962). Intolerance of ambiguity as a personality variable. *Journal of Personality, 30,* 29–50.

Calvin, R., & Lane, P. (1999). Perioperative uncertainty and state anxiety of orthopaedic surgical patients. *Orthopedic Nursing, 18*(6), 61–6.

Carroll, D., Hamilton, G., & McGovern, B. (1999). Changes in health status and quality of life and the impact of uncertainty in patients who survive life-threatening arrhythmias. *Heart and Lung, 28*(4), 251–260.

Charmaz, K. (1994). Identity dilemmas of chronically ill men. *The Sociological Quarterly, 35*(2), 269–288.

Christman, N. J. (1990). Uncertainty and adjustment during radiotherapy. *Nursing Research, 39*(1), 17–20.

Christman, N. J., McConnell, E. A., Pfeiffer, C., Webster, K. K., Schmitt, M., & Ries, J. (1988). Uncertainty, coping, and distress following myocardial infarction: Transition from home to hospital. *Research in Nursing and Health, 11,* 71–82.

Clayton, M. F., Dudley, W. N., & Musters, A. (2006). Communication with breast cancer survivors. *Health Communication, 39,* 175.

Clayton, M. F., Mishel, M. H., & Belyea, M. (2006). Testing a model of symptoms, communication, uncertainty, and well-being, in older breast cancer survivors. *Research in Nursing and Health, 29*(1), 18–39.

Cohen, M. H. (1993a). Diagnostic closure and the spread of uncertainty. *Issues in Comprehensive Pediatric Nursing, 16,* 135–146.

Cohen, M. H. (1993b). The unknown and the unknowable—managing sustained uncertainty. *Western Journal of Nursing Research, 15*(1), 77–96.

Crigger, N. J. (1996). Testing an uncertainty model for women with multiple sclerosis. *Advances in Nursing Science, 18*(3), 37–47.

Davis, L. L. (1990). Illness uncertainty, social support, and stress in recovering individuals and family caregivers. *Applied Nursing Research,* 69–71.

Dombeck, M. (1996). Chaos and self-organization as a consequence of spiritual disequilibrium. *Clinical Nurse Specialist, 10*(2), 69–73; quiz 74–75.

Flemme, I., Edvardsson, N., Hinic, H., Jinhage, B. M., Dalman, M., & Fridlund, B. (2005). Long-term quality of life and uncertainty in patients living with an implantable cardioverter defibrillator. *Heart and Lung, 34*(6), 386–392.

Fleury, J., Kimbrell, L. C., & Kruszewski, M. A. (1995). Life after a cardiac event: Women's experience in healing. *Heart and Lung, 24,* 474–482.

Galloway, S., & Graydon, J. (1996). Uncertainty, symptom distress, and information needs after surgery for cancer of the colon. *Cancer Nursing, 19*(2), 112–117.

Germino, B. B., Mishel, M. H., Belyea, M., Harris, L., Ware, A., & Mohler, J. (1998). Uncertainty in prostate cancer, ethnic and family patterns. *Cancer Practice, 6*(2), 102–113.

Gil, K. M., Mishel, M. H., Belyea, M., Germino, B., Porter, L., & Clayton, M. (2006). Benefits of the uncertainty management intervention for African American and White older breast cancer survivors: 20-month outcomes. *International Journal of Behavioral Medicine, 13*(4), 285–294.

Gil, K. M., Mishel, M. H., Belyea, M., Germino, B., Porter, L. S., LeNey, I. C., et al. (2004). Triggers of uncertainty about recurrence and treatment side effects in long-term older breast African American and Caucasian cancer survivors. *Oncology Nursing Forum, 31*(3), 633–639.

Gil, K. M., Mishel, M. H., Germino, B., Porter, L. S., Carlton-LaNey, I., & Belyea, M. (2005). Uncertainty management intervention for older African American and Caucasian long-term breast cancer survivors. *Journal of Psychosocial Oncology, 23*(2–3), 3–21.

Giurgescu, C., Penckofer, S., Maurer, M. C., & Bryant, F. B. (2006). Impact of uncertainty, social support, and prenatal coping on the psychological well-being of high-risk pregnant women. *Nursing Research, 55*(5), 356–365.

Green, J., & Murton, F. (1996). Diagnosis of Duchenne muscular dystrophy: Parents' experiences and satisfaction. *Child: Care, Health & Development, 22*, 113–128.

Hilton, B. A. (1988). The phenomenon of uncertainty in women with breast cancer. *Issues in Mental Health Nursing, 9*, 217–238.

Hilton, B. A. (1989). The relationship of uncertainty, control, commitment, and threat of recurrence to coping strategies used by women diagnosed with breast cancer. *Journal of Behavioral Medicine, 12*(1), 39–54.

Hilton, B. A. (1993). Issues, problems, and challenges for families coping with breast cancer. *Seminars in Oncology Nursing, 9*(2), 88–100.

Hilton, B. A. (1994). The uncertainty stress scale: Its development and psychometric properties. *Canadian Journal of Nursing Research, 26*(3), 15–30.

Horner, S. (1997). Uncertainty in mothers' care for their ill children. *Journal of Advanced Nursing, 26*, 658–663.

Johnson, L. M., Zautra, A. J., & Davis, M. C. (2006). The role of illness uncertainty on coping with fibromyalgia symptoms. *Health Psychology, 25*(6), 696–703.

Jurgens, C. Y. (2006). Somatic awareness, uncertainty, and delay in care-seeking in acute heart failure. *Research in Nursing and Health, 29*(2), 74–86.

Kang, Y. (2005). Effects of uncertainty on perceived health status in patients with atrial fibrillation. *British Association of Critical Care Nurses, Nursing in Critical Care 2005, 10*(4), 184–191.

Kang, Y. (2006). Effect of uncertainty on depression in patients with newly diagnosed atrial fibrillation. *Progress in Cardiology Nursing, Spring 2006*, 83–88.

Kang, Y., Daly, B. J., & Kim, J. S. (2004). Uncertainty and its antecedents in patients with atrial fibrillation. *Western Journal of Nursing Research, 26*(7), 770–783.

Katz, A. (1996). Gaining a new perspective on life as a consequence of uncertainty in HIV infection. *Journal of the Association of Nurses in AIDS Care, 7*(11), 51–60.

Kreulen, G. L., & Braden, C. J. (2004). Model test of the relationship between self-help-promoting nursing interventions and self-care and health status outcomes. *Research in Nursing & Health, 2004, 27*, 97–101.

Landis, B. J. (1996). Uncertainty, spirituality, well-being, and psychosocial adjustment to chronic illness. *Issues in Mental Health Nursing, 17*, 217–231.

Lazarus, R. S. (1974). Psychological stress and coping in adaptation and illness. *International Journal of Psychiatry in Medicine, 5*, 321–333.

Lee, Y. L. (2006). The relationships between uncertainty and posttraumatic stress in survivors of childhood cancer. *Journal of Nursing Research, 14*(2), 133–142.

Lemaire, G. S. (2004). More than just menstrual cramps: Symptoms and uncertainty among women with endometriosis. *Journal of Obstetric, Gynecologic, and Neonatal Nursing, 33*(1), 71–79.

Lemaire, G. S., & Lenz, E. R. (1995). Perceived uncertainty about menopause in women attending an educational program. *International Journal of Nursing Studies, 32*(1), 39–48.

Light, D. (1979). Uncertainty and control in professional training. *Journal of Health and Social Behavior, 20*, 310–322.

Liu, L., Li, C. Y., Tang, S., Huang, C., & Chiou, A. (2006). Role of continuing supportive cares in increasing social support and reducing perceived uncertainty among women with newly diagnosed breast cancer in Taiwan. *Cancer Nursing, 29*(4), 273–282.

Mandler, G. (1979). Thought processes, consciousness and stress. In V. Hamilton & D. M. Warburton (Eds.), *Human stress and cognition: An information processing approach* (pp. 179–201). New York: Wiley.

Mast, M. E. (1995). Adult uncertainty in illness: A critical review of research. *Scholarly Inquiry for Nursing Practice, 9*(1), 3–24.

Mast, M. E. (1998). Survivors of breast cancer: Illness uncertainty, positive reappraisal, and emotional distress. *Oncology Nursing Forum, 25*(3), 555–562.

McCain, N. L, Munjas, B. A., Munro, C. L., Elswick, R. K., Jr., Robins, J. L., Ferreira-Gonzalez, A., et al. (2003). Effects of stress management on PNI-based outcomes in persons with HIV disease. *Research in Nursing & Health, 26,* 102–117.

McCormick, K. M. (2001). A concept analysis of uncertainty in illness. *Journal of Nursing Scholarship, Second Quarter,* 127–131.

McCormick, K. M., Naimark, B. J., & Tate, R. B. (2006, January/February). Uncertainty, symptom distress, anxiety, and functional status in patients awaiting coronary artery bypass surgery. *Heart & Lung,* pp. 34–44.

Mishel, M. H. (1981). The measurement of uncertainty in illness. *Nursing Research, 30,* 258–263.

Mishel, M. H. (1983). Parents' perception of uncertainty concerning their hospitalized child. *Nursing Research, 32,* 324–330.

Mishel, M. H. (1984). Perceived uncertainty and stress in illness. *Research in Nursing and Health, 7,* 163–171.

Mishel, M. H. (1988). Uncertainty in illness. *Image: Journal of Nursing Scholarship, 20,* 225–231.

Mishel, M. H. (1990). Reconceptualization of the uncertainty in illness theory. *Image: Journal of Nursing Scholarship, 22,* 256–262.

Mishel, M. H. (1993). Living with chronic illness: Living with uncertainty. In S. G. Funk, E. M. Tornquist, M. T. Champagne, & R. A. Wiese (Eds.), *Key aspects of caring for the chronically ill: Hospital and home* (pp. 46–58). New York: Springer Publishing.

Mishel, M. H. (1997a). Uncertainty in acute illness. *Annual Review of Nursing Research, 15,* 57–80.

Mishel, M. H. (1997b). *The efficacy of the uncertainty management intervention for older White and African American women with breast cancer.* Paper presented at the 11th Annual Conference of the Southern Nursing Research Society, Norfolk, VA.

Mishel, M. H. (1999). Uncertainty in chronic illness. *Annual Review of Nursing Research, 17,* 269–294.

Mishel, M. H., Belyea, M., Germino, B. B., Stewart, J. L., Bailey, D. E., Robertson, C., et al. (2002). Helping patients with localized prostate carcinoma manage uncertainty and treatment side effects: Nurse-delivered psychoeducational intervention over the telephone. *Cancer, 94*(6), 1854–1866.

Mishel, M. H., & Braden, C. J. (1987). Uncertainty: A mediator between support and adjustment. *Western Journal of Nursing Research, 9,* 43–57.

Mishel, M. H., & Braden, C. J. (1988). Finding meaning: Antecedents of uncertainty in illness. *Nursing Research, 37,* 98–127.

Mishel, M. H., Germino, B. B., Belyea, M., Stewart, J. L., Bailey, D. E., Mohler, J., et al. (2003). Moderators of an uncertainty management intervention, for men with localized prostate cancer. *Nursing Research, 52*(2), 89–97.

Mishel, M. H., Germino, B., Gill, K. M., Belyea, M., Laney, I. C., Stewart, J., et al. (2005). Benefits from an uncertainty management intervention for African-American and Caucasian older long-term breast cancer survivors. *Psychooncology, 14,* 962–978.

Mishel, M. H., Hostetter, T., King, B., & Graham, V. (1984). Predictors of psychosocial adjustment in patients newly diagnosed with gynecological cancer. *Cancer Nursing,* 7, 291–299.

Mishel, M. H., & Murdaugh, C. L. (1987). Family adjustment to heart transplantation: Redesigning the dream. *Nursing Research, 36,* 332–336.

Mishel, M. H., Padilla, G., Grant, M., & Sorenson, D. S. (1991). Uncertainty in illness theory: A replication of the mediating effects of mastery and coping. *Nursing Research, 40,* 236–240.

Mishel, M. H., & Sorenson, D. S. (1991). Uncertainty in gynecological cancer: A test of the mediating functions of mastery and coping. *Nursing Research, 40,* 167–171.

Mitchell, M. L., Courtney, M., & Coyer, F. (2003). Understanding uncertainty and minimizing families' anxiety at the time of transfer from intensive care. *Nursing & Health Sciences, 5*(3), 207–217.

Moos, R., & Tsu, V. (1977). The crisis of physical illness: An overview. In R. Moos (Ed.), *Coping with physical illness.* New York: Plenum. pp. 3–25.

Mullins, L. L., Cheney, J. M., Balderson, B., & Hommel, K.A. (2000). The relationship of illness uncertainty, illness intrusiveness, and asthma severity to depression in young adults with long-standing asthma. *International Journal of Rehabilitation and Health, 5*(3), 177–185.

Mullins, L. L., Cheney, J. M., Hartman, V. L., Albin, K., Miles, B., & Roberson, S. (1995). Cognitive and affective features of postpolio syndrome: Illness uncertainty, attributional style, and adaptation. *International Journal of Rehabilitation and Health, 1,* 211–222.

Mullins, L., Cote, M., Fuemmeler, B., Jean, V., Beatty, W., & Paul, R. (2001). Illness intrusiveness, uncertainty, and distress in individuals with multiple sclerosis. *Rehabilitation Psychology, 46*(2), 139–153.

Nelson, J. P. (1996). Struggling to gain meaning: Living with the uncertainty of breast cancer. *Advances in Nursing Science, 18*(3), 59–76.

Neville, K. (1998). The relationships among uncertainty, social support, and psychological distress in adolescents recently diagnosed with cancer. *Journal of Pediatric Oncology Nursing, 15*(1), 37–46.

Neville, K. L. (2003). Uncertainty in illness: An integrative review. *Orthopaedic Nursing 22*(3), 206–214.

Northouse, L., Mood, D., Templin, T., Mellon, S., & George, T. (2000). Couples' patterns of adjustment to colon cancer. *Social Science and Medicine, 50*(2), 271–284.

Northouse, L., Walker, J., Schafenacker, A., Mood, D., Mellon, S., Galvin, E., et al. (2002). A family-based program of care for women with recurrent breast cancer and their family members. *Oncology Nursing Forum, 29*(10), 1411–1419.

Norton, R. (1975). Measurement of ambiguity tolerance. *Journal of Personal Assessment, 39,* 607–619.

Nyhlin, K. T. (1990). Diabetic patients facing long-term complications: Coping with uncertainty. *Journal of Advanced Nursing, 15,* 1021–1029.

Padilla, G., Mishel, M., & Grant, M. (1992). Uncertainty, appraisal and quality of life. *Quality of Life Research, 1,* 155–165.

Parry, C. (2003). Embracing uncertainty: An exploration of the experiences of childhood cancer survivors. *Qualitative Health Research, 13*(2), 227–246.

Pelusi, J. (1997). The lived experience of surviving breast cancer. *Oncology Nursing Forum, 24*(8), 1343–1353.

Penrod, J. (2001). Refinement of the concept of uncertainty. *Journal of Advanced Nursing, 34*(2), 238–245.

Porter, L. S., Clayton, M. E., Belyea, J., Mishel, M., Gil, K. M., & Germino, B. B. (2006). Predicting negative mood state and personal growth in African American and

White long-term breast cancer survivors. *Annals of Behavioral Medicine, 31*(3), 195–204.

Prigogine, I., & Stengers, I. (1984). *Order out of chaos: Man's new dialogue with nature.* New York: Bantam Books.

Redeker, N. S. (1992). The relationship between uncertainty and coping after coronary bypass surgery. *Western Journal of Nursing Research, 14,* 48–68.

Righter, B. (1995). Ostomy care. Uncertainty and the role of the credible authority during an ostomy experience. *Journal of Wound and Ostomy Care Nursing, 22*(2), 100–104.

Ritz, L., Nissen, M., Swenson, K., Farrell, J., Sperduto, P., Sladek, M., et al. (2000). Effects of advanced nursing care on quality of life and cost outcomes of women diagnosed with breast cancer. *Oncology Nursing Forum, 27*(6), 923–932.

Rydström, I., Dalheim-Englund, A.-C., Segesten, K., & Rasmussen, B. H. (2004). Relations governed by uncertainty: Part of life of families of a child with asthma. *Journal of Pediatric Nursing, 19*(2 [Print]), 85–94.

Sammarco, A. (2001). Perceived social support, uncertainty, and quality of life of younger breast cancer survivors. *Cancer Nursing, 24*(3), 212–219.

Sanders-Dewey, N., Mullins, L., & Chaney, J. (2001). Coping style, perceived uncertainty in illness, and distress in individuals with Parkinson's disease and their caregivers. *Rehabilitation Psychology, 46*(4), 363–381.

Santacroce, S. (2000). Support from health care providers and parental uncertainty during the diagnosis phase of perinatally acquired HIV infection. *Journal of the Association of Nurses in AIDS Care, 11*(2), 63–75.

Santacroce, S. (2001). Measuring parental uncertainty during the diagnosis phase of serious illness in a child. *Journal of Pediatric Nursing, 16*(1), 3–12.

Santacroce, S. (2002). Uncertainty, anxiety, and symptoms of posttraumatic stress in parents of children recently diagnosed with cancer. *Journal of Pediatric Oncology Nursing, 19*(3), 104–111.

Santacroce, S. J. (2003). Parental uncertainty and posttraumatic stress in serious childhood illness. *Journal of Nursing Scholarship, 35*(1), 45–51.

Santacroce, S. J., & Lee, Y. L. (2006). Uncertainty, posttraumatic stress, and health behavior in young adult childhood cancer survivors. *Nursing Research, 55*(4), 259–266.

Saunders, J. C., & Cookman, C. A. (2005). A clarified conceptual meaning of hepatitis C-related depression. *Gastroenterology Nursing, 28*(2), 123–129; quiz 120–121.

Sexton, D. L., Calcasola, S. L., Bottomley, S. R., & Funk, M. (1999). Adults' experience with asthma and their reported uncertainty and coping strategies. *Clinical Nurse Specialist, 13*(1), 8–17.

Shalit, B. (1977). Structural ambiguity and limits to coping. *Journal of Human Stress, 3,* 32–45.

Sharkey, T. (1995). The effects of uncertainty in families with children who are chronically ill. *Home Healthcare Nurse, 13*(4), 37–42.

Small, S. P., & Graydon, J. E. (1993). Uncertainty in hospitalized patients with chronic obstructive pulmonary disease. *International Journal of Nursing Studies, 30,* 239–246.

Smeltzer, S. C. (1994). The concerns of pregnant women with multiple sclerosis. *Qualitative Health Research, 4,* 497–501.

Sorenson, D. L. S. (1990). Uncertainty in pregnancy. *NAACOG Clinical Issues in Perinatal and Women's Health Nursing, 1*(3), 289–296.

Sterken, D. J. (1996). Uncertainty and coping of fathers of children with cancer. *Journal of Pediatric Oncology Nursing, 13,* 81–90.

Stewart, J. L. (2003). "Getting used to it": Children finding the ordinary and routine in the uncertain context of cancer. *Qualitative Health Research, 13*(3), 394–407.

Stewart, J. L., & Mishel, M. H. (2000). Uncertainty in childhood illness: A synthesis of the parent and child literature. *Scholarly Inquiry for Nursing Practice, 17,* 299–319.

Taylor-Piliae, R. E., & Chair, S. Y. (2002). The effect of nursing intervention utilizing music theory or sensory information on Chinese patients' anxiety prior to cardiac catheterization: A pilot study. *European Journal of Cardiovascular Nursing, 1*, 203–311.

Taylor-Piliae, R., & Molassiotis, A. (2001). An exploration of the relationships between uncertainty, psychological distress and type of coping strategy among Chinese men after cardiac catheterization. *Journal of Advanced Nursing, 33*(1), 79–88.

Tomlinson, P., Kirschbaum, M., Harbaugh, B., & Anderson, K. (1996). The influence of illness severity and family resources on maternal uncertainty during critical pediatric hospitalization. *American Journal of Critical Care, 5*, 140–146.

Turner, M., Tomlinson, P., & Harbaugh, B. (1990). Parental uncertainty in critical care hospitalization of children. *Maternal-Child Nursing Journal, 19*, 45–62.

Van Riper, M., & Selder, F. E. (1989). Parental responses to birth of a child with Down syndrome. *Loss, Grief and Care: A Journal of Professional Practice, 3*(3–4), 59–76.

Walker, L. O., & Avant, K. C. (1989). *Strategies for theory construction in nursing.* Norwalk, CT: Appleton-Century-Crofts.

Webster, K. K., & Christman, N. J. (1988). Perceived uncertainty and coping post myocardial infarction. *Western Journal of Nursing Research, 10*(4), 384–400.

Weems, J., & Patterson, E. T. (1989). Coping with uncertainty and ambivalence while awaiting a cadaveric renal transplant. *ANNA Journal, 16*(1), 27–32.

Weiss, M. E., Saks, N. P., & Harris, S. (2002). Resolving the uncertainty of pre-term symptoms: Women's experiences with the onset of preterm labor. *Journal of Obstetric, Gynecologic, and Neonatal Nursing, 31*(1), 66–76.

Weitz, R. (1989). Uncertainty and the lives of persons with AIDS. *Journal of Health and Social Behavior, 30*, 270–281.

White, R. E., & Frasure-Smith, N. (1995). Uncertainty and psychologic stress after coronary angioplasty and coronary bypass surgery. *Heart & Lung, 24*(1), 19–27.

Wiener, C. L., & Dodd, M. J. (1993). Coping amid uncertainty: An illness trajectory perspective. *Scholarly Inquiry for Nursing Practice, 7*(1), 17–31.

Wineman, N. M. (1990). Adaptation to multiple sclerosis: The role of social support, functional disability, and perceived uncertainty. *Nursing Research, 39*, 294–299.

Wineman, N. M., O'Brien, R. A., Nealon, N. R., & Kaskel, B. (1993). Congruence in uncertainty between individuals with multiple sclerosis and their spouses. *Journal of Neuroscience Nursing, 25*, 356–361.

Wineman, N. M., Schwetz, K. M., Goodkin, D. E., & Rudick, R. A. (1996). Relationships among illness uncertainty, stress, coping, and emotional well-being at entry into a clinical drug trial. *Applied Nursing Research, 9*(2), 53–60.

Wineman, N. M., Schwetz, K. M., Zeller, R., & Cyphert, J. (2003). Longitudinal analysis of illness uncertainty, coping, hopefulness, and mood during participation in a clinical drug trial. *Journal of Neuroscience Nursing, 35*(2), 100–106.

Winters, C. A. (1999). Heart failure: Living with uncertainty. *Progress in Cardiovascular Nursing, 14*, 85–91.

Wonghongkul, T., Dechaprom, N., Phumivichuvate, L., & Losawatkul, S. (2006). Uncertainty appraisal coping and quality of life in breast cancer survivors. *Cancer Nursing, 29*(3), 250–257.

Wonghongkul, T., Moore, S., Musil, C., Schneider, S., & Deimling, G. (2000). The influence of uncertainty in illness, stress appraisal, and hope on coping in survivors of breast cancer. *Cancer Nursing, 23*(6), 422–429.

Wunderlich, R., Perry, A., Lavin, M., & Katz, B. (1999). Patients' perceptions of uncertainty and stress during weaning from mechanical ventilation. *Dimensions of Critical Care Nursing, 18*(1), 8–12.

CHAPTER 5

Theory of Meaning

Patricia L. Starck

A theory of meaning based on the work of Viktor E. Frankl was developed primarily to treat individuals with psychiatric or psychological disorders. It has been expanded to help the average human being cope with everyday stresses of life and catastrophic, life-changing events. It has also evolved past the individual level for use with groups and applies to the level of community/society.

PURPOSE OF THE THEORY AND HOW IT WAS DEVELOPED

In Europe during Frankl's professional era, a precise set of assumptions and philosophy was called a school of thought rather than a theory. Thus, Frankl, as a Viennese psychiatrist and neurologist, studied in the First School of Viennese Psychiatry, known as the Will to Pleasure, espoused by Sigmund Freud. Later, the Second School, or the Will to Power, developed by Alfred Adler, came into vogue.

Frankl (1978) acknowledged the worth of Freud and Adler, as well as behaviorists who followed, but he believed that man can no longer be seen as a being whose basic concern is to satisfy drives and gratify instincts or, for that matter, to reconcile id, ego, and superego; nor can the human reality be understood merely as the outcome of conditioning processes or conditioned reflexes. Here man is revealed as a being in search of meaning—a search whose futility seems to account for many of the ills of our age (p. 17).

Frankl called his theory the Will to Meaning, and it became known as the Third School of Viennese Psychiatry. He postulated that human beings are motivated to seek answers to such questions as: Why am I here? He went on to develop treatment, which he termed *logotherapy,* the practice of helping people find meaning and purpose in life, no matter what their life circumstances.

There is a common misperception that Frankl's theory emerged as a result of his internment in German concentration camps during World War II. This misperception was a source of irritation to Frankl as he clarified that in actuality he formulated his ideas about meaning in life when he was a young child, with his first clear understanding at age 5. After his medical education he planned to write a book about the theory. However, the plan was interrupted when he was seized by the Nazis in Germany and imprisoned (Fabry, 1991). During the concentration camp experience, he validated the theory.

He found that in spite of great suffering, survival behaviors were more evident in those who had a strong reason to live than in those who did not. Frankl preserved the theory by recreating a manuscript he had lost when he was imprisoned. During his internment at four different concentration camps over a 2½-year period, he wrote on scraps of paper to keep his mind focused on his reason to survive. After his release at the end of World War II, he published the book that was later titled *Man's Search for Meaning,* under the title *From Death Camp to Existentialism.* In the book he described his experience in prison, detailing the unimaginable sufferings of the imprisoned. He began to develop his concept of human suffering by defining suffering as a challenge. In the experience of suffering, the challenge to the individual is to decide how to respond to unavoidable, deplorable life circumstances. It is an opportunity to show courage and to behave decently in spite of circumstances. He coined the term *logotherapy* from the Greek word, *logos,* denoting meaning. Logotherapy is the practice of the theory, intended to assist individuals to find purpose in life regardless of circumstances.

Frankl's work has been examined in light of Kerlinger's (1973) criteria for a theory that describes, explains, and predicts human behavior (Starck, 1985a). The postulates are the central core of the theory and are generalized statements of truth that serve as essential underpinnings for this body of knowledge. The postulates follow:

A person's search for meaning is the primary motivation of life. This meaning is unique and specific in that it must and can be fulfilled by the person alone. (Frankl, 1984, p. 121)

A person is free to be responsible, and is responsible for the realization of the meaning of life, the *logos* of existence. (Frankl, 1961, p. 9)

A person may find meaning in life even when confronted with a hopeless situation, when facing a fate that cannot be changed. (Frankl, 1984, p. 135)

A person's life offers meaning in every moment and in every situation. (Fabry, 1991, p. 130)

The theory of meaning is a framework that lends itself to interdisciplinary endeavors. Frankl's work has been used as the basis for research and practice in many fields, including medicine, psychology, counseling, education, ministry, and nursing. Travelbee (1966, 1969, 1972) was the first nurse to use Frankl's work in practice. She used parables and other stories to help psychiatric patients realize that human suffering comes to all and that we have the means to combat life problems no matter the circumstances.

I had the great privilege of knowing Viktor E. Frankl over a 20-year period beginning when I was a doctoral student seeking ways to promote rehabilitation of spinal cord–injured patients. I came upon Frankl's work and wrote to him. He responded and encouraged me, saying I would be the first to apply his theory and practice to physically disabled individuals.

I met him in 1979 when I presented my dissertation, including the logotherapeutic nursing intervention I had designed, to the first World Congress of Logotherapy. I was deeply honored when he quoted my work in his publications and presentations.

I later received further training in logotherapy from his protégé, Elizabeth Lukas, a logotherapist from Munich, Germany. I visited with Dr. and Mrs. Frankl in their home in Vienna and received several treasured mementos—a photograph of him and me together, his sketches of our two profiles, and a reprint of one of his early publications.

I was pleased to invite him to come to the University of Texas Health Science Center at Houston in 1985, where he gave a 90-minute lecture to a packed auditorium. We made a videotape of this lecture and another tape in which I interviewed him about human suffering. In this latter tape, we were joined by Jerry Long, a quadriplegic who became a doctorally prepared logotherapist after his injury at age 17. I saw Dr. Frankl at several more World Congresses until health prevented his travel. Their only child, a daughter, became a logotherapist and carries on his work in Vienna. His two grandchildren have also developed their careers in ways to enhance his work.

Dr. Frankl died in 1997, the same week that Princess Diana of England and Mother Theresa of India died. His work goes on as educators, practitioners, and researchers from various disciplines continue to broaden and enrich his theory.

CONCEPTS OF THE THEORY

Three major concepts from Frankl's works are the building blocks of the theory: life purpose, freedom to choose, and human suffering. These concepts are supported by three human dimensions: the physical or soma, the mental or psyche, and the spiritual or noos (Frankl, 1969). The physical and the mental dimensions can become ill and the spiritual dimension can become blocked or frustrated. To explain this three-dimensional assumption, Frankl (1969) described laws of dimensional ontology. He sought to illustrate the simultaneous ontological differences and the anthropological unity of these three dimensions by using geometrical structures as an analogy to show qualitative differences while not destroying the unity of the structure. Dimensional ontology rests on two laws:

1. "One and the same phenomenon projected out of its own dimension into different dimensions lower than its own is depicted in such a way that the individual pictures contradict one another" (p. 23). For example, a cylinder when projected vertically would be perceived as a rectangle from the vertical view (from the side), but as a circle when projected as a horizontal view (from above). The meaning ascribed to the shape is relative to one's position in relation to the cylinder view. Therefore, this law articulates complexity emerging from unique perspectives of a single phenomenon.
2. "Different phenomena projected out of their own dimension into one dimension lower than their own are depicted in such a manner that the pictures are ambiguous" (p. 23). This second law articulates the quality of potential sameness occurring when multiple distinct levels of phenomena are viewed in relation to each other. For example, a cylinder, a cone, and a sphere all cast shadows as a circle when projected above onto a horizontal plane. It would be possible to ascribe the same or different meaning to each of these distinct shapes given a particular perspective.

Frankl's point is that while we have these three dimensions of soma, psyche, and noos, we can be both parts and a whole. From different points of view, different impressions and, therefore, different meanings, reveal themselves. He called attention to the fact that a problem in one dimension may show up as a symptom in another. For example, spiritual emptiness may manifest in a physiological symptom such as intense headaches. An important understanding when considering dimensional ontology is Frankl's emphasis on the human spirit, the noos, and the "defiant" power of the noos. Fabry (1991) interpreted this conceptualization as, "You *have* a body and a psyche, but you *are* your noos (spirit)" (p. 127). The human spirit can defy the odds and rise above the other dimensions.

Examples of the power of the noos will be provided throughout this chapter as vignettes are shared and stories are told about people who excelled beyond expectations to accomplish extraordinary feats. The noos is essential to the pursuit of life purpose.

Life Purpose

Life purpose is the central concept of the theory of meaning. It is the summary of reasons for one's existence, answering the questions: Who am I? and Why am I here? A sense of life purpose brings satisfaction with one's place in the world. Life purpose is that to which one may feel called and to which one is dedicated. There is a theme to one's life purpose—making a contribution, leaving the world a better place. The major premise of Frankl's theory is that the search for meaning in one's life is an overriding search for purpose. Life purpose flows from the "uniqueness of the person and the singularity of the situation" (Frankl, 1973, p. 63). Every person is "indispensable and irreplaceable" (Frankl, 1973, p. 117).

Fabry (1991) explained meaning from various existential viewpoints. The French existentialists, Sartre and Camus, believed that life itself had no meaning other than the meaning that humans gave to it. In contrast, the German existentialists, including Frankl, maintained that meaning exists and the task is to discover it, and in discovering meaning one also discovers life purpose. Fabry emphasized that our human spirits are the instruments for finding a purpose in life through tapping the spiritual treasure in each of us.

Frankl asserts that each person must discover his or her own meaning. It cannot be prescribed by another. A professional caregiver working with a person who has recently suffered a loss cannot tell the person how to look for meaning in another dimension of life, but the caregiver can help guide the person to find new avenues of meaning through shifting views of soma, psyche, and noos. "And meaning is something to be found rather than to be given, discovered rather than invented" (Frankl, 1969, p. 62).

Frankl (1984) postulated that meaning in life always changes but never ceases to be. He specified three different ways to find meaning on the path to uncovering life purpose: (1) creating a work or doing a deed that moves beyond self, (2) experiencing something or encountering someone, and (3) choosing our attitude toward our own fate. In the first way, a strong sense of purpose or meaning in life may be seen when a terminally ill person hangs on tenaciously to the achievement of some goal such as a child graduating from college. This will to meaning is a strong life force that can defy the odds given by the most expert clinician. Frankl (1984) also emphasized that our past achievements are monuments of meaning in our lives. "All we have done, whatever great thoughts we may have had, and all we have suffered, all this is not lost, though it is past; we have brought it into being. Having been is also a kind of being, and perhaps the surest kind" (p. 104). Fabry (1980) distinguished between "meaning of the moment" in everyday choices we make and "universal meaning," or the bigger picture that we may not completely understand at this time. Meaning of the moment is the everyday situation where one has a chance to act in a meaningful way through action, experiences, and the stand one takes.

Ultimate meaning is the trust that there is order in the universe and that humans are part of that order; it is the opposite of seeing the world as chaotic and humans as the victims of whim.

Self-transcendence (Frankl, 1969) is related to life purpose. It is described as getting outside the self for a cause greater than the self. It is creating a work or doing a deed that reaches beyond one's egocentricity toward others, even though it may be difficult to do when life has been cruel (Fabry, 1991). Self-transcendence is contrasted with self-awareness. In self-awareness, the focus is internal, such as guilt, past traumas, or other feelings. By contrast, self-transcendence is distancing from oneself. In the distancing, a different view of the situation comes to light along with a changed meaning of the situation. For example, parents who have lost a child to violence may put energy toward getting new legislation passed that will protect children and prevent the type of loss they have suffered from happening to others. The hardship is deliberately endured so that others may benefit. Self-transcendence should not be confused with self-actualization as defined by Maslow (1968). Frankl (1975) stated that "what is called 'self-actualization' is ultimately an effect, the unintentional by-product of self-transcendence" (p. 78).

A second way to find meaning and enable life purpose is through experiences like loving or encountering another human being. Frankl believed that love goes beyond an individual and is long lasting. "Love is so little directed toward the body of the beloved that it can easily outlast the other's death, can exist in the lover's heart until his own death" (Frankl, 1973, p. 138).

The third way to find meaning on the path of life purpose is by choosing one's own attitude to whatever life presents. Choosing to remain positive, brave, or optimistic in spite of difficult circumstances illustrates this way of finding meaning. Purpose in life can come when a choice is made to deliberately change one's attitude and view the situation in a different way.

Frankl identified two states that describe a lack of meaning: existential frustration and existential vacuum. Existential frustration is searching for meaning in which there is a state of being unsettled, of wanting more from life (Frankl, 1969). Existential vacuum is a sense of utter despair, of hopelessness, that life has no meaning and all is of no use (Frankl, 1969). This is an inner emptiness where one feels trapped in unhappiness. Times of transition may lead to an existential vacuum, such as when a person is dissatisfied with work but is afraid of risking change. Existential vacuum may also occur during times of loss, such as the sudden, unexpected death of a child, when one does not trust values that have formerly been a guide. Fabry (1980) believed that lack of meaning is a major problem in society because people repress their natural desire to find meaning, causing them to feel that life has no purpose, no challenges, and no obligations. This problem is experienced as a crisis among the rich and the poor, the old and the young, the successful and those who have failed. Fabry (1980) identified unhealthy ways that people cope, including drugs, workaholism, thrill-seeking, and overeating. This crisis experience may also serve as a stimulus to find a more meaningful existence.

A poignant example of finding meaning and accomplishing life purpose, even at the end of life, is a story that will live in history as one in which individuals transcended self for the good of others. On September 11, 2001, passengers on United Airlines flight #93 found that fate had placed them on a plane hijacked by terrorists intent on a suicide mission to destroy innocent lives and symbols of American democracy. With the aid of cell phone technology, some passengers learned there had already been terrorist attacks by other flights that morning and there was no doubt what their fate was to be. Many talked to family members about the things that gave meaning to their lives—the love they had, the expressed wish for the family to go on to complete meaningful lives. Yet, in the face of their own deaths, they had freedom of choice. They had a chance to transcend their own fears, one last chance to do something good for humanity. In the last moments of their lives they could and did perform a selfless act—they made sure the plane did not reach its intended target but rather crashed in a nonpopulated area in Pennsylvania. In accomplishing this unexpected life purpose, they gave meaning to their lives and left a legacy of heroism, not only for their loved ones, but for every American citizen. Even if among this group there was one whose life had been meaningless, when that one exercised his freedom to act and to transcend his own needs, by this one act in the final moments, his life was flooded with meaning and purpose.

Freedom to Choose

Freedom to choose is the second concept of the theory of meaning. It is the process of selecting among options over which one has control.

In enduring the most intense imaginable hardship, that of the Holocaust, Frankl (1973) pointed out that there is value to be found in a person's attitude toward the limiting factors of life. Being confronted by an unalterable destiny where one can act only by acceptance provides a unique opportunity to choose one's attitude. "The way in which he accepts, the way in which he bears his cross, what courage he manifests in suffering, what dignity he displays in doom and disaster, is the measure of his human fulfillment" (Frankl, 1973, p. 44). One can be subjected to torture, humiliation, and worse, and yet retain the attitude to face one's fate with courage. It is the attitude of the sufferer that drives the behavior, not the actions of the persecutor. The right to choose one's own attitude may be thought of as spiritual freedom or independence of mind.

> We who lived in concentration camps can remember the men who walked through the huts comforting others, giving away their last piece of bread. They may have been few in number, but they offer sufficient proof that everything can be taken from a man but one thing: the last of the human freedoms—to choose one's attitude in any given set of circumstances, to choose one's own way. (Frankl, 1984, p. 86)

Freedom to be self-determining within the limits of endowment and environment was validated during Frankl's experiences in the concentration camps.

> In this living laboratory and on this testing ground, we watched and witnessed some of our comrades behave like swine while others behaved like saints. Man has both potentialities within himself; which one is actualized depends on decisions but not on conditions. (Frankl, 1984, p. 157)

Fabry (1991) offered practical guidelines for modifying attitudes by considering that something positive can be found in all situations. Some sample questions to stimulate one's attitude change are: "What am I still able to do that would benefit someone? Whom do I love and wish to protect in this situation?" (p. 43). By asking these questions, one shifts the attention away from what has been lost and from self to others. Fabry (1991) suggested that one's attitude can begin to change by "acting as if" one has the attribute. For example, if a person wanted to be courageous, then to act "as if" would beget a change in attitude.

Lukas (1984, 1986) introduced several ideas important to Frankl's work. She expanded understanding of one's freedom to choose by indicating that life events can be classified as either fate or freedom. Fate is when we cannot change the situation; freedom includes what one can do, including choosing what attitude to adopt. When confronting a problem, the person should ask, Where are my areas of freedom? Which possible choices do I have, and which one do I want to actualize?

Human Suffering

Human suffering is the third concept of the theory of meaning. It is a subjective experience that is unique to an individual and varies from simple transitory discomfort to extreme anguish and despair (Starck & McGovern, 1992). Frankl did not define suffering but rather described it as a subjective, all-consuming human experience. He believed that "the meaning of suffering . . . is the deepest possible meaning" (Frankl, 1969, p. 75), and that the ultimate meaning of life or of human suffering can never be found. He used the following comparison:

> If I point to something with my finger, the dog does not look in the direction in which I point, it looks at my finger and sometimes snaps at it. And what about man? Is not he, too, unable to understand the meaning of something, say the meaning of suffering, and does not he, too, quarrel with his fate and snap at its finger? (Frankl, 1969, p. 145)

Frankl was clear that there is no meaning *in* suffering. For example, there is no meaning in cancer. However, one can find meaning *in spite of* having cancer. Suffering is a part of the human experience. Things happen to us that are undeserved, unexplainable, and unavoidable. We do not need to look for meaning in these events; rather, meaning comes from stances we take toward the suffering, for example, the courageous way a person chooses to live with the cancer. Frankl (1975) described the worst kind of suffering as "despair, suffering without meaning" (p. 137).

RELATIONSHIPS AMONG THE CONCEPTS: THE MODEL

The relationships among the concepts of the theory are depicted in Figure 5.1. This illustration suggests that meaning is a journey toward life purpose with the freedom to choose one's path in spite of inevitable suffering.

USE OF THE THEORY IN NURSING RESEARCH

Instruments

A number of instruments have been developed by protégés of Frankl. These tools have been used in both research and clinical practice. All are available from the Viktor E. Frankl International Institute for Logotherapy in Abilene, Texas. Instruments that quantify meaning and instruments

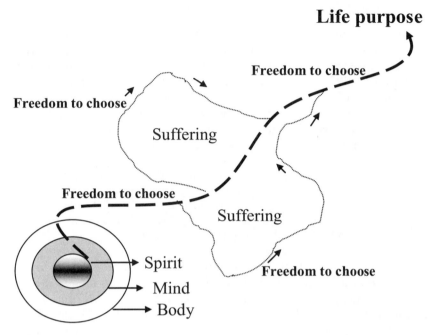

FIGURE 5.1   Meaning.

that can serve as a clinical guide to planning interventions include the Purpose in Life (PIL) test (Crumbaugh, 1968; Crumbaugh & Maholick, 1976), the Seeking of Noetic Goals (SONG) test (Crumbaugh, 1977), and the Meaning in Suffering Test (MIST) (Starck, 1985b). Another useful instrument is the List of Values created by Crumbaugh (1980). This is a list of 20 values. The person is directed to choose his or her top five values in life.

There are various other instruments available, including the Logotest developed by Elizabeth Lukas, PhD, in Munich for use in the practice of logotherapy, and the Life Purpose Questionnaire developed by Hutzell and Peterson (1986). Table 5.1 compares the most frequently used instruments, distinguishing the purpose of each instrument and providing psychometric information. The reader may contact the Institute for more information.

Nursing Research

Several nursing researchers who have referenced Frankl's work have made significant contributions in the area of suffering and the search for

TABLE 5.1 Instruments Used to Measure Meaning and Purpose

	Purpose (What the instrument captures)	Samples (General)	Reliability	Validity	Example Citation
PIL	Degree of existential vacuum	Adults	.85 Pearson correlation Spearman–Brown corrected to .92	Construct and criterion	Crumbaugh, 1968
SONG	Degree of strength/ motivation to find life meaning	Adults	.71 Pearson correlation Spearman–Brown corrected to .83	Construct	Crumbaugh, 1977
MIST	Degree of meaning found in un-avoidable suffering	Adults	.82 split-half; .81 Chronbach's Alpha	Logical construct	Kuuppelomaki, and Lauri, 1998
Life Purpose Questionnaire	Degree of life-meaning	Adults	.90	Construct and criterion	Hutzell and Peterson, 1986

meaning with a variety of groups. Using qualitative research, Kahn and Steeves (1986, 1994, 1995) and Steeves and Kahn (1987) have described the concept of suffering as an individual's experience of threat to self and as meaning given to events such as pain or loss.

They cited the ability of hospice patients and families to find meaning in spite of suffering through discrete experiences during which they were affected by something greater than themselves (Steeves & Kahn, 1987). They identified the goal of nursing care in such situations as helping to establish and maintain the conditions necessary to experience meaning. They identified eight aphorisms of suffering (Kahn & Steeves, 1995) that characterize the experience. The aphorisms note the individual encompassing nature of suffering, the recognition of suffering through its expression rather than the experience itself, and the influence of a caring environment on the suffering process (Kahn & Steeves, 1995).

Steeves, Kahn, and Benoliel (1990) investigated how nurses experience and react to a person's suffering, with themes progressing from understanding suffering from the perspective of the patient's medical condition and ending with nurses personalizing the suffering as their own. With bone marrow transplant patients, Steeves (1992) investigated the process of "meaning making" and "life interpretation." A change in the social position of the patient was influenced by protective isolation and communication problems. Patients described searching for understanding with examples of experiences of meaningfulness. Steeves (1996) illustrated the use of storytelling in helping individuals and families find meaning in loss and grief.

Nurse researchers (Coward, 1991, 1994, 1995, 1996, 1998; Coward & Dickerson, 2003; Coward & Kahn, 2004, 2005; Coward & Lewis, 1993; Coward & Reed, 1996), have studied meaning and purpose in life as well as the phenomenon of self-transcendence. The approach Coward and Kahn (2004, 2005) have used combines the work of several authors, including Frankl, in defining self-transcendence and helping patients overcome spiritual disequilibrium.

Starck (1979) was the first person to apply Frankl's theory and practices to a physically disabled population with a permanent spinal cord injury (SCI). Starck conducted a study to determine whether a logotherapeutic nursing intervention could favorably influence the perception of meaning and purpose in life for persons disabled with SCI.

A model using Frankl's theory, Travelbee's (1969) approaches to interpersonal communication, and Maslow's (1968) hierarchy of needs was developed and applied with the subjects. Both the PIL and the SONG were used as pre- and posttests to measure the effectiveness of the intervention. The patients ($N = 25$) were referred from a regional spinal cord injury center, and home visits were conducted for both the control and the experimental groups. The nursing intervention involved use of written parables or provocative thoughts to stimulate reflective thinking and application to the patient's life. For example, one parable described two frogs that fell into a churn of milk. One gave up and drowned; the other fought his fate and splashed around. Soon the milk had turned to butter and he was afloat on top. In relation to this parable, study participants discussed how they might rally the human spirit to cope with permanent paralysis.

Although there was evidence that some clients increased their sense of meaning and purpose in life, there was no support for the effectiveness of the nursing intervention at a statistically significant level. However, there were several findings of clinical importance not heretofore found in the literature. These findings included the following: (a) patients could not stand on scales to monitor weight, and insidious weight gain complicated health problems inherent to their limited mobility; (b) fear in their environment thwarted seeking to flee from danger and safety was of great concern; and (c) the telephone was viewed as a means of physical protection as well as emotional comfort. One of the clients objected to having a wheelchair ramp on the house for fear that it would alert burglars that a handicapped person might be alone in the house. The study findings suggest that there were many factors that could interfere with attainment of goals for a meaningful life.

Many SCI patients had found meaning in spite of severe physical limitations. For example, a girl who was seriously injured in a random shooting typed letters with her mouthstick to offer words of encouragement and motivation for others. Another quadriplegic, who was the first in his family to graduate from high school, took on the role of tutoring younger relatives.

Starck (1992) studied suffering in a nursing home environment and found that suffering was operationally defined as loss. Although there were physical, social/emotional, and economic losses, the greatest losses were in the spiritual domain. These were loss of autonomy, loss of freedom of choice, and loss of a sense of purpose in life. Furthermore, it was found that the nursing home staff responded with negative sanctions to those who complained about the suffering inherent in their condition and with a caring response to those who were quiet and passive sufferers.

A Web-based logotherapy research forum has been established for professional and student researchers to encourage international interaction. This Web site posts research projects and lists all known research instruments. The Web site address is http://www.viktorfrankl.org/research.

USE OF THE THEORY IN NURSING PRACTICE

Fabry (1980) has described logotherapy as "guiding people toward understanding themselves as they are and *could be* and their place in the totality of living" (p. xiii). When contrasted with traditional psychotherapy, it is less retrospective and introspective (Frankl, 1984). Other comparisons between psychotherapy and logotherapy are found in Table 5.2.

The goal of logotherapy is to help persons separate themselves from their symptoms, to tap into the resources of their noetic dimension, and to arouse the dynamic power of the human spirit. Helping another find meaning may be described as promoting an unfolding of what is already there. It is helping the other discover his or her values and facilitating awareness of subconscious beliefs and commitments.

Frankl does not advocate techniques in a routine procedural sense but rather encourages creativity based on the situation at hand. Frankl (1969) has described *three* logotherapeutic approaches. These approaches are dereflection, paradoxical intention, and Socratic dialogue. Both dereflection and paradoxical intention "rest on two essential qualities of human existence, namely, man's capacities of self-transcendence and self-detachment" (Frankl, 1969, p. 99).

Dereflection

Dereflection is the act of de-emphasizing or ceasing to focus on a troublesome phenomenon, issue, or problem; it is putting this issue aside. Dereflection strengthens the capacity for self-transcendence.

Obsessions are recognized as hyperreflection or excess attention, described as the "compulsion to self-observation" (Frankl, 1973, p. 253). The urge for better sexual performance is an example. "Sexual performance or experience is strangled to the extent to which it is made either an object of attention or an objective of intention" (Frankl, 1969, p. 101).

TABLE 5.2   Contrast of Psychotherapy and Logotherapy

Psychotherapy	Logotherapy
Depth psychology	Height psychology
Sees life in terms of problems	Sees life in terms of solutions
Focuses on obstacles	Focuses on goals
Is reductionistic	Is holistic
Emphasis on uncovering	Emphasis on discovering
Analytical style	Uniqueness and improvisational style
Psychiatrist listens	Logotherapist talks

Complaining is an example of hyperreflection, as an excessive amount of attention is given to the self. Dereflection helps the person stop fighting an anxiety, a neurosis, or a psychosis, and spares the person the reinforcement of additional suffering. If a person is depressed, dereflection can help achieve distance between the person and the depression, "to see himself—not as a person who is depressed but—as a full human being who has depressions with the capacity to find meaning despite the depressions" (Fabry, 1991, p. 136).

Paradoxical Intention

Paradoxical intention is intentionally acting the opposite to one's desired ends, thereby confronting one's fears and anxieties. Paradoxical intention strengthens the capacity for self-distancing. By distancing from the triggers of problems, these triggers become ineffective. Paradoxical intention is helpful in dealing with the problem of anticipatory anxiety. The object of the person's fear is fear itself. The underlying dynamic is apprehension about the potential effects of the anxiety attacks. And, of course, the fear of the fear increases the fear, producing precisely what the person is afraid of. The person is caught in a restricting cycle. The aim of therapy is to break the cycle, to interfere with the feedback mechanism. In logotherapy, one is asked to replace fear with a paradoxical wish, to wish for the very thing one fears. By this treatment, Frankl said, "the wind is taken out of the sails of the anxiety" (1984, p. 147).

This approach makes use of the specific human capacity for self-detachment. For example, in sleep disturbances when a person worries that he or she will not be able to get to sleep and focuses on trying to go to sleep, sleep will not come. The fear of sleeplessness results in the hyperintention to fall asleep, which inevitably leads to sleeplessness. Paradoxical intention advises the person not to try to sleep, but rather to try to do the opposite, stay awake as long as possible. The person who has been trying to stay awake wakes up to find that he or she has been asleep.

Paradoxical intention can be used to change unwanted behavior patterns. This does not depend upon understanding how and why the behavior started. It simply breaks the cycle of fear.

Socratic Dialogue

Socratic dialogue is a conversation of questions and answers, probing deeply into existential issues such as one's values. It is rhetorical debate to trigger a change in attitude, behavior, or both. Socratic dialogue is self-discovery discourse and seeks to get rid of masks that have been put on to please or to be accepted. The therapist poses questions so that patients become aware of their unconscious decisions, their repressed hopes, and their unadmitted self-knowledge. In Socratic dialogue, experiences of the past are explored as well as fantasies for the future to modulate attitude (Fabry, 1980). Socratic dialogue requires improvisation and intuition and asks probing questions like the following:

Was there a time when life had meaning?
Who do you know who leads a meaningful life? What keeps you from living like this person?
Who are the people who need you?
Tell me about an experience that made you see things differently.
Tell me something you said you couldn't do but you did it.

As an example, Lukas (1984), working with a patient who had strong values in physical ability and who had undergone a leg amputation, asked the question, "Does the value of human existence depend on the use of two legs?" (p. 47).

Fabry (1991) proposed five guideposts to probe areas of meaning. These are self-discovery, choice, uniqueness, responsibility, and self-transcendence. He also identified a number of creative methods and exercises to illustrate choice, where family members act out the role of others in the way they wish the others had responded. The flashlight technique can be useful in self-discovery and in aggressive discussion. The facilitator shines the flashlight on the partner who says something offensive to the other, indicating that the person must rephrase what has been said without hostility or sarcasm, thus helping reshape attitudes and behaviors. Fabry (1991) also has guidelines for groups, wherein the Socratic dialogue becomes a multilogue.

Other Practices Using Logotherapy

Pearce (2005), a parish nurse, declared that Frankl was a forerunner to integrative medicine and holistic nursing, contrasting this with today's fragmented system of healers specializing in healing only a part of the whole. Patients with a complex interaction of physical, psychological, and spiritual suffering often find their way to logotherapy after being disappointed with the existing health care system. Logotherapy provides tools to tap into inner resources to emerge as a stronger and more joyous self.

Winters and Schulenberg (2006) pointed out that diagnosis is a necessary evil in practice. Diagnosis is inherently reductionistic and focuses on defeats. To address this problem, the authors developed a holistic, logotherapeutic model of diagnosis. The diagnostic process is a bio-psycho-social-spiritual one and incorporates an assessment of one's inner strength.

For example, the provider might include a positive history of emotional balance and a history of making it through previous difficult times as noetic resources. Logotherapy is aimed at empowering the patient by emphasizing choice, responsibility, and hope.

CONCLUSION

The theory of meaning can be a useful guide in research and practice. The theory focuses on discovering meaning when facing life challenges that threaten one's purpose in relation to unique circumstances. Nurse researchers and practitioners can draw on the theory to understand ordinary life stresses, as well as life-changing events and human suffering.

For more information about continuing work being done with Viktor Frankl's ideas contact: The Viktor E. Frankl International Institute for Logotherapy, Box 15211, Abilene, TX 79698-5211. http://www.logotherapyinstitute.org/

REFERENCES

Coward, D. D. (1991). Self-transcendence and emotional well-being in women with advanced breast cancer. *Oncology Nursing Forum, 18,* 857–863.

Coward, D. D. (1994). Meaning and purpose in the lives of persons with AIDS. *Public Health Nursing, 11,* 331–336.

Coward, D. D. (1995). The lived experience of self-transcendence in women with AIDS. *Journal of Obstetric, Gynecologic and Neonatal Nursing, 24,* 314–318.

Coward, D. D. (1996). Self-transcendence and correlates in a health population. *Nursing Research, 45*(2), 116–121.

Coward, D. D. (1998). Facilitation of self-transcendence in a breast cancer support group. *Oncology Nursing Forum, 25*(1), 75–84.

Coward, D. D., & Dickerson, D. (2003). Facilitation of self-transcendence in breast cancer support group: II. *Oncology Nursing Forum, 30*(2), 291–300.

Coward, D. D., & Kahn, D. L. (2004). Resolution of spiritual disequilibrium by women newly diagnosed with breast cancer. *Oncology Nursing Forum, 31*(2), E24–31.

Coward, D. D., & Kahn, D. L. (2005). Transcending breast cancer: Making meaning from diagnosis and treatment. *Journal of Holistic Nursing, 23*(3), 264–283.

Coward, D. D., & Lewis, F. M. (1993). The lived experience of self-transcendence in gay men with AIDS. *Oncology Nursing Forum, 20,* 1363–1368.

Coward, D. D., & Reed, P. G. (1996). Self-transcendence: A resource for healing at the end of life. *Issues in Mental Health Nursing, 17,* 275–288.

Crumbaugh, J. C. (1968). Cross-validation of purpose in life test based on Frankl's concepts. *Journal of Individual Psychology, 24,* 74–81.

Crumbaugh, J. C. (1977). The Seeking of Noetic Goals test (SONG): A complementary scale to the Purpose in Life test (PIL). *Journal of Clinical Psychology, 33,* 900–907.

Crumbaugh, J. C. (1980). *Logotherapy—new help for problem drinkers.* Chicago: Nelson-Hall.

Crumbaugh, J. C., & Maholick, L. T. (1976). *Purpose in Life test*. Abilene, TX: Viktor Frankl Institute for Logotherapy.

Fabry, J. B. (1980). *The pursuit of meaning*. New York: Harper & Row.

Fabry, J. B. (1991). *Guideposts to meaning: Discovering what really matters*. Oakland, CA: New Harbinger.

Frankl, V. E. (1961). Dynamics, existence, and values. *Journal of Existential Psychiatry, 11*(5), 5–16.

Frankl, V. E. (1969). *The will to meaning*. New York: New American Library.

Frankl, V. E. (1973). *The doctor and the soul*. New York: Vintage.

Frankl, V. E. (1975). *The unconscious God*. New York: Simon & Schuster.

Frankl, V. E. (1978). *The unheard cry for meaning*. New York: Simon & Schuster.

Frankl, V. E. (1984). *Man's search for meaning: An introduction to logotherapy*. Boston: Beacon.

Hutzell, R. R., & Peterson, T. J. (1986). Use of the Life Purpose Questionnaire with an alcoholic population. *International Journal of Addiction, 22*, 51–57.

Kahn, D. L., & Steeves, R. H. (1986). The experience of suffering: Conceptual clarification and theoretical definition. *Journal of Advanced Nursing, 11*, 623–631.

Kahn, D. L., & Steeves, R. H. (1994). Witnesses to suffering: Nursing knowledge, voice, and vision. *Nursing Outlook, 42*, 260–264.

Kahn, D. L., & Steeves, R. H. (1995). The significance of suffering in cancer care. *Seminars in Oncology Nursing, 11*(1), 9–16.

Kerlinger, F. H. (1973). *Foundations of research* (2nd ed.). New York: Holt, Rinehart, and Winston.

Kuuppelomaki, M. & Lauri, S. (1998). Cancer patients' reported experiences of suffering. *Cancer Nursing, 21*. pp. 364–369.

Lukas, E. (1984). *Meaningful living: A logotherapeutic guide to health*. Cambridge, MA: Schenkman.

Lukas, E. (1986). *Meaning in suffering: Comfort in crisis through logotherapy*. Berkeley, CA: Institute of Logotherapy Press.

Maslow, A. (1968). *Toward a psychology of being*. New York: Van Nostrand.

Pearce, M. (2005). Appeal and application of logotherapy in parish nursing practice. *The International Forum of Logotherapy: Journal of Search for Meaning, 28*(1), 26–30.

Starck, P. L. (1979). Spinal cord injured clients' perception of meaning and purpose in life, measurement before and after nursing intervention. *Dissertation Abstracts International, 40*(10), 4741. (UMI No. 8007891)

Starck, P. L. (1985a). Logotherapy comes of age: Birth of a theory. *The International Forum of Logotherapy: Journal of Search for Meaning, 8*(2), 71–75.

Starck, P. L. (1985b). *The Meaning in Suffering Test*. Berkeley, CA: Institute of Logotherapy Press.

Starck, P. L. (1992). Suffering in a nursing home: Losses of the human spirit. *The International Forum of Logotherapy: Journal of Search for Meaning, 15*(2), 76–79.

Starck, P. L., & McGovern, J. P. (1992). The meaning in suffering. In P. L. Starck & J. P. McGovern (Eds.), *The hidden dimension of illness: Human suffering* (pp. 25–42). New York: National League for Nursing Press.

Steeves, R. H. (1992). Patients who have undergone bone marrow transplantation: Their quest for meaning. *Oncology Nursing Forum, 19*, 899–905.

Steeves, R. H. (1996). Loss, grief, and the search for meaning. *Oncology Nursing Society, 23*, 897–903.

Steeves, R. H., & Kahn, D. L. (1987). Experience of meaning in suffering. *Journal of Nursing Scholarship, 19*(3), 114–116.

Steeves, R. H., Kahn, D. L., & Benoliel, J. Q. (1990). Nurses' interpretation of the suffering of their patients. *Western Journal of Nursing Research, 12*(6), 715–731.

Travelbee, J. (1966). *Interpersonal aspects of nursing*. Philadelphia: F. A. Davis.

Travelbee, J. (1969). *Intervention in psychiatric nursing: Process in the one-to-one relationship*. Philadelphia: F. A. Davis.

Travelbee, J. (1972). To find meaning in illness. *Nursing, 72*(2), 6–7.

Winters, M., & Schulenberg, S. (2006). Diagnosis in logotherapy: Overuse and suggestions for appropriate use. *The International Forum of Logotherapy: Journal of Search for Meaning, 29*(1), 16–24.

CHAPTER 6

Theory of Self-Transcendence

Pamela G. Reed

The theory of self-transcendence is an empirical theory of nursing. It was created from recognition of the developmental nature of human beings and the relevance of developmental phenomena for well-being. The word, developmental, is used to emphasize the ongoing and innovative change that occurs among human beings in their environmental contexts. Nursing is not only a human science but a developmental science as well. The theory was initially created out of an interest in acknowledging the developmental nature of older adults as integral to mental health and well-being. Although the role of development had long been an accepted perspective in work with children and adolescents, little attention was given to its significance among adults and especially among older adults.

PURPOSE OF THE THEORY AND
HOW IT WAS DEVELOPED

The purpose of the theory of self-transcendence is to enhance understanding about well-being in later adulthood. The theory is also applicable to any person whose life situation increases awareness of vulnerability and personal mortality. It is consistent with life span development theory, which posits that development is influenced less by chronological age and the passage of time and more by normative and nonnormative life events and the accruement of life experiences.

The idea for a theory of self-transcendence was influenced by three major events. First, the life span movement of the 1970s in developmental psychology provided philosophic awareness and empirical evidence that development did indeed continue beyond adolescence, into adulthood, and throughout processes of aging and dying (Reed, 1983). Second, Martha Rogers's (1970) early postulations about the nature of change in human beings provided further inspiration for development of the theory (Reed, 1997b). Third, the theory of self-transcendence was encouraged by clinical experiences in applying developmental theories in child and adolescent psychiatric–mental health care. A nursing approach to fostering mental health and well-being required an understanding of patients' developmental processes. Self-transcendence facilitates integration of complex and conflicting elements of living, aging, and dying.

Health events in particular confront people with increased complexity in terms of new people in their lives, new information, and new feelings and concerns. For example, the diagnosis of a chronic illness necessitates relationships with new people (health care providers) and community resources. It introduces strange, new information and terminology about the illness itself, medications, and other treatments and self-care activities. Chronic illness also initiates, if not intensifies, patient and family concerns about the future and raises fears about pain and mortality. Self-transcendence can help the person organize these challenges into some meaningful system to sustain well-being and a sense of wholeness across the trajectory of the illness.

CONCEPTS OF THE THEORY

The theory of self-transcendence rests on two major assumptions. First, it is assumed that human beings are integral with their environments, as postulated in Rogers's science of unitary human beings. Human beings are "pandimensional" (Rogers, 1980, 1994), coextensive with their environment, and capable of an awareness that extends beyond physical and temporal dimensions (Reed, 1997a). This awareness may be experienced through altered states of consciousness, but more often it is found in everyday practices in reaching deeper within the self and reaching out to others, to nature, to one's God, or other sources of transcendence. Self-transcendence embodies experiences that connect rather than separate a person from self, others, and the environment. It is a concept that enables description and study of the nature of human pandimensionality within everyday contexts of living. It focuses on the local and personal realm, whether or not there is something universal about self-transcendence.

The second assumption is that self-transcendence is a developmental imperative, meaning that it is a human characteristic that demands expression, much like other developmental processes such as walking in toddlers, abstract reasoning in adolescents, and grieving in those who have suffered a loss. These resources are a part of being human and realizing one's potential for well-being. As such, the person's participation in self-transcendence is integral to well-being, and nursing should have a role in facilitating this process.

Self-Transcendence

Self-transcendence is the major concept of the theory. It is the capacity to expand self-boundaries intrapersonally (toward greater awareness of one's philosophy, values, and dreams), interpersonally (to relate to others and one's environment), temporally (to integrate one's past and future in a way that has meaning for the present), and transpersonally (to connect with dimensions beyond the typically discernible world). Self-transcendence is a characteristic of developmental maturity in terms of an enhanced awareness of the environment and an orientation toward broadened perspectives about life.

Neo-Piagetian theories about development in adulthood and later life were foundational in formulating the concept of self-transcendence. Beginning in the 1970s, life span development researchers discovered patterns of thinking in older adults that extended beyond Piaget's formal operations, once thought to be the final stage of cognitive development. Life span developmental theories on social–cognitive development extended Piaget's original theory on reasoning, which had identified formal operations (abstract and symbolic reasoning) in youth and young adulthood as the apex of cognitive development. Researchers identified abilities in older adults indicating that cognitive development continued well into later life beyond the phase of formal operations. Arlin's (1975) problem-finding stage, Riegel's (1976) and Basseches's (1984) dialectic operations, and Koplowitz's (1984) unitary stage are examples of these patterns. Theorists described these abilities as postformal thinking.

It is now widely recognized that older adults use postformal patterns of thought in reasoning about their world. In contrast to patterns used by young adults, postformal thought is more contextual, more pragmatic, more spiritual, and more tolerant of ambiguity and the paradoxes inherent in living and dying (Commons, Demick, & Goldberg, 1996; Sinnott, 1998, 2003). Postformal reasoning incorporates personal experience and pragmatics as well as scientific evidence and an awareness of the larger social and temporal contexts that extend beyond the self and immediate situation. The adult who uses postformal thinking does not seek absolute answers to questions in life but rather seeks meaning of life events as integrated within a moral, social, and historical context. The person has an appreciation of the greater environment and things unseen, as well as an inner knowledge of self. A perspective of relativism from multiple, sometimes conflicting views is balanced by the ability to make a commitment to one's beliefs.

Self-transcendence was conceptualized as a correlate of postformal thinking. Older adults and others facing end-of-life issues acquire an expanded awareness of self and environment. With this mature approach to life and death, people reflect strivings more in line with generativity and ego integrity than with more self-focused strivings for identity and intimacy characteristic of earlier developmental phases (Sheldon & Kasser, 2001). Self-transcendence is expressed through various behaviors and perspectives such as sharing wisdom with others, integrating the physical changes of aging, accepting death as a part of life, and finding spiritual meaning in life.

Well-Being

A second major concept of the theory is well-being. Well-being is a sense of feeling whole and healthy, in accord with one's own criteria for wholeness and health. It is theorized that self-transcendence, as a basic human pattern of development, is logically linked with positive, health-promoting experiences and is therefore a correlate if not a predictor and resource for well-being. Well-being may be defined in many ways, depending upon the individual or patient population. Indicators of well-being are as diverse as human perceptions of health and wellness. Examples of indicators of well-being include life satisfaction, positive self-concept, hopefulness, happiness, and sense of meaning in life. Well-being is a correlate and an outcome of self-transcendence.

Vulnerability

Another key concept of the theory is vulnerability. Vulnerability is awareness of personal mortality and the likelihood of experiencing difficult life events. It is theorized that self-transcendence, as a developmental capacity (and perhaps as a survival mechanism), emerges naturally in health experiences that confront a person with issues of mortality and immortality. Life events that heighten one's sense of mortality, inadequacy, or vulnerability can—if they do not crush the individual's inner self—trigger developmental progress toward a renewed sense of identity and expanded self-boundaries (Corless, Germino, & Pittman, 1994; Erikson, 1986; Frankl, 1963; Marshall, 1980). Examples of these life events include serious or chronic illness, disability, aging, parenting, childbirth, loss of a loved one, career difficulties, and other life crises. Self-transcendence is evoked through such events and may enhance well-being by transforming losses and difficulties into healing experiences (Reed, 1996).

RELATIONSHIPS AMONG THE CONCEPTS: THE MODEL

The model of the theory of self-transcendence is presented in Figure 6.1. Three basic sets of relationships exist among the concepts in the theory. First, it is expected that there is a relationship between the experience of vulnerability and self-transcendence such that increased levels of vulnerability, as brought on by health events, for example, influence increased levels of self-transcendence. However, this may hold only within certain levels of experienced vulnerability. The relationship between vulnerability and self-transcendence is best characterized as a nonlinear relationship in that very low and very high levels of vulnerability are not expected to relate to increased levels of self-transcendence, or at least not without the influence of other factors in that relationship.

A second relationship exists between self-transcendence and well-being. This relationship is posited to be direct and positive with positive

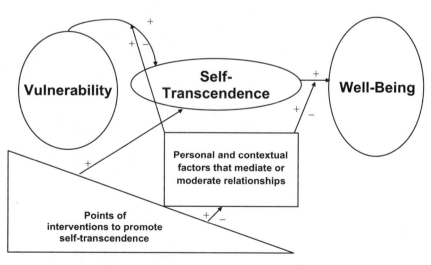

FIGURE 6.1   Self-transcendence.

indicators of well-being. For example, self-transcendence relates positively to sense of well-being and morale but relates negatively to level of depression as an indicator of well-being.

Third, there is a diversity of personal and contextual factors that may moderate these two central relationships.

A wide variety of personal and contextual factors and their interactions influence the process of self-transcendence as it relates to well-being. Examples of these factors are age, gender, cognitive ability, health status, past significant life events, and the sociopolitical environment. As moderators, these factors either enhance or diminish the strength of the relationships. For example, a recent and significant loss may diminish the positive relationship between an experience of vulnerability and self-transcendence. Advanced age or education may potentiate the relationship between self-transcendence and well-being. Continued research into other personal and contextual factors is needed to better understand the potential role of these variables in the theory and their interrelationships.

Other concepts and relationships can be identified to extend the theory of self-transcendence. The theory was initially constructed to better understand the role of self-transcendence at the end of life. Since then, researchers' findings have extended the boundaries of theory beyond later life and end-of-life illness experiences to include other experiences of vulnerability. For example, end-of-life health experiences were found to be significant correlates of self-transcendence among younger adults. In another study, middle-aged adults were studied using the variables of parenting and self-acceptance as indicators of self-transcendence.

Because of my nursing commitment toward gaining better understanding of the inherent resources that foster human well-being, I have approached the study of self-transcendence as an independent variable, a contributor to well-being, and possible predictor of well-being outcomes, rather than as the dependent or outcome variable. Nursing interventions that support the person's inner resource for self-transcendence may focus directly on facilitating self-transcendence. Interventions may also focus on influencing some of the personal and contextual factors that mediate or moderate the relationships between vulnerability and self-transcendence and between self-transcendence and well-being (see Figure 6.1).

In contrast to self-transcendence as an independent variable, some scholars have conceptualized it as an outcome (or dependent) variable of interest (Coward, 1998; Haase, Britt, Coward, Leidy, & Penn, 1992). In these cases, self-transcendence is regarded more as an indicator of well-being rather than as a correlate or facilitator of well-being. In addition, other antecedents of self-transcendence may be identified. For example, in Haase and colleagues' (1992) concept analysis, spiritual perspective was identified as an "antecedent" of self-transcendence. This is congruent with Reed's model in that spirituality may broadly represent the person's pandimensional nature, which facilitates emergence of self-transcendence as it is defined in the theory. Others may not view spirituality and self-transcendence as two separate concepts. More research on the model is needed to identify empirical support for the various relational statements that have been proposed.

Self-transcendence is a concept relevant to the discipline of nursing. Themes of self-transcendence are evident in foundational nursing theories (Reed, 1996). In Watson's (1985/1999) theory of human caring, as written and revised since 1985, transcendence is integral to understanding the essence of patients and nurses and their inner strivings toward greater self-awareness and inner healing.

In Parse's (1992) theory of human becoming, cotranscending is a major theme underlying the philosophical assumptions of her theory. Cotranscending involves a relational process of developing new ways of living and transforming the self that incorporate yet reach beyond the old ways. Mobilizing transcendence is an exemplary nursing practice within Parse's paradigm.

Newman's (1994) theory of health postulates a transcendence of time and space as one reaches beyond illness to develop an awareness of one's patterns, self-identity, and higher level of consciousness. Through this process, there is health and well-being in even the most difficult of illness experiences. Although all of these theorists present unique views of transcendence, theorists generally share the idea of expanding awareness beyond the immediate or constricted views of oneself and the world to transform life experiences into healing (Reed, 1996).

Self-transcendence is also congruent with Newman's (1992) unitary–transformative paradigm, which presents human beings as embedded in an ongoing developmental process of changing complexity and organization, a process integrally related to well-being. Further, self-transcendence is an example of Reed's (1997a) redefinition of "nursing process," that is a process of self-organizing inherent among human systems and related to well-being.

Other disciplines, particularly transpersonal psychology and psychiatry, have addressed the concept of self-transcendence. Cloninger and his colleagues (Cloninger, Svrakic, & Svrakic, 1997) conceptualized self-transcendence as a factor in the organization of the personality and in development of psychopathology. Cloninger measured self-transcendence as one of three dimensions in his instrument, the Temperament and Character Inventory (TCI). Psychologists Frankl (1963) and Maslow (1969) are frequently cited for their emphasis on the self-transcendent capacity of human beings. Psychologists' conceptualizations of self-transcendence, however, diverge from nursing in their emphasis on self-transcendence as involving an elevation or a separation of self from the environment.

USE OF THE THEORY IN NURSING RESEARCH

There is an increasing number of studies that provide empirical support for Reed's theory. Nevertheless, it is expected that ongoing research will lead to extensions, modifications, or refinements of the theory, since all theories undergo change as they are tested or challenged. In general, however, the results to date indicate that self-transcendence is a resource that accompanies serious life experiences that intensify one's sense of vulnerability or mortality. Findings also support the theorized relationship between self-transcendence and various indicators of well-being across groups of study participants facing a wide variety of health experiences.

The Self-Transcendence Scale

Reed's (1991b) Self-Transcendence Scale (STS) has been used in much of the research that most directly relates to the theory. The STS is a 15-item one-dimensional scale. It originated from a 36-item instrument, the Developmental Resources of Later Adulthood (DRLA) scale (Reed, 1986, 1989), which measured the level of developmentally based psychosocial resources in a person. The DRLA was constructed from an extensive review of theoretical and empirical literature on adult development and aging, selected nursing conceptual models and life span theories, and clinical encounters with older adults.

A self-transcendence factor, which explained nearly half of the variance in the instrument and had good internal consistency, was identified within the scale. The STS was developed around this empirically based factor. The STS was subsequently used in research to measure intrapersonal, interpersonal, temporal, and transpersonal experiences that reflect expanded boundaries of the self in developmentally mature adults. The STS has demonstrated reliability and construct validity and is brief and easy to administer as a questionnaire or in an interview format. Many researchers and graduate students have used the instrument in studying self-transcendence as it relates to various health experiences and outcomes.

Initial Research

The initial research used to build the theory of self-transcendence focused on well elders and elders hospitalized for psychiatric treatment of depression (Reed, 1986, 1989). Elders were selected as a group potentially facing end-of-life issues. Correlational and longitudinal studies were designed to examine the nature and significance of the relationship between self-transcendence and mental health outcomes. It was found consistently that self-transcendence was a correlate and predictor of mental health in these elders. Correlations were significant and of moderate magnitude. Reed's (1986) longitudinal study provided empirical evidence for a potential link between self-transcendence and subsequent occurrence of depression among mentally healthy adults; this link approached statistical significance and was in the expected direction among clinically depressed adults.

Self-transcendence was next examined for its relevance to mental health among the oldest-old, adults 80 to 100 years of age (Reed, 1991a). Quantitative and qualitative data generated further support for the theory. Significant inverse correlations of moderate magnitude were found between self-transcendence and both depression and overall mental health symptomatology. In addition, four conceptual clusters representing different aspects of self-transcendence were generated from a content analysis: generativity, introjectivity, temporal integration, and body transcendence. Elders who scored high on depression reflected weak patterns in these four areas, particularly in body-transcendence, inner-directed activities, and positive integration of present and future. These qualitative findings provided further support for the theory, which posited the salience of self-transcendence as a correlate of well-being in later adulthood or other critical times of life.

Basic and Practice-Based Research by Coward

Coward, who as a doctoral student studied with Reed, continued research into self-transcendence with a focus on middle-aged adults confronting their mortality through serious illness, advanced cancer, and AIDS. Coward (1990, 1995) initially studied the lived experience of self-transcendence in women with advanced breast cancer. Results from her phenomenological study were consistent with findings from quantitative studies. Self-transcendent perspectives were salient in this group, which had a heightened awareness of personal mortality; self-transcendence was expressed in terms of reaching out beyond self to help others, to permit others to help them, and to accept the present, unchangeable events in time.

This research validated Reed's (1989) quantitative measure of self-transcendence. In subsequent phenomenological research, Coward and Lewis (1993) explored self-transcendence in women and men with AIDS. Despite increased fear and sadness at the prospect of death, all participants indicated self-transcendent perspectives, which in turn helped them find meaning and achieve emotional well-being.

Findings from a study in which structural equation modeling was used to analyze responses in a sample of women with advanced breast cancer indicated that self-transcendence led to decreased illness distress through the mediating effect of emotional well-being. Self-transcendence had a significant and direct positive effect on emotional well-being (Coward, 1991).

Coward (1996) also studied healthy adults, who ranged in age from 19 to 85 years. She was interested in extending the theory of self-transcendence by examining its salience in a group of adults who were not as actively confronted with end-of-life issues as other seriously ill populations. Self-transcendence was again found to be a significant and strong correlate of well-being indicators, namely coherence, self-esteem, hope, and other variables assessing emotional well-being. Coward concluded that while her research supported the hypothesized relationship between self-transcendence and mental health variables, the findings, as generated from a sample of healthy adults, did not necessarily support the theoretical link between awareness of end-of-life issues and self-transcendence. Coward cited Frankl (1969) in proposing that self-transcendence is an essential human characteristic that may surface at any time in the life span.

Although Coward's interpretation of the results may expand the boundaries of the theory in terms of populations where self-transcendence may be salient, her results do not necessarily dispute the idea that some awareness of human mortality is integral to self-transcendence. Awareness of mortality is a basic characteristic of the human condition among both healthy and ill adults. This awareness may emerge slowly from the accumulation of life experiences as well as suddenly by a health crisis event.

Intervention research by Coward and Kahn (2004, 2005) focused on the experiences and functions of self-transcendence in women newly diagnosed with breast cancer. Self-transcendent practices and perspectives were particularly effective in helping women resolve spiritual disequilibrium often experienced after diagnosis of breast cancer (Coward & Kahn, 2004). In their 2005 study, the investigators compared a traditional community cancer support group with a self-transcendence theory-based group on outcomes regarding the experiences of self-transcendence and physical and emotional well-being. Women in the treatment group were able to attain a better sense of community with their support group. However, the most striking finding was that women in both groups had self-transcendent experiences as described in Reed's theory, which sustained them through the diagnosis and treatment of their illness. They expressed themes of outward, inward, and temporal expansion of self-boundaries such as reaching out for support and information, finding inner strength to endure, and constructing meaning out of past experiences and future hopes. The authors interpreted this finding as support for the idea that the capacity for transcending an adverse event is a universal trait that motivates a person to expand one's conceptual boundaries in multiple and beneficial ways.

In summary, Coward's program of research has provided empirical evidence to support and possibly extend the theory of self-transcendence. Her findings from various studies have consistently indicated that self-transcendence is a resource that accompanies serious illness and is significantly related to indicators of well-being. This was found with women facing the end of life through advanced breast cancer and AIDS and through men's experience with AIDS. Her research with a healthy population provided further support for the theory of self-transcendence while raising new questions about the significance of awareness of personal mortality in the emergence of self-transcendence.

Research by Colleagues and Reed

In an attempt to examine the theory in a group of adults that was healthy and younger than the elders typically studied, Ellermann and Reed (2001) reported on their study of self-transcendence in middle-aged adults. Theorizing as Coward did several years earlier that self-transcendence was a life span phenomenon and not confined to later life, they sought evidence that extended applications of the theory of self-transcendence. They identified parenting, self-acceptance, and spirituality as expressions of self-transcendence in middle-aged adults in particular and related these experiences to mental health. The results indicated a strong inverse relationship between self-transcendence and level of depression in this group, particularly among women.

In comparing their findings to those from other studies, Ellermann and Reed (2001) found that self-transcendence was higher among groups of older participants although still salient among the middle-aged participants. Gender differences were identified, including the finding that self-transcendence was more predominant among women than men. Their research not only supported the theory of self-transcendence but also introduced questions about the role of human experiences such as parenting and spirituality in the theory; that is, do they function as indicators, correlates, or antecedents of self-transcendence?

Decker and Reed (2005) studied self-transcendence and moral reasoning within the context of several contextual and developmental factors to better understand end-of-life treatment preferences among older adults. Self-transcendence was found to be significantly and positively related to level of integrated moral reasoning, that is reasoning that includes both the autonomous and social domains of moral decision making. This was expected based on life span developmental theory on adult thinking processes. Self-transcendence did not relate significantly to desired level of aggressiveness of end-of-life treatment, although investigators argued that more research is needed into the role of self-transcendence and end-of-life decisions. The results help explain why reasoning about end-of-life treatment options reflects a complex and integrated approach among some elders.

Runquist and Reed (2007) reported on findings from Runquist's master's thesis research in which self-transcendence along with the variables of spiritual perspective, fatigue, and health status were measured to identify significant correlates of well-being in 61 homeless men and women. Self-transcendence coupled with physical health factors were theorized to be statistically independent correlates (resources) for well-being in this sample. A strong positive relationship between self-transcendence and well-being was found, as theorized. In addition, two variables, self-transcendence and health status, together explained a significant 60% of the variance in well-being, with self-transcendence having the greater correlation with well-being. These findings suggest that an effective clinical approach with homeless persons does not necessarily require extensive clinical applications to enhance well-being. The investigators concluded that attention to the spiritual side of living, in addition to physical health, may be equally important in fostering well-being among homeless persons.

Research by Other Investigators

Other research conducted over the past 15 years has provided support for the theory of self-transcendence. In most of the quantitative studies reported here, researchers measured self-transcendence with Reed's Self-Transcendence Scale. In the case of qualitative studies, researchers worked from a conceptualization of self-transcendence congruent with Reed's definition unless or until the findings indicated something different. Research has focused on various populations including older adults with chronic illness and adults with life-threatening illness.

Chronic Illness and Aging. Several researchers in addition to Reed have studied self-transcendence in older adults. These studies include older adults who have chronic or serious illness, mental illness, and older adults who are relatively healthy.

Walton and colleagues (1991) reported one of the earliest studies. They explored self-transcendence as measured by a 58-item scale based upon Peck's (1968) developmental stages of old age. They identified a significant inverse relationship between self-transcendence and loneliness among 107 healthy older adults.

Billard (2001) examined the role of self-transcendence in the well-being of aging Catholic sisters for her doctoral research. Specifically, she combined Reed's (1987) Spiritual Perspective Scale with Reed's (1991a) Self-Transcendence Scale to measure the concept of spiritual transcendence and its relationship to the variable of emotional intelligence in a sample of 377 elder Catholic sisters. She found that spiritual transcendence, along with selected personality and demographic factors, contributed significantly to explaining emotional intelligence. Fostering spiritual transcendence was recommended as a resource for helping aging sisters transform their own lives and the lives of others in positive ways.

In research into suicide by Buchanan, Farran, and Clark (1995), the findings supported the hypothesis that self-transcendence was integral to older adults coping with the changes in later life. Other important factors in coping were loss of spouse and friends, loss of work, and state of finances. In studying 35 elders hospitalized for depression, the researchers found that desire for death and self-transcendence (as measured by the STS) were significantly and inversely related at $r = -.55, p < .001$. All other relationships between self-transcendence and suicide ideation were in the expected direction but were not significant, likely due to the small sample size.

Klaas (1998) studied self-transcendence and depression in 77 depressed and nondepressed elders. Her results in both groups supported the theory of self-transcendence. Significant negative correlations were found between depression and self-transcendence. In addition, self-transcendence was significantly and positively correlated with meaning in life in this group. Last, the depressed group of elders scored significantly lower on the STS as well as on Meaning in Life. Scores on the STS and Purpose in Life test were significantly and positively related, supporting the construct validity of the STS.

A significant positive relationship was found between self-transcendence and activities of daily living among 88 chronically ill elders in research by Upchurch (1999). She proposed a theoretical model in which self-transcendence, as a developmental strength and part of human essence, may partly explain why some elders continued to remain independent while others did not, regardless of health status.

Walker (2002) measured self-transcendence and mastery of stress in testing his theory of transformative aging. His study was based upon the idea that stressful events can bring about transformative change that enables the person to deal with the losses and challenges that accompany aging. Self-transcendence was conceptualized as a process of transforming among middle-aged adults and older adults. Results of the study lent support to the hypothesized relationships derived from his theory; self-transcendence was significantly and positively related to mastery of stress and significantly inversely related to stress of aging. His findings have implications for engaging the resource of self-transcendence to assist middle-aged and older adults in mastering stress and existential anxiety over the aging process. Similarly, in a study of older women living with rheumatoid arthritis, Neill (2002) found that transcendence of self-boundaries and personal transformation represented a process of living successfully with a chronic illness.

In a correlational study of oldest-old adults, a group of Swedish researchers studied self-transcendence and similar variables as related to mental and physical health outcomes in later life (Nygren et al., 2005). They found significant, positive relationships of moderate magnitude between self-transcendence and several variables in both the men's and women's groups including resilience, sense of coherence, and purpose in life. Self-transcendence was also positively related to indicators of mental health but significantly so only in the women's group. The results overall indicated that oldest-old adults were capable of experiencing levels of self-transcendence and other positive factors comparable to those in younger adults. The investigators concluded that the impact of aging on inner strength and other spiritually related and psychological variables may differ between men and women and suggested further research. More knowledge about gender differences would help refine the theory of self-transcendence.

Elderly nursing home residents were studied for their perceptions on what personal qualities allowed them to rise above the difficulties faced in their advanced age (Bickerstaff, Grasser, & McCabe, 2003). Results from this qualitative study were consistent with patterns of self-transcendence identified earlier by Reed (1991a) in her study of community-dwelling oldest-old adults: generativity, introjectivity, temporal integration, body-transcendence, and one not previously identified, "relationship with self/others/higher being." Many participants exhibited more than one pattern of self-transcendence. The researchers concluded that caregivers of older adults in long-term care facilities and at home should look beyond custodial care to incorporate activities that build upon the residents' capacity for self-transcendence that can help them cope with the losses of later life.

In a study of factors related to self-care in older African Americans, Upchurch and Mueller (2005) found that self-transcendence was significantly and positively related to the ability to carry out instrumental activities of daily living (IADLs). They also found a significant interaction effect between self-transcendence and education, which related positively to IADLs among the least-educated elders. The investigators recommended that caregivers consider interventions designed to enhance self-transcendence to help caregivers support self-care abilities of older adults.

The dissertation and thesis studies of graduate students (e.g., Draur, 1997; Kamienski, 1997) have also provided creative and consistent evidence to support the theory of self-transcendence in samples of older adults.

Serious and Life-Threatening Illness in Adults. Several researchers in addition to Coward have studied self-transcendence in people who have life-threatening illnesses. Stevens (1999) examined the relationships between self-transcendence and depression in young adults with AIDS and found the two variables to be significantly and inversely related, consistent with the theory of self-transcendence.

Wright (2003) studied the relationship between quality of life and self-transcendence in liver transplant recipients. She found a significant positive relationship between self-transcendence and quality of life ($r = .51$, $p < .01$). Self-transcendence was also significantly and inversely related to fatigue in this sample ($r = -.20$, $p < .01$). Women scored significantly higher on self-transcendence than men. They concluded that self-transcendence, illness distress, fatigue, and age are important factors related to quality of life.

In a phenomenological study of eight women who had completed breast cancer therapy, Pelusi (1997) found that surviving breast cancer very much involved self-transcendence. In this population, self-transcendence was expressed as setting life priorities, finding meaning in life, and looking within self. Similar findings occurred in a study by Kinney (1996), who reported on her own journey through breast cancer. A process of listening to and trusting one's inner voice facilitated transcendence. Self-transcendence in turn was central to reconstruction of self.

Self-transcendence and quality of life were studied in 46 HIV-positive adults by Mellors, Riley, and Erlen (1997). Data analysis revealed a significant moderate positive relationship between self-transcendence and quality of life for the group, particularly for those who were the most seriously ill. The dimensions of quality of life that related most significantly to self-transcendence were health and functioning and psychological/spiritual dimensions.

Chin-A-Loy and Fernsler (1998) examined self-transcendence among 24 men, aged 61 to 84, attending a prostate cancer support group. The participants scored fairly high on the STS, averaging 50 of a possible 15 to 60. The high level of self-transcendence in this group indicated that group members had developed ways to expand beyond the limitations posed by their cancer, despite or perhaps because of aging and living with prostate cancer. Results from other research also attest to the capacity for seriously ill individuals to transcend their illness. In a study of persons with AIDS, researchers found evidence that they were able to transcend the suffering associated with their illness (Mellors, Erlen, Coontz, & Lucke, 2001). The participants demonstrated three dominant patterns indicative of self-transcendence: creating a meaningful life pattern, achieving a sense of connectedness, and engaging in self-care.

A group of investigators (Ramer, Johnson, Chan, & Barrett, 2006) interested in quality of life among persons with HIV/AIDS studied 420 mostly Hispanic, male patients to determine the relationships of self-transcendence and spirituality to demographic, cultural, and clinical factors. Among the findings was a significant positive relationship between self-transcendence and level of energy in the patients. In addition, researchers found that levels of acculturation and self-transcendence were significantly related, suggesting that the meaning of self-transcendence may be influenced by cultural factors. Their study not only provided support for the relevance of self-transcendence among these patients, it also suggested that acculturation may moderate the relationship between self-transcendence and health outcome variables in people with HIV/AIDS.

Research on Nurses and Other Caregivers

Self-transcendence has also been studied as it occurs in family caregivers, nurses, and others providing care to patients. This area of research has been increasing in recent years.

Enyert and Burman (1999) conducted a qualitative study of self-transcendence in caregivers of terminally ill persons. They found that caregivers' self-transcendent behaviors, such as being with and doing for their loved one as death approached, provided personal growth and other positive consequences for them. They found new meaning, a new view of life, and were able to reach out to help others besides their family member.

Poole (1999) found that self-transcendence was an important phase in being a caregiver. Using the grounded theory method, Poole studied 19 family caregivers in the process of being a caregiver for frail older adults at home. Three phases of caregiving were identified by which the caregiver became able to work with health care personnel as a partner instead of perpetuating conflict in the relationship. The three phases were: connecting, discovering self, and transcending self.

Acton and Wright (2000) and Acton (2002) addressed self-transcendence in family caregivers of adults with dementia. Based on the literature they found it to be a relevant and potentially therapeutic experience for family caregivers and identified strategies to facilitate self-transcendence in family caregivers. However, when Acton (2002) conducted a naturalistic field study of family caregivers, she found that caregivers of adults with dementia had little opportunity to nurture self-transcendence; instead they experienced social isolation, ambivalence, emotional fragility, and burden of caring for their family member. She concluded that some of these negative experiences associated with caregiving may inhibit development of self-transcendence in caregivers and interfere with their continued growth and well-being.

Reese and Murray (1996) examined the role of self-transcendence in great-grandmothering in a qualitative study of African American and White groups of great-grandmothers. From interviews of 16 great-grandmothers, they identified five domains of self-transcendence: connectedness, religion, being wise, values, and stories. These domains reflect dimensions in the definition of self-transcendence in Reed's theory. The authors considered great-grandparents vital in facilitating self-transcendence and good relationships among family members.

As part of her study of spiritual growth in nurses, Kilpatrick (2002) studied the relationships between self-transcendence, spiritual perspective, and spiritual well-being among female nursing students and faculty. She found positive correlations between these variables in students and faculty. Nursing students and faculty differed significantly on level of self-transcendence and spiritual well-being, suggesting that self-transcendence may increase with development.

More recently, McGee (2004) reported on her creative dissertation research into self-transcendence in nursing. She employed the method of interpretive phenomenology to examine self-transcendence and its impact on nurses' practice. Among the results from the moving stories of nurses, McGee found self-transcendence an important mechanism of healing for nurses who have experienced difficult and traumatic personal life experiences. Her work expands the theory of self-transcendence by revealing the role of self-transcendence in healing the *nurse* and in enriching the practice of nurses for the mutual benefit of both patient and nurse.

Along a similar line of thinking, Hunnibell (2006) conducted dissertation research based upon self-transcendence theory. She studied self-transcendence as related to burnout syndrome in hospice and oncology nurses. Both groups of nurses face death and life-threatening illness through their work with patients. However, she hypothesized that because of the philosophy of their health care setting and opportunities to process loss, hospice nurses would demonstrate higher levels of self-transcendence and lower levels of burnout than oncology nurses. Hunnibell's findings provided statistically significant support for the hypothesis and for an inverse relationship between self-transcendence and burnout. She concluded that self-transcendence is a resource for nurses and may protect them against burnout.

This review of research on self-transcendence provides consistent evidence of the significance of this variable on the well-being of nurses and other caregivers. Nurses and caregivers experience vulnerability and related health experiences through the challenges of their work as well as in their personal lives. It is important not to overlook the importance of research to gain a better understanding of self-transcendence as a resource for well-being in caregivers.

USE OF THE THEORY IN NURSING PRACTICE

Research findings have shown that self-transcendence is integral to well-being across a diversity of health experiences that confront a person with end-of-life issues. Nursing practices that facilitate self-transcendence result in healing outcomes during these health events, as in, for example, diminished depression over time among clinically depressed elders, increased hopefulness and care of self among chronically ill elders, sense of well-being among persons with advanced breast cancer or with HIV/AIDS, and decreased suicidal ideation among hospitalized depressed elders. Although these particular health events have been the focus of self-transcendence research, many if not most health events confront a person with vulnerability and mortality and therefore are potential contexts for promoting healing and well-being through self-transcendence.

Encouraged by these results, nurses continue to identify other health experiences in which they can promote well-being by facilitating self-transcendence: for example, in bereavement (Joffrion & Douglas, 1994), family caregiving (Acton & Wright, 2000), and in maintenance of sobriety and well-being (McGee, 2000).

With the rise of managed care, advanced practice nurses increasingly had to provide spiritual care to specialty populations; this care extends beyond that typically provided by primary care practitioners (McCormick, Holder, Wetsel, & Cawthon, 2001). This care includes an integrative approach to spiritual care that includes facilitating self-transcendence.

Theory-Guided Strategies for Practice

Intrapersonal strategies help the person expand inward and make room to integrate loss in all its diverse experiences. Meditation, prayer, visualization, life review, and journaling are techniques of self-transcendence that nurses can guide and facilitate (Acton & Wright, 2000; McGee, 2000).

These approaches help a person look inward to clarify and expand knowledge about self and find or create meaning and purpose in the experience. Encouraging patients to keep a journal, for example, helps them become more aware of their process of transformation and transcendence. Recognition of the process and the pattern of their own healing is empowering for patients. The nurse may also encourage cognitive strategies that help patients integrate a health event into their lives. Acquiring information about the illness, using positive self-talk, and engaging in meaningful and challenging activities are all techniques that can help a person integrate and grow from the illness experience (Coward & Reed, 1996).

Interpersonal strategies for facilitating self-transcendence focus on connecting the person to others through formal or informal means, including face-to-face, telephone, or through the Internet. Maintaining meaningful relationships and strengthening affiliations with civic groups and with a supporting faith community are also strategies that the nurse can facilitate (McCormick et al., 2001). Nurse visits, peer counseling, informal networks, and formal support groups are examples of interpersonal strategies that the nurse can help arrange for the person (Acton & Wright, 2000).

Support groups are often cited as an effective way to connect people facing a difficult life situation. Groups that bring together people of similar health experiences can facilitate self-transcendence by connecting the person to others who can share the loss and exchange information and wisdom about coping with the experience and by providing an opportunity to reach beyond the self to help another. Joffrion and Douglas (1994) reported that nurses can facilitate self-transcendence during bereavement by helping the person participate in church or civic groups, develop or resume a hobby, share personal experiences of grief with others, and support others who have experienced loss. In pre-experimental and quasi-experimental studies, Coward (1998, 2003) developed and refined a series of support group sessions to facilitate self-transcendence. These sessions provided a variety of activities designed to support self-transcendence in women facing breast cancer: orientation and information sessions, sharing cancer stories, problem-solving, assertive communication training, relaxation training, values clarification, ongoing educational components, constructive thinking and self-instructional training, feelings management, and pleasant activity planning. The self-transcendence based sessions resulted in expanded perspectives and views, and in improved sense of well-being at the end of treatment, although this did not hold 1 year later. Ongoing group support based on self-transcendence theory may be helpful to women, depending upon their available resources.

Altruistic activities facilitate self-transcendence. They provide a context for learning new things and expanding awareness about oneself and one's world (Coward & Reed, 1996). Altruism also enhances a person's inner sense of worth and purpose. McGee (2000) explained that practicing humility and providing service to others are tools of self-transcendence that can empower individuals to maintain a healthy lifestyle. Connections between people, whether to receive or provide support, are key strategies for enhancing self-transcendence.

Group psychotherapy is another intervention strategy for enhancing self-transcendence. Young and Reed (1995) found that this intervention approach was effective in generating a variety of outcomes for a group of elders: for example, intrapersonally in terms of achieving self-enrichment, self-esteem, and self-affirmation; interpersonally in terms of bonding with and helping others, enabling self-disclosure, and overcoming self-absorption; and temporally in terms of gaining acceptance of one's past and feeling empowered about the future.

Similarly, Stinson and Kirk (2006) reported research in which they tested the effect of group reminiscing on depression (measured by the Geriatric Depression Scale) and self-transcendence (measured by the STS) in a group of older women living in an assisted living facility. Given previous findings that consistently supported the relationship between self-transcendence and depression, it was logical to examine interventions that may increase self-transcendence as well as decrease depression. Results indicated a nonsignificant decrease in depression and an increase in self-transcendence after 6 weeks of reminiscence group sessions. Findings also indicated a significant inverse relationship between depression and self-transcendence as theorized.

Schumann (1999) found that self-transcendence enhanced well-being in ventilated patients. Spiritual connections enabled patients to use temporal perspectives of past and future to empower themselves; they synchronized their lives with the realities of being on a ventilator and anticipating extubation and were then better able to manage this life-threatening health experience.

Diener (2003) conducted a randomized, clinical trial to examine the effectiveness of personal narrative as an intervention for enhancing self-transcendence in women with HIV, multiple sclerosis, and systemic lupus erythematosus. The STS scores increased significantly in the intervention groups, suggesting that the intervention was successful in helping the women address issues related to having a life-threatening or life-altering illness.

Transpersonal strategies are designed to help the person connect with a power or purpose greater than self. The nurse's role in this process is often one of creating an environment in which transpersonal exploration can occur. For example, to foster self-transcendence in family caregivers of adults with dementia, Acton and Wright (2000) identify the importance of helping arrange for in-home assistance or day care so the family members have the time and energy to engage in activities that promote transpersonal awareness. Religious activities and prayer in particular are frequently identified as significant to the well-being of persons facing life crises. McGee (2000) explains the need for the nurse to provide an environment in which patients can look beyond themselves toward a higher power for help and be inspired to help others. In addition, several of the strategies that foster intrapersonal growth also can foster a sense of transpersonal connection, such as meditation, visualization, and journaling.

CONCLUSION

Professional nurses are defined in large part by their ability to engage the human capacities for healing and well-being. Self-transcendence was presented as a human capacity for well-being. It represents "both a human capacity and a human struggle that can be facilitated by nursing" (Reed, 1996, p. 3). A goal in developing the theory was to gain better understanding of the dynamics of self-transcendence as it relates to health and well-being. This knowledge, in addition to that acquired through personal and ethical knowing and practice experience, can be used by nurses to foster well-being through strategies of self-transcendence.

Rogerian and life span principles of development external to the theory influenced the theory's development. Philosophic views include the pandimensionality of human beings and the human potential for healing and well-being. Several nursing theories were also foundational to the theory of self-transcendence.

There is consistency among the elements internal to the theory—the concepts, their definitions, and proposed relationships. Positive relationships were identified between vulnerability and self-transcendence and between self-transcendence and well-being. However, new twists in the stated relationships may yet be discovered. A number of researchers have studied self-transcendence as an outcome or a process of well-being in its own right, disregarding the third key relationship identified in the theory between self-transcendence and well-being. In other research, self-transcendence functions as a resource, correlate, or facilitator of specific indicators of well-being. In addition, recent research findings provide evidence to support the role of mediators and moderators in the process of self-transcendence as proposed in the theory. For example, variables such as acculturation, age, education, gender, time span and nature of group support, physical health status, type of occupation, and caregiver burden are among those factors that may moderate relationships proposed by the theory.

The theory now reaches beyond the initial focus on elders to include adults of all ages who experience vulnerability. Future research may further broaden the scope to include other normative life transitions and developmental events among youth and children, whose processes of self-transcendence have yet to be explored. The scholarship of advanced practice nurses, graduate students, and researchers can continue to offer new insights into personal, contextual, and cultural factors that influence the process of self-transcendence.

The theory is significant in that it is a theory for the present. Self-transcendence reflects a nursing perspective of human beings and proposes a mechanism by which human beings generate well-being in times of vulnerability. This process has been supported by research. Nursing, through its theories and practices that inspire human transcendence, can make a significant contribution to sustaining human beings within the context of their everyday experiences.

Self-transcendence may very well be a developmental imperative for younger as well as older people, for those healthy and ill. If so, nursing must be there to generate the knowledge and provide the expert support that facilitates this cost-effective and holistic process of well-being.

REFERENCES

Acton, G. J. (2002). Self-transcendent views and behaviors: Exploring growth in caregivers of adults with dementia. *Journal of Gerontological Nursing, 28*(12), 22–30.

Acton, G. J., & Wright, K. B. (2000). Self-transcendence and family caregivers of adults with dementia. *Journal of Holistic Nursing, 18,* 143–158.

Arlin, P. K. (1975). Cognitive development in adulthood: A fifth stage? *Developmental Psychology, 11,* 602–606.

Basseches, M. (1984). *Dialectical thinking and adult development.* Norwood, NJ: Ablex.

Bickerstaff, K. A., Grasser, C. M., & McCabe, B. (2003). How elderly nursing home residents transcend losses of later life. *Holistic Nursing Practice, 17*(3), 159–165.

Billard, A. (2001). *The impact of spiritual transcendence on the well-being of aging Catholic sisters.* Unpublished doctoral dissertation, Loyola College, Baltimore, MD.

Buchanan, D., Farran, C., & Clark, D. (1995). Suicidal thought and self-transcendence in older adults. *Journal of Psychosocial Nursing, 33*(10), 31–34.

Chin-A-Loy, S. S., & Fernsler, J. I. (1998). Self-transcendence in older men attending a prostate cancer support group. *Cancer Nursing, 21,* 358–363.

Cloninger, C. R., Svrakic, N. M., & Svrakic, D. M. (1997). Role of personality self-organization in development of mental order and disorder. *Development and Psychopathology, 9,* 881–906.

Commons, M., Demick, J., & Goldberg, C. (1996). *Clinical approaches to adult development.* Norwood, NJ: Ablex.

Corless, I. B., Germino, B. B., & Pittman, M. (1994). *Dying, death, and bereavement: Theoretical perspectives and other ways of knowing.* Boston: Jones and Bartlett.

Coward, D. (1990). The lived experience of self-transcendence in women with advanced breast cancer. *Nursing Science Quarterly, 3,* 162–169.

Coward, D. (1991). Self-transcendence and emotional well-being in women with advanced breast cancer. *Oncology Nursing Forum, 18,* 857–863.

Coward, D. (1995). Lived experience of self-transcendence in women with AIDS. *Journal of Obstetric, Gynecologic, and Neonatal Nursing, 24,* 314–318.

Coward, D. (1996). Self-transcendence and correlates in a healthy population. *Nursing Research, 45,* 116–122.

Coward, D. (1998). Facilitation of self-transcendence in a breast cancer support group. *Oncology Nursing Forum, 25,* 75–84.

Coward, D. D. (2003). Facilitation of self-transcendence in a breast cancer support group: Part II. *Oncology Nursing Forum, 30*(2), 291–300.

Coward, D. D., & Kahn, D. L. (2004). Resolution of spiritual disequilibrium by women newly diagnosed with breast cancer. *Oncology Nursing Forum, 31*(2), E1–E8.

Coward, D. D., & Kahn, D. L. (2005). Transcending breast cancer: Making meaning from diagnosis and treatment. *Journal of Holistic Nursing, 23*(3), 264–283.

Coward, D., & Lewis, F. (1993). The lived experience of self-transcendence in gay men with AIDS. *Oncology Nursing Forum, 20,* 1363–1369.

Coward, D., & Reed, P. G. (1996). Self-transcendence: A resource for healing at the end of life. *Issues in Mental Health Nursing, 17,* 275–288.

Decker, I. M., & Reed, P. G. (2005). Developmental and contextual correlates of elders' anticipated end-of-life treatment decisions. *Death Studies, 29,* 827–846.

Diener, J. E. S. (2003). *Personal narrative as an intervention to enhance self-transcendence in women with chronic illness.* Unpublished doctoral dissertation. University of Missouri, St. Louis.

Draur, G. A. (1997). *Intrinsic religious motivation, adverse life events, coping practices, and the development of self-transcendence in older women.* Unpublished doctoral dissertation, University of Nebraska, Lincoln.

Ellermann, C. R., & Reed, P. G. (2001). Self-transcendence and depression in middle-aged adults. *Western Journal of Nursing Research, 23,* 698–713.

Enyert, G., & Burman, M. E. (1999). A qualitative study of self-transcendence in caregivers of terminally ill patients. *American Journal of Hospice and Palliative Care, 16*(2), 455–462.

Erikson, E. H. (1986). *Vital involvement in old age.* New York: Norton.

Frankl, V. E. (1963). *Man's search for meaning.* New York: Pocket Books.

Frankl, V. E. (1969). *The will to meaning.* New York: New American Library.

Haase, J. E., Britt, T., Coward, D. D., Leidy, N. K., & Penn, P. E. (1992). Simultaneous concept analysis of spiritual perspective, hope, acceptance and self-transcendence. *Image: Journal of Nursing Scholarship, 24,* 141–147.

Hunnibell, L. S. (2006). *Self-transcendence and the three aspects of burnout syndrome in hospice and oncology nurses.* Unpublished doctoral dissertation, Case Western Reserve University, Cleveland, OH.

Joffrion, L. P., & Douglas, D. (1994). Grief resolution: Facilitating self-transcendence in the bereaved. *Journal of Psychosocial Nursing, 32*(3), 13–19.

Kamienski, M. C. (1997). *An investigation of the relationship among suffering, self-transcendence, and social support in women with breast cancer.* Unpublished doctoral dissertation, Rutgers, the State University of New Jersey, Newark.

Kilpatrick, J. A. W. (2002). *Spiritual perspective, self-transcendence, and spiritual well-being in female nursing students and female nursing faculty.* Unpublished doctoral dissertation, Widener University, Wilmington, DE.

Kinney, C. K. (1996). Transcending breast cancer: Reconstructing one's self. *Issues in Mental Health Nursing, 17*(3), 201–216.

Klaas, D. (1998). Testing two elements of spirituality in depressed and non-depressed elders. *The International Journal of Psychiatric Nursing Research, 4,* 452–462.

Koplowitz, H. (1984). A projection beyond Piaget's formal operational stage: A general systems stage and a unitary stage. In M. L. Commons, F. A. Richards, & C. Armon (Eds.), *Beyond formal operations: Late adolescence and adult cognitive development* (pp. 272–296). New York: Praeger.

Marshall, V. M. (1980). *Last chapter: A sociology of aging and dying.* Monterey, CA: Brooks-Cole.

Maslow, A. H. (1969). Various meanings of transcendence. *Journal of Transpersonal Psychology, 1,* 56–66.

McCormick, D. P., Holder, B., Wetsel, M. A., & Cawthon, T. W. (2001). Spirituality and HIV disease: An integrated perspective. *Journal of the Association of Nurses in AIDS Care, 12*(3), 58–65.

McGee, E. M. (2000). Alcoholics Anonymous and nursing. *Journal of Holistic Nursing, 18*(1), 11–26.

McGee, E. M. (2004). *I'm better for having known you: An exploration of self-transcendence in nurses.* Unpublished doctoral dissertation, Boston College, Boston.

Mellors, M. P., Erlen, J. A., Coontz, P. D., & Lucke, K. T. (2001). Transcending the suffering of AIDS. *Journal of Community Health Nursing, 18*(4), 235–246.

Mellors, M. P., Riley, T. A., & Erlen, J. A. (1997). HIV, self-transcendence, and quality of life. *Journal of the Association of Nurses in AIDS Care, 2,* 59–69.

Neill, J. (2002). Transcendence and transformation in the life patterns of women living with rheumatoid arthritis. *Advances in Nursing Science, 24*(4), 27–47.

Newman, M. (1992). Prevailing paradigms in nursing. *Nursing Outlook, 40,* 10–13.

Newman, M. (1994). *Health as expanding consciousness* (2nd ed.). New York: National League for Nursing.

Nygren, B., Alex, L., Jonsen, E., Gustafson, Y., Norberg, A., & Lundman, B. (2005). Resilience, sense of coherence, purpose in life and self-transcendence in relation to perceived physical and mental health among the oldest old. *Aging & Mental Health, 9*(4), 354–362.

Parse, R. (1992). Human becoming: Parse's theory of nursing. *Nursing Science Quarterly, 5,* 35–42.

Peck, R. C. (1968). Psychological development in the second half of life. In B. L. Neugarten (Ed.), *Middle age and aging* (pp. 88–92). Chicago: University of Chicago Press.

Pelusi, J. (1997). The lived experience of surviving breast cancer. *Oncology Nursing Forum, 24*(8), 1343–1353.

Poole, D. K. (1999). *Partnering with a formal program: Expanding the boundaries of family caregiving for frail older adults.* Unpublished doctoral dissertation, Medical College of Georgia, Augusta.

Ramer, L., Johnson, D., Chan, L., & Barrett, M. T. (2006). The effect of HIV/AIDS disease progression on spirituality and self-transcendence in a multicultural population. *Journal of Transcultural Nursing, 17*(3), 280–289.

Reed, P. G. (1983). Implications of the life-span developmental framework for well-being in adulthood and aging. *Advances in Nursing Science, 6,* 18–25.

Reed, P. G. (1986). Developmental resources and depression in the elderly: A longitudinal study. *Nursing Research, 35,* 368–374.

Reed, P. G. (1987). Spirituality and well-being in terminally ill hospitalized adults. *Research in Nursing and Health, 10*(5), 335–344.

Reed, P. G. (1989). Mental health of older adults. *Western Journal of Nursing Research, 11*(2), 143–163.

Reed, P. G. (1991a). Self-transcendence and mental health in oldest-old adults. *Nursing Research, 40,* 7–11.

Reed, P. G. (1991b). Toward a theory of self-transcendence: Deductive reformulation using developmental theories. *Advances in Nursing Science, 13*(4), 64–77.

Reed, P. G. (1996). Transcendence: Formulating nursing perspectives. *Nursing Science Quarterly, 9*(1), 2–4.

Reed, P. G. (1997a). Nursing: The ontology of the discipline. *Nursing Science Quarterly,* *10*(2), 76–79.

Reed, P. G. (1997b). The place of transcendence in nursing's science of unitary human beings: Theory and research. In M. Madrid (Ed.), *Patterns of Rogerian knowing* (pp. 187–196). New York: National League for Nursing.

Reese, C. G., & Murray, R. B. (1996). Transcendence: The meaning of great-grandmothering. *Archives of Psychiatric Nursing, 10*(4), 245–251.

Riegel, K. F. (1976). The dialectics of human development. *American Psychologist, 31,* 631–647.

Rogers, M. E. (1970). *Introduction to the theoretical basis of nursing.* Philadelphia: F. A. Davis.

Rogers, M. E. (1980). A science of unitary man. In J. P. Riehl & C. Roy (Eds.), *Conceptual modes for nursing practice* (2nd ed., pp. 329–337). New York: Appleton-Century-Crofts.

Rogers, M. E. (1994). The science of unitary human beings: Current perspectives. *Nursing Science Quarterly, 7*(1), 33–35.

Runquist, J. J., & Reed, P. G. (2007). Self-transcendence and well-being in homeless adults. *Journal of Holistic Nursing, 25*(1), 5–13; discussion, 14–15.

Schumann, R. R. (1999). *Intensive care patients' perceptions of the experience of mechanical ventilation.* Unpublished doctoral dissertation, Texas Women's University, Denton.

Sheldon, K. M., & Kasser, T. (2001). Getting older, getting better? Personal strivings and psychological maturity across the life span. *Developmental Psychology, 37,* 491–501.

Sinnott, J. D. (1998). *The development of logic in adulthood: Postformal thought and its applications.* New York: Plenum.

Sinnott, J. D. (2003). Postformal thought and adult development: Living in balance. In J. Demick & C. Andreoletti (Eds.), *Handbook of adult development* (pp. 221–238). New York: Kluwer Academic/Plenum.

Stevens, D. D. (1999). *Spirituality, self-transcendence and depression in young adults with AIDS.* Unpublished doctoral dissertation. University of Miami, Coral Gables, FL.

Stinson, C. K., & Kirk, E. (2006). Structured reminiscence: An intervention to decrease depression and increase self-transcendence in older women. *Journal of Clinical Nursing, 15*(2), 208–218.

Upchurch, S. (1999). Self-transcendence and activities of daily living: The woman with the pink slippers. *Journal of Holistic Nursing, 17,* 251–266.

Upchurch, S., & Mueller, W. H. (2005). Spiritual influences on ability to engage in self-care activities among older African Americans. *International Journal of Aging and Human Development, 60*(1), 77–94.

Walker, C. A. (2002). Transformative aging: How mature adults respond to growing older. *The Journal of Theory Construction & Testing, 6*(2), 109–116.

Walton, C. G., Shultz, C., Beck, C. M., & Walls, R. C. (1991). Psychological correlates of loneliness in the older adult. *Archives of Psychiatric Nursing, 5*(3), 165–170.

Watson, J. (1985/1999). *Nursing: Human science and human care.* Sudbury, MA: Jones & Bartlett. (Original work published 1985)

Wright, K. B. (2003). *Quality of life, self-transcendence, illness distress, and fatigue in liver transplant recipients.* Unpublished doctoral dissertation, University of Texas at Austin.

Young, C., & Reed, P. G. (1995). Elders' perceptions of the effectiveness of group psychotherapy in fostering self-transcendence. *Archives of Psychiatric Nursing, 9,* 338–347.

CHAPTER 7

Theory of Community Empowerment

Cynthia Armstrong Persily and Eugenie Hildebrandt

The community empowerment theory was developed to give direction to improving health in communities. The first conceptualization of the theory came out of participatory action research using an exploratory design. The middle range theory is a merging of empowerment and community development theory for promoting health by building relationships both at individual and community levels (Hildebrandt, 1994, 1996).

PURPOSE OF THE THEORY AND HOW IT WAS DEVELOPED

The community empowerment middle range theory provides a framework for research and practice through development of effective interventions at individual and community levels. As such, it explicates for nursing the direct transfer of knowledge and expertise from nurse professionals to lay people to promote health. The theory was designed to structure a community involvement approach that enables community people to increase their knowledge and health care decision-making capabilities.

Persily has been involved for the past 20 years in the area of women's health and childbearing as a practitioner, educator, and researcher. Her research has emphasized nursing care with high-risk pregnancy. Beginning in 1987, Persily participated as a research clinical nurse specialist at the University of Pennsylvania School of Nursing in the project entitled "Early Discharge and Nurse Specialist Transitional Care of Women With

131

Diabetes in Pregnancy," funded by the National Center for Nursing Research. In this randomized clinical trial of early discharge, she provided early discharge and follow-up intervention being tested as the independent variable. Her dissertation research came directly from the study and examined the relationship among women's perceptions of the impact of diagnosis and treatment of high-risk pregnancy and treatment adherence, help-seeking from professionals, and clinical practice. It was found that women who perceived a high life impact from their pregnancy were more likely to seek help from care providers for social, psychological, and economic issues than for how to care for themselves. This finding led to the idea that it may not be necessary for nurses to provide all interventions with an at-risk group of pregnant women; rather, a combination of professionals and other providers may be more appropriate (Persily, 1995). Persily built on her dissertation research, and began to design a study in which lay providers worked with health care professionals to offer services to pregnant women in rural communities. After a pilot study, it was determined that there was a need for broader community involvement. Thus, she began her search for a model to guide that involvement. In searching the literature relative to community involvement in health promotion, Persily discovered Hildebrandt's work on a model for community participation (Hildebrandt, 1996). Persily made contact with Hildebrandt, who had tested the model in a postapartheid city of 100,000 people in South Africa. Hildebrandt's published model had been used to guide community-based participatory research (CBPR) for four community-based interventions. Through a series of discussions, Persily and Hildebrandt agreed that adaptation of the Hildebrandt model could provide useful guidance if developed as a middle range theory of community empowerment.

CONCEPTS OF THE THEORY

The middle range theory of community empowerment includes three major concepts: involvement, lay workers, and reciprocal health. Community empowerment is the involvement or participation of community-based lay workers in the promotion of reciprocal health. The theory propositions address relationships between (a) community lay workers and the community, (b) lay-worker involvement/actions in the community and the health of the community, and (c) community involvement/interactions with lay health workers and health for the community (reciprocal health).

The community is the entity from which the nature and scope of a public health problem, as well as the capacity to respond to that problem, evolves (American Public Health Association, 1991). That is, the answers to community health problems lie within the community. This premise is made clear in the *Healthy People 2010* goals, charging individuals, organizations, and communities to take responsibility for determining how they will work individually and collectively to achieve goals by the year 2010 (U.S. Department of Health and Human Services, 2000).

Involvement or participation occurs when community people identify their common ground of needs, resources, and barriers, and are able to build support or coalitions to mount a response to a problem through planning, implementing, and intervening. Health care professionals facilitate involvement when they share information and control with community residents by teaching and supporting consumers in identifying and participating in the management of health problems for self, family, and community.

Lay workers are trained persons who share backgrounds with the families they visit. Unlike professional health care workers, lay workers are indigenous to the community in which they live and work and are from similar cultural backgrounds. Their knowledge of community resources and values and firsthand life experiences enable them to reach out to families not easily accessible to outsiders. Lay workers are a vital link to community programs for families at risk. They assist with access to health and social services, offer guidance, provide counseling, and share learned life skills with families. The use of lay workers to promote community health has been incorporated into developing countries with limited health resources and personnel. The success of this approach has been attributed in part to the lay workers being indigenous to the communities they serve. This approach has since proved successful even in the resource-rich United States and has been tested and formalized through lay visiting programs. Home visiting using a variety of providers including lay workers increases the use of preventive services and encourages healthy behaviors (Blondel & Breart, 1995; McElmurry, Park, & Buseh, 2003; Olds et al., 1997; Rogers, Peoples-Sheps, & Suchindran, 1996; Zotti & Zahner, 1995). Lay visiting programs are one means of meeting individual and community health care needs (Julnes, Konefal, Pindur, & Kim, 1994; LaPierre, Perreault, & Goulet, 1995; Mahon, McFarlane, & Golden, 1991; McFarlane & Wriist, 1997; Rogers, Peoples-Sheps, & Sorenson, 1995).

Reciprocal health is defined as the actualization of inherent and acquired human potential (Pender, Murdaugh, & Parsons, 2002) and is a desired outcome of community empowerment where the community and professionals engage to promote proactive healthy behaviors. Reciprocal health emerges when professionals and community residents work together, respecting and sharing what each has to offer, thereby magnifying the potential for participants to manage their own health (World Health Organization, 1991a, 1991b). In contrast to reactive approaches that derive from an illness model, the concept of reciprocal health is positive and proactive because communities participate in ways to attain their highest potential (Israel, Checkoway, Schulz, & Zimmerman, 1994).

Community development literature proposes that individuals and groups grow through community participatory action and achieving identified goals. Community development is guided by models that advocate the support of people and communities to develop their strength and confidence while working on problems they have identified as important (Facet, Paine-Andrews, Francisco, & Schultz, 1995; Fiske, Hill, Krouskos, Legged, & Seagull, 1989). Community development models have been tested with varying results. Farley (1993) worked with an impoverished community in Alabama in a multigenerational project. Her intervention study explored strategies of inclusion that fostered professional–citizen partnership. She focused on the problems that mattered most to community people. Farley's results indicated that traditional power structures and stakeholder desire to maintain the status quo were barriers to health promotion. She proposed that these results support the need to empower community people so that sustainability of care delivery systems is built into the traditional power structure. Then when outside care delivery personnel leave the community, the new services will be maintained.

Several authors have proposed community interventions that facilitate enhanced health through enhanced empowerment. Swider and McElmurry (1990) developed a community empowerment intervention for use in two densely populated urban settings; it was subsequently extended to an urban immigrant outreach program (McElmurry et al., 2003). Community health workers were trained to help mobilize community residents to improve health. The Community Health Worker curriculum included problem solving, exercises in group dynamics, skill development for working within political systems, and strategies to build self-reliance in order to facilitate change and empower participants.

Building on this original empowerment intervention, McElmurry, Tyska, Gugenheim, Misner, and Poslusny (1995) used a leadership development approach where low- to middle-level agency staff people were educated to deliver the intervention and facilitate change. Findings in both studies indicated that traditional power structures in communities made change difficult to sustain.

Flynn and colleagues (Flynn, Ray, & Rider, 1994; Flynn, Rider, & Bailey, 1992) tested a community development model using participatory action research. The assumptions underlying their model were the empowerment process can be learned, experiencing the process best accomplishes learning it, and broad-based leadership from the community is more likely to be successful than localized–restrictive leadership. Flynn emphasized community leadership development addressing the weaknesses described in previous studies of community development. Further work with this model has yielded additional lessons essential to successful community development. In a study of rural community development through a nurse-managed clinic, Krothe, Flynn, Ray, and Goodwin (2000) found that community priorities may not always match quantitative data, successes must frequently be shared, and clear communication relative to accountability within communities must occur for community development models to succeed.

Zakus (1998) gathered data from 40 health centers to evaluate the community participation strategy that had been adopted by the Mexican government, which used volunteers to staff town-based centers and health outposts. Here, too, the power structure and status quo were barriers. The findings suggest that the communities were not encouraged to organize themselves, but instead the national Ministry of Health co-opted the resources of the communities to meet their objectives for expanding health services. The process increased rather than decreased community dependence on the Ministry of Health, thereby decreasing empowerment of the people.

Hildebrandt (2002) trained and used interviewers indigenous to an impoverished Midwest urban community in a study including women enrolled in the federal work-based welfare program enacted to replace Aid to Families With Dependent Children (AFDC). Findings showed benefits of working with people familiar with the community as well as barriers for impoverished single mothers balancing work and family responsibilities.

While community capacity building, community empowerment, and community participation have continued to emerge as strategies to improve health in communities, Chino and DeBruyn (2006) caution that few of these models have been specifically developed by or with indigenous communities. Chino and DeBruyn hold that many of these models fail to recognize that professional definitions of success and expected community benefits may differ greatly from indigenous community benefits. These authors provide implications for community development for indigenous, and specifically tribal, communities that can be applied across vulnerable populations. For example, the development of a positive collective identity and trust in each other are common values across many communities. Additionally, Chino and DeBruyn believe that indigenous people can come together in a way that is respectful of different cultures and traditions. Finally, they point out that models must integrate the past, present, and future vision of the community. They advocate for programs that are "community-based" rather than "community-placed" (p. 599).

Empowerment has been defined in a number of ways in the professional and lay literature. In this theory, empowerment is defined as the process of developing problem-solving capacity and self-competence by which people gain mastery over their lives. It is applicable at individual, family, and community levels. Empowerment is consistently emphasized by the World Health Organization (WHO, 1978) and widely advocated in primary health care as a critical component to improve the general health of vulnerable populations worldwide.

In nursing literature, individual empowerment has been defined relative to the nurse–client dyad and as related to changes in health behaviors. Ellis-Stoll and Popkess-Vawter (1998) define individual empowerment as a "participative process through a nurse–client dyad designed to assist in changing unhealthy behaviors" (p. 64). They further add that this process is designed to help the client develop proactive, healthy behaviors. Clifford (1992) believes empowerment is a process closely linked to caring and that caring for clients is intrinsic to the profession and important for the process to be successful. Rafael (1995) also links empowerment to participation, defining it as "a process in which clients participate with nurse facilitators, with the desired outcome of client control toward authentic self-determination" (p. 25).

Because the concepts of empowerment and health are closely linked, an empowering partnership between health care providers and communities is vital for effective community health. When considering the concept of empowerment, it is important to recognize different views. Some sources distinguish between the process of empowering and the process of becoming empowered. Others consider these processes one and the same, and still others consider them as a cause-and-effect relationship. For example, the World Health Organization notes that community empowerment occurs when professionals share information and control (empowering) with community residents in ways that result in neighborhoods and communities where people are effective participants in managing their own health care (empowered) (WHO, 1991a, 1991b). This is a cause–effect view, suggesting that becoming empowered is a result of an empowering process. Israel and colleagues (1994), on the other hand, do not distinguish between the two processes when they define community empowerment as "the ability of people to gain understanding and control over personal, social, economic and political forces in order to take action to improve their life situations" (p. 152).

Participatory research in these areas is moving forward under the umbrella term of Community-Based Participatory Research (CBPR), which is defined as involving the community of interest in every phase of the research: needs assessment, planning, designing the study, implementation, and evaluation. Israel and colleagues (2001) apply the knowledge gained through community development models to community-based participatory research and practice. Specifically, they note that there is significant evidence to suggest that resources, strengths, and skills are available in communities that may be useful for addressing problems and promoting health. They present several premises upon which community-based participatory research are built. These are recognizing community as a unit of identity, building on strengths and resources existing in the community, facilitating collaboration and equitable involvement of all partners, promoting a colearning and empowering process, and addressing health from a variety of perspectives. The authors believe these principles are as essential to community practice as they are to research.

RELATIONSHIPS AMONG THE CONCEPTS: THE MODEL

The concepts, when considered together, describe empowerment of community people through the involvement of lay workers in promoting reciprocal health (see Figure 7.1). Within any community, lay workers serve as resources that can be used in addition to traditional health care providers, thereby increasing access and extending opportunities for health promotion. In some rural communities and in developing countries, the lay worker is the only health care resource within the community. Lay workers and the health promotion opportunities they provide work with health care providers to facilitate community involvement to promote reciprocal health.

USE OF THE THEORY IN NURSING RESEARCH

In Hildebrandt's (1994) participatory action studies in South Africa, she used an exploratory descriptive design to develop self-care strategies to meet the health needs of Black South Africans in a township setting.

Data were gathered through interviews by trained, paid persons who were indigenous to the community. The use of indigenous workers helped diminish barriers engendered by distrust, race, and language. The intent of the study was to gather information about the growing elderly population and develop self-care strategies directed to that group. The strategies involved the multigenerational families of the elderly and were designed from the perspective of the elderly as a part of the community and not as an isolated group. A process model of strategies used to develop resources was designed based on the assumption that trust can be built on shared information, interaction, and partnership. The eight steps of

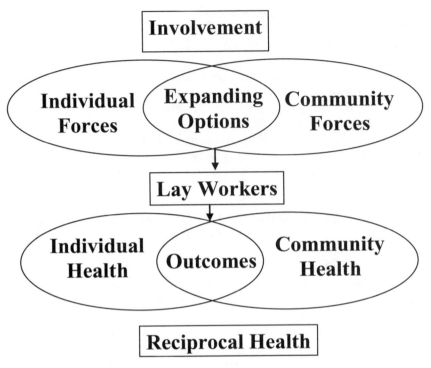

FIGURE 7.1   Community empowerment.

the model include (1) seek information, (2) seek support, (3) establish a work group to determine a plan and goals, (4) determine tasks, deadlines, and person responsible, (5) determine interim and start-up dates, (6) nurture the new program, (7) measure goals accomplished, and (8) keep community informed of progress. Needs identified in the study clustered around health and nutrition, roles and status, economic resources, and community amenities. Once the needs were identified, the community prioritized them and chose programs in partnership with the researcher. Four programs were developed and implemented. They included a health education and screening program to provide diabetes and hypertension screening and health education to the elderly community members; a literacy program with a library story hour run by older adults for the young to demonstrate new roles for the elderly through intergenerational helping behaviors; a food gardening program to address the move away from traditional food growing patterns experienced by the urban poor when they left their rural settings; and a nutrition education program to give community homemakers needed information about nutritionally sound, low-cost foods. Outcomes indicated lay workers and health care personnel could effectively respond to basic human needs of all age groups in the community. There was a considerable investment of time and resources to introduce community involvement, and it was appropriate to empower lay people in the promotion of community health.

We will describe an example of a randomized clinical trial based on the community empowerment theory that focuses on rural community empowerment to change perinatal outcomes and costs. The purpose of the study would be to compare maternal and infant outcomes and cost of care between two groups of rural women. The control group would receive routine prenatal care and the intervention group would receive care based on the community empowerment middle range theory. The intervention would be introduced in two stages. In the first stage (years 1–2½) Resource Mothers would serve as lay workers providing services to pregnant women. In the second stage (years 2½–4½), a Community Mentoring Board would be added to the Resource Mother intervention. Both the control and the intervention groups in both stages would be composed of rural pregnant women who seek care at a rural health site. Resource Mothers would visit women in their homes monthly throughout pregnancy and the first 6 months of the infant's life. In the second stage of implementation, Resource Mother services would be guided by a Community Mentoring Board that would partner with health care providers to assure that individual and community needs are met. Strategies would be shared across sites through quarterly meetings so that lay workers can learn from each other. Process evaluation would analyze the type of services provided by Resource Mothers in the first stage and analyze the level of involvement of the community in the program in the second stage. The proposition to be addressed in the study would be that involvement of lay workers (Resource Mothers) would lead to reciprocal health (improved maternal and infant outcomes, strengthened Resource Mothers and Community Mentoring Board), thus leading to community empowerment.

Specific questions that would be answered in each stage of this study include:

1. What are the effects of an intervention guided by community empowerment theory on

   a. *Maternal Outcomes:* Adequacy of prenatal care (month of prenatal care registration, gestational age, and number of prenatal care visits), changes in risk behaviors (smoking, nutritional status), incidence of preterm delivery, attendance at follow-up postpartum/family planning visits, maternal affect (anxiety, hostility, and depression), satisfaction with prenatal care, repeat pregnancies at 6 months after delivery,

b. *Infant Outcomes:* Gestational age, infant birth weight, well-child checkups, immunization status, health status at 6 months of age,

c. *Cost of Care:* Hospitalization (maternal and infant), prenatal/postnatal and infant care services, Resource Mothers program costs (intervention group)?

2. What are the major issues addressed during Resource Mothers' contacts with pregnant women?
3. What is the level of community and health professional involvement and responsibility in the Resource Mothers program over time?
4. Does the perceived level of empowerment among Resource Mothers and Community Mentoring Board members change over time?

The Community Mentoring Board (introduced in stage 2 of the intervention) would guide the transfer of knowledge and information from health care professionals to lay women workers from the community (Resource Mothers), who, in turn, would teach and support pregnant women who are at risk for reasons that include education deficits, poverty, race, gender or social bias, or living in deprived environments. Health professionals would work with the Community Mentoring Board and the Resource Mothers to implement interventions for improving individual and community health outcomes. Resource Mothers involve the entire family in the interventions through home visiting and are viewed as providers at the intersection of traditional health care and individual/community forces. As a critical interface between health-promoting forces, Resource Mothers offer the possibility for managing barriers to obtaining health care. Interventions carried out by the Resource Mothers are targeted to individual problems with the intention of effecting intermediate and long-term health outcomes guided by the Community Mentoring Board and health care providers. Study outcomes would provide important data about lay worker effects on perinatal outcomes, cost, major issues addressed, and interventions used by lay workers.

USE OF THE THEORY IN NURSING PRACTICE

There are many opportunities for use of the middle range theory of community empowerment in nursing practice. For example, this theory has been used to drive the development of school health programs in rural West Virginia. Through the West Virginia Rural Health Education Partnerships (WVRHEP) program, West Virginia health science students from the disciplines of nursing, medicine, pharmacy, dentistry, and allied health rotate in rural areas of the state (divided geographically into consortia) gaining valuable experience in rural clinical care. A major component of this program is the integration of service learning opportunities in rural communities. Each consortium is governed by a board of directors made up of community members and health care providers. In one consortium of the WVRHEP program, the board of directors and students have been engaged with several rural communities—systematically working with those communities to perform detailed community assessments, presenting those assessments to key stakeholders in the community, and subsequently working along with community members to plan and implement projects based on identified community needs, with the full support and inclusion of community stakeholders.

The purpose of these activities is to involve the community in identifying needs by getting the community involved through meetings with key informants, surveys of community members, and analysis of community-level data. Consistently identified needs include healthy lifestyle programs for children, nutrition education, exercise opportunities, and obesity prevention. In the spring of 2006, WVRHEP students from the disciplines of nursing, medicine, and pharmacy spent the semester working with local schools to develop a school-specific ideal healthy lifestyle program, considering the realities of the school and the community. The WVRHEP students spent the spring semester researching current obesity intervention/prevention programs; working with school personnel to ascertain school successes, limitations, and barriers for program planning and implementation; and surveying parents and children to determine their preferences for intervention programs.

The programs the WVRHEP students designed with the school communities during the spring were implemented in the fall. The 5-2-1-0 program was implemented at two elementary schools in one rural county. 5-2-1-0 stands for 5 fruits and vegetables a day, 2 hours or less of screen time, 1 hour or more of physical activity, and 0 or no soda pop or sugar-sweetened beverages per day. With full support from the school principal and school staff, this program involved the presentation of a curriculum based around the *My Pyramid for Kids* (U.S. Department of Agriculture, 2006) program. After a program presentation, children were given a 5-2-1-0 log book where they were asked to chart their progress over a month. Each day the children were asked to chart whether they met their 5-2-1-0 goal for that day. Fifty-one percent of the children returned logs and were given a jump-rope for their effort.

An after-school physical activity and nutrition program at another elementary school provided the children with a brief 10-minute nutrition lesson, rotation through a variety of different physical activity stations, and a healthy snack before they went home. Since transportation is an issue when any type of program takes place after school, 35 children who walked to school in second through fifth grades were invited to participate in this program. All 35 returned permission slips for participation. During the 6-week after-school program, the number of elementary students attending never dropped below 30.

Key components of the middle range theory of community empowerment were used to plan and implement these programs. Involvement is linking a group of community people to identify their common ground of needs, resources, and barriers, and to build support or coalitions to mount a response to a problem through planning, implementing, and maintaining interventions. Health care professionals, and in this case, health sciences students, facilitated involvement when they shared information and control with community residents by teaching and supporting consumers in identifying and participating in the management of health problems for self, family, and community. The answer to community health problems does in fact lie in communities. By including the community in designing programs that meet the needs of the community, a high degree of success can be realized in developing strategies that work. Lay workers in these exemplars, while not specifically designated as such, include the consortium community board members, the indigenous middle and high school students, and the school personnel who supported the programs in many ways.

Reciprocal health is promoted when professionals and community residents work together, respecting and sharing what each has to offer, and thereby magnifying the potential for participants to manage their own health (WHO, 1991a, 1991b). Actualizing these opportunities means increased community competence. The community is empowered to move to a new level of accomplishment.

CONCLUSION

The community empowerment middle range theory highlights theory, practice, and research links to develop more effective nursing interventions. It is adapted from Hildebrandt's Community Involvement in Health Empowerment model that was designed and successfully pilot-tested in primary health care research with a vulnerable Black population in South Africa and is the basis for research with vulnerable populations in the United States (Hildebrandt, 1994). Both the original conceptual model and the middle range theory incorporate the components of community empowerment and citizen participation that are central to Flynn's Healthy Cities work (Flynn et al., 1992, 1994). The community empowerment theory structures community participation with lay workers to promote reciprocal health. The theory's potential lies in its dual approach of reducing the effect of limited access and limited health care resources in caring for vulnerable populations and using unique, nontraditional ways to promote health. Application of the theory in practice provides opportunities to maximize the potential of a community through achievements of outcomes related to the health of individuals and groups. Research questions derived from the theory will structure studies to examine relationships among the concepts that will lead to refinement of the theory.

REFERENCES

American Public Health Association. (1991). *Healthy communities 2000: Model standards for community attainment of the year 2000 national health objectives.* Washington, DC: Author.

Blondel, B., & Breart, G. (1995). Home visits during pregnancy: Consequences on pregnancy outcome, use of health services and women's situations. *Seminars in Gerontology, 19,* 263–271.

Chino, M., & DeBruyn, L. (2006). Building true capacity: Indigenous models for indigenous communities. *American Journal of Public Health, 96,* 596–599.

Clifford, P. (1992). The myth of empowerment. *Nursing Administration Quarterly, 16,* 1–5.

Ellis-Stoll, C., & Popkess-Vawter, S. (1998). A concept analysis on the process of empowerment. *Advances in Nursing Science, 21,* 62–68.

Facet, S., Paine-Andrews, A., Francisco, V., & Schultz, J. (1995). Using empowerment theory in collaborative partnerships for community health and development. *American Journal of Community Psychology, 23,* 677.

Farley, S. (1993). The community as partner in primary health care. *Nursing and Health Care, 14,* 244–249.

Fiske, G., Hill, A., Krouskos, D., Legged, D., & Seagull, O. (1989). The community development in health project. *Community Health Studies, 8,* 93–99.

Flynn, B., Ray, D., & Rider, M. (1994). Empowering communities: Action research through healthy cities. *Health Education Quarterly, 21,* 395–405.

Flynn, B., Rider, M., & Bailey, W. (1992). Developing community leadership in healthy cities: The Indiana model. *Nursing Outlook, 40,* 121–126.

Hildebrandt, E. (1994). A model for community involvement in health (CIH) program development. *Social Science Medicine, 39,* 247–254.

Hildebrandt, E. (1996). Building community participation in health care: A model and example from South Africa. *Image, 28,* 155–159.

Hildebrandt, E. (2002). The health effects of work-based welfare. *Journal of Nursing Scholarship, 34*(4), 363–368.

Israel, B., Checkoway, B., Schulz, A., & Zimmerman, M. (1994). Health education and community empowerment: Conceptualizing and measuring perceptions of individual, organizational and community control. *Health Education Quarterly, 2,* 149–170.

Israel, B., Schulz, A., Parker, E., & Becker, A. (2001). Community based participatory research: Policy recommendations for promoting a partnership approach in health research. *Education for Health, 14,* 182–197.

Julnes, G., Konefal, M., Pindur, W., & Kim, P. (1994). Community based perinatal care for disadvantaged adolescents: Evaluation of the resource mothers program. *Journal of Community Health, 19*, 41–53.

Krothe, J., Flynn, B., Ray, D., & Goodwin, S. (2000). Community development through faculty practice in a rural nurse managed clinic. *Public Health Nursing, 17*, 264–272.

LaPierre, J., Perreault, M., & Goulet, C. (1995). Prenatal peer counseling: An answer to the persistent difficulties with prenatal care for low income women. *Public Health Nursing, 12*, 53–60.

Mahon, J., McFarlane, J., & Golden, K. (1991). Demadresamadres: A community partnership for health. *Public Health Nursing, 8*, 15–19.

McElmurry, B. J., Park, C. G., & Buseh, A. G. (2003). Health policy and systems. The nurse-community health advocate team for urban immigrant primary health care. *Journal of Nursing Scholarship, 35*, 275–281.

McElmurry, B. J., Tyska, C., Gugenheim, A. M., Misner, S., & Poslusny, S. (1995). Leadership for primary health care. *Nursing and Health Care: Perspectives on Community, 16*, 229–233.

McFarlane, J., & Wriist, W. (1997). Preventing abuse to pregnant women: Implementation of a mentor mother advocacy model. *Journal of Community Health Nursing, 14*, 237–249.

Olds, D., Eckenrode, J., Henderson, C., Kitzman, H., Powers, J., Cole, R., et al., (1997). Long term effects of home visitation on maternal life course and child abuse and neglect. *Journal of the American Medical Association, 278*, 637–643.

Pender, N. J., Murdaugh, C. L., & Parsons, M. A. (2002). *Health promotion in nursing practice.* Upper Saddle River, NJ: Prentice Hall.

Persily, C. (1995). Helpseeking in high risk pregnancy: The role of the CNS. *CNS: The Journal of Advanced Practice, 9*, 207–220.

Rafael, A. (1995). Advocacy and empowerment: Dichotomous or synchronous concepts? *Advances in Nursing Science, 18*, 25–32.

Rogers, M., Peoples-Sheps, M., & Sorenson, J. (1995). Translating research into MCH service: Comparison of a pilot project and a large-scale resource mothers program. *Public Health Reports, 110*, 563–569.

Rogers, M., Peoples-Sheps, M., & Suchindran, C. (1996). Impact of a social support program on teenage prenatal care use and pregnancy outcomes. *Journal of Adolescent Health, 19*, 132–140.

Swider, S. M., & McElmurry, B. (1990). A women's health perspective in primary health care: A nursing and community health worker demonstration project in urban America. *Family and Community Health, 13*, 1–17.

United States Department of Agriculture. (2006). Retrieved October 10, 2006, from http://www.mypyramid.gov/kids/index.html

United States Department of Health and Human Services. (2000). *Healthy people 2010* (conference edition, in two volumes). Washington, DC: Author.

World Health Organization. (1978). Declaration of Alma-Ata. *WorldHealth*, 28–29.

World Health Organization. (1991a). *Environmental health in urban development.* Technical Report Series, No. 807. Geneva: Author.

World Health Organization. (1991b). *Community involvement in health development: Challenging health services.* Technical Report Series, No. 809. Geneva: Author.

Zakus, J. (1998). Resource dependency and community participation in primary health care. *Social Science & Medicine, 46*, 475–494.

Zotti, M., & Zahner, S. (1995). Evaluation of public health nursing home visits to pregnant women on WIC. *Public Health Nursing, 12*, 294–304.

CHAPTER 8

Theory of Symptom Management

Janice Humphreys, Kathryn A. Lee, Virginia Carrieri-Kohlman, Kathleen Puntillo, Julia Faucett, Susan Janson, Bradley Aouizerat, DorAnne Donesky-Cuenco, and the UCSF School of Nursing Symptom Management Faculty Group

A symptom is defined as a subjective experience reflecting changes in the biopsychosocial functioning, sensations, or cognition of an individual. In contrast, a sign is defined as any abnormality indicative of disease that is detectable by the individual or others (Dodd, Janson et al., 2001). Signs and symptoms are important aspects of health and illness that disrupt physical, mental, and social functioning. An acute or unrelenting symptom is often what brings the patient into the health care system, particularly after self-care management strategies have failed. The presence of a symptom or cluster of symptoms may be the first indication to the patient or provider of a developing illness. Symptoms can also be brought on by prescribed pharmacologic or medical therapy. Whether the goal is to eliminate the symptom or to minimize the distress of the symptom experience, the theory of symptom management provides useful information. The middle range theory serves to guide symptom assessment and treatment in nursing practice and questions and hypotheses for nursing research.

PURPOSE OF THE THEORY AND
HOW IT WAS DEVELOPED

The faculty at the University of California, San Francisco (UCSF) School of Nursing first introduced the symptom management model in 1994 (Larson et al., 1994). That original model provided a framework to allow faculty involved in symptom research and clinical practice to improve collaboration and to move forward in a more organized way of thinking about the symptom experience, management strategies, and outcomes of symptom management. The conceptualization at that time was based upon models that had been developed by nurses such as Orem's self-care model (1971, 1980, 1985) and Sorofman, Tripp-Reimer, Lauer, and Martin's (1990) model of symptoms of self-care, as well as related models from anthropology, sociology, and psychology. UCSF faculty concluded that none of these frameworks adequately addressed the patient's role in self-care *and* the "patient's experience, his or her tested management strategies, or the desired outcomes" (Larson et al., 1994, p. 273). With further testing of the model and its components and ongoing discussion among UCSF faculty and students, the UCSF symptom management model was revised in 2001 (Dodd, Janson et al., 2001). Selected published research studies were used to build an evidence-based foundation and to compare and contrast the concepts across symptoms. With this revision the concept labels and nature of the relationships among the concepts was slightly altered. In addition, the influence of person, environment, and health and illness domains was made explicit by situating the entire model within these spheres. With this chapter we have further revised our thinking and now propose the symptom management theory (SMT). As depicted in Figure 8.1, the three components of symptom experience, management strategies, and outcomes continue to form the conceptual basis of the SMT for research and practice. The SMT addresses specific phenomena but does not necessarily limit application to one narrow group. The SMT also proposes explicit and testable relationships among the three concepts, provides a structure for understanding the connections among these concepts, and provides a framework for considering interventions and outcomes. As will be shown later in this chapter, the SMT provides a strong basis for research and has also begun to inform practice as well as education in nursing.

CONCEPTS OF THE THEORY

The three essential concepts of the symptom management theory are symptom experience, symptom management strategies, and symptom status outcomes. The concepts are framed within the dimensions of nursing science (person, environment, and heath/illness) to serve as a reminder of the contextual considerations for nursing research. For instance, a woman's symptom experience will vary by age and reproductive status as well as by her genetic risk factors (person dimension), her cultural beliefs about the meaning of a symptom or whether she is assessed in the laboratory, clinic, home, or job (environmental dimension), and her current state of health or diagnosis (health and illness dimension).

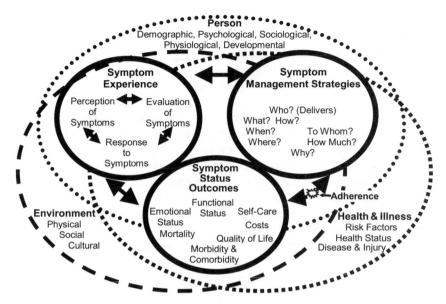

FIGURE 8.1   Symptom management.

Note: Reprinted with permission from: Dodd, M., Janson, S., Facione, N., Faucett, J., Froelicher, E. S., Humphreys, J., Lee, K., Miaskowski, C., Puntillo, K., Rankin, S., & Taylor, D. (2001). Advancing the science of symptom management. *Journal of Advanced Nursing, 33,* 668–676.

Symptom experience is a simultaneous perception, evaluation, and response to a change in one's usual feeling. For example, a woman may suddenly feel hot and diaphoretic. In order to cool her body temperature down to relieve the symptom, she can either remove some clothing or begin to fan herself. This symptom perception and response differs depending on whether it occurs during an important meeting or during the night while asleep. If it continues with sufficient frequency and severity over time and is perceived as distressing and interfering with her life, her response is likely to include seeking help and more effective strategies to eliminate or minimize the symptom. The authors of the "Theory of Unpleasant Symptoms" (Lenz, Pugh, Milligan, Gift, & Suppe, 1997) acknowledge that the symptom experience may include not just one but several synergistic symptoms. Some of the investigators who developed the SMT have explored this phenomenon by studying individuals who experience clusters of symptoms (Dodd, Miaskowski, & Lee, 2004; Dodd, Miaskowski, & Paul, 2001; Voss, Portillo, Holzemer, & Dodd, 2007).

Symptom management strategies are efforts to avert, delay, or minimize the symptom experience. The strategy can be effective in three ways: (1) reducing the frequency of the symptom experience, (2) minimizing the severity of the symptom, or (3) relieving the distress associated with the symptom (Portenoy et al., 1994). A framework for the study and development of management strategies includes the specifications of who, how, where, and when, and what the intervention strategy entails.

Increasing attention is being given to self-management strategies used by patients (Bodenheimer, Lorig, Holman, & Grumbach, 2002). An outcome of this effort is to shift more of the responsibility of managing symptoms to the individual. Patients essentially become their own primary caregivers and manage their symptoms themselves on a day-to-day basis. Where an intervention strategy is tested or used, such as in the laboratory or in the home, can impact or modulate the symptom. The "what" is viewed as the strategy itself; one strategy might be a medical therapy that also needs provider input while another may involve a complementary therapy or relaxation technique that the patient or family can carry out on a daily basis. Yet another may involve alteration of the hospital room, home, or work environment. Patients and providers may also attempt more than one strategy and use a combination of interventions that have a greater effect on the symptom or cluster of symptoms. Tailoring the management strategy to the person or the family has been shown to be important in bringing about behavior change (Committee on Quality of Health Care in America, 2001) as well as symptom reduction.

The dose (i.e., how much) and the timing (i.e., when) aspects of interventions or strategies are also important to modulate symptoms in nursing practice and research. The dose of a strategy is an important consideration, particularly when implementing a behavioral intervention. Dose could include actual time spent exercising, number of times a stress reduction session was attended, or amount of educational material provided. The dose of time spent by the health care provider or family member administering the intervention is also critical to consider in terms of how much time and support is actually provided to the person experiencing the symptom. One example of dose in terms of environmental management may be the degree of job or disability accommodation that a workplace provides.

Symptom status outcomes are clear and measurable outcomes to assess following the implementation of a strategy. Outcomes include the obvious change in symptom status, whereby the symptom is less frequent, less intense, or less distressing. This improvement in symptoms can lead to better physical and mental functioning, improved quality of life, shorter hospital stay, quicker return to work, and less cost to the individual, family, health care system, or employer.

RELATIONSHIPS AMONG THE CONCEPTS: THE MODEL

The SMT has three major concepts. The concepts are: symptom experience, symptom management strategies, and symptom status outcomes. The bidirectional arrows within the model of SMT are meant to indicate a simultaneous interaction among all three concepts. The symptom experience is conceptualized as influencing and being influenced by both symptom management strategies and symptoms status outcomes. As individuals become aware of symptoms, initiate strategies, and assess symptom outcomes, their symptom perception is affected. This interaction can take place in a matter of moments as is often the case in common symptom self-care management (e.g., minor colds, rashes, stomach upset, etc.). However, when symptoms are more pronounced and/or distressing, other sources of symptom management strategies may be sought and symptom status outcomes may be assessed in a more formal fashion. This iterative process continues until symptoms resolve and/or are stabilized. However, the process of managing symptoms goes amiss when adherence (i.e., whether the intended recipient of the strategy actually receives or uses the strategy prescribed) becomes a problem. This breakdown is illustrated by the broken arrow between the symptom management strategies and symptoms status outcomes components of the SMT. Within the SMT, nonadherence occurs when interventions are too demanding, are not applied, or are applied inconsistently. In addition, factors situated in the person, environment, and health and illness domains may contribute to nonadherence in managing symptoms.

USE OF THE THEORY IN NURSING RESEARCH

The SMT has evolved as more research studies have contributed to the understanding and development of relationships among the three concepts of the theory. Likewise, the study of symptom experiences and responses, both with individual and clusters of symptoms, has continued to flourish using the SMT as a conceptual guide. The work of Carrieri, Janson-Bjerklie, and colleagues provides an illustration of the systematic development of knowledge for clinical practice that has been possible with the SMT. Their initial research sought to explore patient symptom experience and responses to dyspnea (Carrieri & Janson-Bjerklie, 1986; Carrieri, Kieckhefer, Janson-Bjerklie, & Souza, 1990; Janson-Bjerklie & Carrieri, 1986; Janson-Bjerklie, Ferketich, Benner, & Becker, 1992). Their research uncovered the diverse symptom experience of individuals as well as the variety of terms patients used to describe their experience. Subsequent testing of the effect of management strategies on symptom experience as well as other multivariate outcomes, such as exercise performance, depression, self-efficacy for managing dyspnea, health-related quality of life, and health care utilization (Carrieri-Kohlman et al., 2005; Davis, Carrieri-Kohlman, Janson, Gold, & Stulbarg, 2006; Nguyen & Carrieri-Kohlman, 2005) has provided an understanding of how patients manage their symptoms and how those symptoms and their management affect functional status.

Similarly, application of this research trajectory to asthma revealed the distinct role of symptoms in monitoring asthma control. Increasing chronic asthma symptoms or the sudden onset of acute symptoms signals the loss of asthma control and requires actions to preserve life, yet many adults delay seeking urgent medical care when asthma worsens (Janson & Becker, 1998). Interventions designed to increase self-management skills for responding to acute episodes and controlling chronic asthma produced improved adherence to anti-inflammatory therapy and improved control of asthma (Janson, Fahy, Covington, Gold, & Boushey, 2003).

The SMT has seen increasing use since the 2001 revision. A search of both research and practice-focused literature from 2002–2006 produced 35 publications that explicitly address the theory, four additional citations were located through Web searches and professional contacts. Among these documents, 20 reported on research that used the theory as the conceptual basis. Two documents discussed the model as part of a focused review of the literature (Holzemer, 2002; Portillo, Holzemer, & Chou, 2007).

Two other articles used it as part of a theoretical synthesis (Henly, Kallas, Klatt, & Swenson, 2003; Maag, Buccheri, Capella, & Jennings, 2006) or in a comparison with another framework to determine which provided the best framework for future research (Voss, Dodd, Portillo, & Holzemer, 2006). In addition, three grants funded by NIH were found that explicitly use the SMT (Aouizerat, 2006; Lee, 2004, 2006).

Research Studies Using the SMT

Research has varied in the extent of use of the SMT as a conceptual basis, and no study has sought to actually test the entire theory. However, the research findings are remarkably similar and supportive of the theory across diverse study populations. In particular, the patients' varied symptom experiences, diverse management strategies, and the influence of person, environment, and health and illness domains were confirmed in every study where they were included.

The symptom experience dimension has been the most often studied. Heilemann, Coffey-Love, and Frutos (2004) used qualitative and quantitative methods to explore the symptom experience of 107 women of Mexican descent with a history of depression. They explored women's perceptions of the causation of their depression and found that half were related to problems with relationships. They concluded that health care providers must explore women's perceptions of the cause of their symptoms if they are to develop meaningful strategies.

Battered women's symptom experience was explored in two descriptive, correlational studies (Humphreys, 2003; Humphreys & Lee, 2005). In the first, abused women's symptom severity and intensity was found to be correlated with the severity and frequency of intimate partner violence. In the second study, Humphreys and Lee (2005) noted that the majority of abused women in transitional housing programs suffered from disturbed sleep. They concluded that further study of context-specific symptom management strategies was needed to improve sleep.

Aouizerat is working in collaboration with Dodd, Lee, and Miaskowski to identify genetic predictors of symptoms (e.g., sleep disturbance, fatigue, pain) that play a role in interindividual variation in symptom levels that are either disease-specific (e.g., HIV disease) or general determinants of symptoms that operate across chronic diseases (Aouizerat, 2006; Lee, 2004, 2006; Miaskowski, Aouizerat, Dodd, & Cooper, in press; Miaskowski et al., 2006). The role of genetics in human disease occupies the person domain of the SMT. However, Aouizerat is quick to note that genetics can occupy both the environment and health and illness domains as well.

The sensation of bronchoconstriction experienced by people with asthma from different ethnic groups was studied by Hardie, Janson, Gold, Carrieri-Kohlman, and Boushey (2000). They identified ethnic differences in the symptoms and sensations experienced and reported by African Americans as compared to Whites. The verbal descriptions were distinctly different between these two ethnic groups at the same level of induced bronchoconstriction.

Several other studies have examined symptom experiences in diverse populations and symptom management strategies. Most often these studies also consider the influence of person, environment, and health and illness domains on key variables. Tsai, Hsiung, and Holzemer (2002) studied 134 HIV+ patients and 31 health care providers to determine the degree to which research results in the United States were applicable in Taiwan. Their findings confirmed that persons with HIV/AIDS report a variety of symptoms using a range of terms. They also note that similar to other studies in the United States, providers have limited knowledge about actual patient self-care strategies, and patients acquire knowledge from diverse sources. They conclude that symptom management strategies are an under-explored issue.

Hudson, Taylor, Lee, and Gilliss (2005) drew a similar conclusion in their study of the symptom experience of 87 community-based African American midlife women. They found that participants were more likely to use passive rather than active management strategies and that these findings were likely due to ethnic differences in the samples. However, they also concluded that providers must inquire about these strategies to make sure that women know about strategies that have been shown to be most beneficial.

Coleman and colleagues (2006) explored the relationship between symptom experience and the use of prayer as a management strategy in a community-based sample of HIV+ African Americans ($N = 448$). They found that prayer was used by the majority of participants as a way of managing fatigue, nausea, and depression and that while there were gender-based differences in its use, 50% rated prayer as highly efficacious.

Three studies focused solely on the symptom management strategies dimension (Chou, Holzemer, Portillo, & Slaughter, 2004; Kirksey et al., 2002; Nicholas et al., 2002). Their findings, along with those of Faucett, Meyers, Tejeda et al. (2001), also documented that patients used a variety of approaches to manage their symptoms and that those approaches often included complementary therapies. The totality of research on symptom management provides strong evidence that providers need to foster open communication with patients if they are to learn patients' self-care strategies and to increase the likelihood that patients are aware of approaches that have been shown to be most beneficial.

Three studies examined the relationship between symptom experience and outcomes in HIV+ individuals (Hudson, Kirksey, & Holzemer, 2004; Rivero-Méndez, Holzemer, Portillo, Solís-Báez, & Wantland, in review; Voss, 2005). Once again, patients reported a variety of symptoms that were associated with varied outcomes affecting patients' lives. However, all noted that person, environment, and health/illness domains were highly influential. Hudson and colleagues (2004) also suggest that functional status as a symptom status outcome may fail to capture the full range of role impairment that some HIV+ individuals experience. They suggest that the symptoms status dimension within the model might be expanded to include role strain, enhancement, limitations, and satisfaction. Faucett and colleagues also suggest that workplace changes may significantly alter employees' symptom experiences and subsequently their work performance (Faucett, Meyers, Miles, Janowitz, & Fathallah, et al., 2007; Meyers et al., 2001).

Six studies include measures of the three dimensions: symptom experience, symptom management strategies, and symptom status outcomes (Eller et al., 2005; Fuller, Welch, Backer, & Rawl, 2005; Hearson,

2006; Janson et al., 2003; Tsai, Holzemer, & Leu, 2005). Hearson is currently using the SMT to study sleep disturbances in family caregivers of terminally ill persons with advanced stage cancer in the home. While Eller and colleagues studied 34 HIV+ individuals with depressive symptoms and Fuller's research team studied constipation in women with a history of pelvic floor disorders, their findings are remarkably similar. Both studies again noted that patients' symptom experience was much broader than that previously reported in the literature and that patients used a variety of strategies acquired from varied sources to attempt to manage their symptoms. However, they also found that many patient self-care strategies were of questionable effectiveness. Thus, patients' lives continued to be affected by their ongoing and poorly managed symptoms. Eller and colleagues note that only 28% of the strategies reported by patients were suggested by providers and that 31% of the strategies were found by patients through trial and error.

In the attempt to improve HIV+ Taiwanese patients' symptom management, Tsai, Holzemer, and Leu (2005) prepared a manual that provided symptom management information. In a pretest–posttest single group study they noted that symptom intensity diminished with the use of the manual; however, quality of life did not improve. The authors conclude that information about how to manage symptoms alone is not enough to improve symptom status outcomes.

An intriguing area of interest is the study of symptom clusters. While the original SMT focused on how a single symptom can be studied, the symptom experience is likely to involve more than one symptom. Dodd and colleagues (2004) define symptom clusters as two or more symptoms that are both related to one another and occur concurrently. Commonly occurring clusters are symptoms like nausea, vomiting and poor appetite, or pain, depression, and disturbed sleep. There is only limited research that addresses symptom clusters (Dodd, Miaskowski et al., 2001; Voss, Portillo, Holzemer, & Dodd, 2007) and there are considerable methodological issues that must be resolved (Miaskowski, 2006). However, the concept of a symptom cluster is consistent with the SMT. Miaskowski (2006) suggests that research into symptom clusters may provide new insights into the underlying mechanisms. "If common biological mechanisms are found for specific symptom clusters, this knowledge may lead to the development of novel symptoms management strategies" (p. 793). In asthma, symptom clusters occur commonly: chest tightness, shortness of breath, wheeze, and cough often occur together when asthma flares. These symptoms have been measured together on separate visual analog or numerical rating scales (Janson et al., 2003; Janson, Hardie, Fahy, & Boushey, 2001; Janson-Bjerklie & Shnell, 1988).

USE OF THE THEORY IN NURSING PRACTICE

Reports of the use of the SMT in practice are found less frequently in the literature. Jablonski and Wyatt (2005) applied the model to end-of-life care as a means of expanding understanding of the needs of dying patients and environmental barriers that prevent them from getting necessary care. Ahlberg (2005) used the SMT to illustrate a framework for dealing with cancer-related fatigue. Finally, Maag, Buccheri, Capella, and Jennings (2006) synthesized the SMT with other theories to form a conceptual framework for a clinical nurse leader education program. They include the theory to assure that the clinical nurse leader graduate will effectively evaluate patient symptoms, develop and implement management intervention strategies, thus achieving optimal outcomes.

CONCLUSION

The body of knowledge acquired from research using the SMT is growing. Across multiple studies with diverse samples and methods, the results are remarkably similar. Patients experience a wide range of symptoms and use a variety of terms and phrases to describe these sensations. They largely attempt to manage these symptoms themselves using strategies that have evidence-based support as well as those of questionable value. Providers are seen as an important source for information about symptoms, but so are family, friends, employers, and the media. There is clear evidence that providers must establish and maintain good patient–provider communication if they are to understand the patients' symptom perception, accept symptom experience and implement management strategies. It is also essential for providers to consider the strengths and limitations imposed upon patients within the person, environment, and health and illness dimensions. When symptoms are not adequately addressed, patients continue to suffer reduced quality of life and altered functional status.

However, the SMT may also be in need of reconsideration and possible revision. The temporal dimension of time is largely missing from the model. This is increasingly apparent as more sophisticated studies use longitudinal designs. The need to consider changes in symptoms over time is also important to understand patient adherence to prescribed strategies and to determine what and when management strategies are best received and most beneficial. Henley, Kallas, Klatt, and Swenson (2003) have attempted to address this limitation by synthesizing a new theory that includes four temporal dimensions of symptoms. However, in so doing they have created a far more linear framework that fails to consider the multidimensional nature of symptoms. However, their efforts may provide some insight into future versions of the SMT.

Donesky-Cuenco has also noted that adherence, currently situated in the SMT between symptom management strategies and symptom status outcomes, may need reconsideration. In research with patients with chronic obstructive pulmonary disease, Donesky-Cuenco and Carrieri-Kohlman have found a bidirectional relationship between adherence and all three concepts of the symptom management theory as well as the person, environment, and health/illness dimensions of nursing science (Donesky-Cuenco, Janson, Neuhaus, Nielands, & Carrieri-Kohlman, 2007). For example, a person who is less short of breath (SOB) will walk more or a person who has cognitively restructured their experience of SOB will walk more; and walking more will decrease the SOB experience over the long-term. These researchers further note that not only does adherence influence the relationship between intervention and outcome, but the characteristics of the intervention will also influence adherence (for example, desirability of the intervention will influence whether a person adheres). They have concluded that placement of adherence solely at the intervention–outcome link may be too restrictive.

Ongoing discussion with UCSF faculty and trainees in our T32 Nurse Research Training in Symptom Management has noted that the model itself is somewhat difficult to see. It has often been suggested that the ideal figure would involve a holographic, 3-dimensional representation that depicts the three suspended concepts of symptom management theory within three revolving spheres representing the person, environment, and health/illness dimensions. Revision of the SMT to make it clearer and more parsimonious may also increase its usefulness to researchers and clinicians.

In the decade since the SMT was originally introduced, it has gained acceptance as a valuable theory for organizing research and clinical practice, especially in the symptom experience domain within the person, environment, and health/illness dimensions of nursing science. The management strategies domain of the theory provides guidance in evaluating self-management strategies in addition to clinician-prescribed strategies, and the symptom status outcomes domain underscores the importance of measuring the symptom as an outcome following an intervention as well as distinguishing other important outcomes related to the symptom experience. The SMT has brought together researchers and clinicians from diverse backgrounds and populations around the shared interest in managing symptoms, with the result that knowledge is expanding in the areas of symptom clusters and extrapolating knowledge gained in one symptom area to similarities of assessment, management, and evaluation strategies with other symptoms. Research related to the SMT supports its current value and encourages continuing efforts to refine the theory for ongoing research and application to clinical practice.

REFERENCES

Ahlberg, K. (2005). The symptom management model is used to illustrate a framework for dealing with cancer-related fatigue. In N. Kearney & A. Richardson (Eds.), *Nursing patients with cancer: Principles and practice* (pp. 657–674). London: Churchill Livingstone.

Aouizerat, B. E. (2006). *NIH roadmap for medical research* (KL2 RR024130). National Center for Research Resources.

Bodenheimer, T., Lorig, K., Holman, H., & Grumbach, K. (2002). Patient self-management of chronic disease in primary care. *JAMA, 288,* 2469–2475.

Carrieri, V. K., & Janson-Bjerklie, S. (1986). Strategies patients use to manage the symptom of dyspnea. *Western Journal of Nursing Research, 8,* 284–305.

Carrieri, V. K., Kieckhefer, G., Janson-Bjerklie, S., & Souza, J. (1990). The sensation of pulmonary dyspnea in school-age children. *Nursing Research, 40,* 81–85.

Carrieri-Kohlman, V., Nguyen, H. Q., Cuenco, D., Neuhaus, J., Demir-Deviren, S., & Stulbarg, M. S. (2005). Impact of brief or extended exercise training on the benefit of a dyspnea self-management program in COPD. *Journal of Cardiopulmonary Rehabilitation, 25,* 275–284.

Chou, F. Y., Holzemer, W. L., Portillo, C. J., & Slaughter, R. (2004). Self-care strategies and sources of information for HIV/AIDS symptom management. *Nursing Research, 53,* 332–339.

Coleman, C. L., Holzemer, W. L., Eller, L. S., Corless, I., Reynolds, N., Nokes, K. M., et al. (2006). Gender differences in use of prayer as a self-care strategy for managing symptoms in African Americans living with HIV/AIDS. *The Journal of the Association of Nurses in AIDS Care, 17*(4), 16–23.

Committee on Quality of Health Care in America (2001). *Crossing the quality chasm.* Washington, DC: National Academy Press.

Davis, H. T., Carrieri-Kohlman, V., Janson, S. L., Gold, W. M., & Stulbarg, M. S. (2006). Effects of treatment on two types of self-efficacy in people with chronic obstructive pulmonary disease. *Journal of Pain and Symptom Management, 32,* 60–70.

Dodd, M., Janson, S., Facione, N., Faucett, J., Froelicher, E. S., Humphreys, J., et al. (2001). Advancing the science of symptom management. *Journal of Advanced Nursing, 33,* 668–676.

Dodd, M. J., Miaskowski, C., & Lee, K. A. (2004). Occurrence of symptom clusters. *Journal of the National Cancer Institute Monographs, 32,* 76–78.

Dodd, M. J., Miaskowski, C., & Paul, W. M. (2001). Symptom clusters and their effect on the functional status of patients with cancer. *Oncology Nursing Forum, 28,* 465–470.

Donesky-Cuenco, D., Janson, S., Neuhaus, J., Nielands, T., & Carrieri-Kohlman, V. (2007). Adherence to a home-walking prescription in patients with COPD. *Heart and Lung, 36*(5), 348–363.

Eller, L. S., Corless, I., Bunch, E. H., Kemppainen, J., Holzemer, W., Nokes, K., et al. (2005). Self-care strategies for depressive symptoms in people with HIV disease. *Journal of Advanced Nursing, 51*(2), 119–130.

Faucett, J., Meyers, J., Miles, J., Janowitz, I., & Fathallah, F. (2007). Rest break interventions in stoop labor tasks. *Applied Ergonomics, 38,* 219–226.

Faucett, J., Meyers, J., Tejeda, D., Janowitz, I., Miles, J., & Kabashima, J. (2001). An instrument to measure musculoskeletal symptoms among immigrant Hispanic farmworkers: Validation in the nursery industry. *Journal of Agricultural Safety & Health, 7*(3), 185–198.

Fuller, E., Welch, J. L., Backer, J. H., & Rawl, S. M. (2005). Symptom experience of chronically constipated women with pelvic floor disorders. *Clinical Nurse Specialist, 19,* 34–40.

Hardie, G., Janson, S. L., Gold, W., Carrieri-Kohlman, V., & Boushey, H. A. (2000). Ethnic differences. Word descriptors used by African American and White asthma patients during induced bronchoconstriction. *Chest, 117,* 935–943.

Hearson, B. (2006). Sleep disturbance in family caregivers: Application of the Revised Symptom Management Model. *Journal of Palliative Care, 22*(3), 216.

Heilemann, M. V., Coffey-Love, M., & Frutos, L. (2004). Perceived reasons for depression among low income women of Mexican descent. *Archives of Psychiatric Nursing, 18,* 185–192.

Henly, S. J., Kallas, K. D., Klatt, C. M., & Swenson, K. K. (2003). The notion of time in symptom experiences. *Nursing Research, 52,* 410–417.

Holzemer, W. L. (2002). HIV and AIDS: The symptom experience. *American Journal of Nursing, 102*(4), 48–52.

Hudson, A., Kirksey, K., & Holzemer, W. (2004). The influence of symptoms on quality of life among HIV-infected women. *Western Journal of Nursing Research, 26,* 9–23.

Hudson, A. L., Taylor, D., Lee, K. A., & Gilliss, C. L. (2005). Symptom experience and self-care strategies among healthy, midlife African-American women. *Journal of National Black Nurses Association, 16*(2), 6–14.

Humphreys, J. (2003). Resilience in sheltered battered women. *Issues in Mental Health Nursing, 24*(2), 137–152.

Humphreys, J., & Lee, K. A. (2005). Sleep disturbance in battered women living in transitional housing. *Issues in Mental Health Nursing, 25,* 771–780.

Jablonski, A., & Wyatt, G. K. (2005). A model for identifying barriers to effective symptom management at the end of life. *Journal of Hospice and Palliative Nursing, 7*(21), 23–36.

Janson, S. L., & Becker, G. (1998). Reasons for delay in seeking treatment for acute asthma. *Journal of Asthma, 35,* 427–435.

Janson, S. L., Fahy, J. V., Covington, J. K., Gold, W., & Boushey, H. A. (2003). Effects of individual self-management education on clinical, biological and adherence outcomes in asthma. *American Journal of Medicine, 115,* 620–626.

Janson, S. L., Hardie, G., Fahy, J. V., & Boushey, H. A. (2001). Use of biological markers of airway inflammation to detect the efficacy of nurse delivered asthma education. *Heart & Lung, 30,* 39–46.

Janson-Bjerklie, S., & Carrieri, V. K. (1986). The sensations of pulmonary dyspnea. *Nursing Research, 35,* 154–159.

Janson-Bjerklie, S. L., Ferketich, S., Benner, P., & Becker, G. (1992). Clinical markers of asthma severity and risk: Importance of subjective as well as objective factors. *Heart & Lung, 21,* 265–272.

Janson-Bjerklie, S., & Shnell, S. (1988). Effect of peak flow information on patterns of self-care in adult asthma. *Heart Lung, 17,* 543–549.

Kirksey, K. M., Goodroad, B. K., Kemppainen, J. K., Holzemer, W. L., Bunch, E. H., Corless, I. B., et al. (2002). Complementary therapy use in persons with HIV/AIDS. *Journal of Holistic Nursing, 20*(3), 264–278.

Larson, P. J., Carrieri-Kohlman, V., Dodd, M. J., Douglas, M., Faucett, J., Froelicher, E. S., et al. (1994). A model for symptom management. *Image: Journal of Nursing Scholarship, 26,* 272–276.

Lee, K. (2004). *Biomarkers of insomnia and fatigue in HIV/AIDS* (5 R01 MH074358-02). National Institute of Mental Health.

Lee, K. (2006). *Nursing research training in symptom management* (2 T32 NR07088-11). National Institute of Nursing Research.

Lenz, E. R., Pugh, L. C., Milligan, R. A., Gift, A., & Suppe, F. (1997). The middle-range theory of unpleasant symptoms: An update. *ANS. Advances in Nursing Science, 19*(3), 14–27.

Maag, M. M., Buccheri, R., Capella, E., & Jennings, D. L. (2006). A conceptual framework for the clinical nurse leader program. *Journal of Professional Nursing, 22,* 367–372.

Meyers, J., Miles, J., Faucett, J., Janowitz, I., Tejeda, D., Weber, E., et al. (2001). Priority risk factors for back injury in agricultural field work. *Journal of Agromedicine, 8*(1), 37–52.

Miaskowski, C. (2006). Symptom clusters: Establishing the link between clinical practice and symptom management research. *Supportive Care in Cancer, 14*(8), 792–794.

Miaskowski, C., Aouizerat, B. E., Dodd, M., & Cooper, B. (in press). Conceptual issues in symptom clusters research and their implications for quality of life assessment in patients with cancer. *Journal of the National Cancer Institute.*

Miaskowski, C., Cooper, B. A., Paul, S. M., Dodd, M., Lee, K., Aouizerat, B. E., et al. (2006). Subgroups of patients with cancer with different symptom experiences and quality-of-life outcomes: A cluster analysis. *Oncology Nursing Forum, 33*(5), E79–89.

Nguyen, H. Q., & Carrieri-Kohlman, V. (2005). Dyspnea self-management in patients with chronic obstructive pulmonary disease: Moderating effects of depressed mood. *Psychosomatics, 46,* 402–410.

Nicholas, P. K., Kemppainen, J. K., Holzemer, W. L., Nokes, K. M., Eller, L. S., Corless, I. B., et al. (2002). Self-care management for neuropathy in HIV disease. *AIDS Care, 14*(6), 763–771.

Orem, D. E. (1971). *Nursing: Concepts of practice.* New York: McGraw-Hill.

Orem, D. E. (1980). *Nursing: Concepts of practice* (2nd ed.). New York: McGraw-Hill.

Orem, D. E. (1985). *Nursing: Concepts of practice* (3rd ed.). New York: McGraw-Hill.

Portenoy, R. K., Thaler, H. T., Kornblith, A. B., McCarthy Lepore, J., Friedlander-Klar, H., Kiyasu, E., et al. (1994). The memorial symptom assessment scale: An instrument for the evaluation of symptom prevalence, characteristics and distress. *European Journal of Cancer, 30A,* 1326–1336.

Portillo, C. J., Holzemer, W. L., & Chou, F. (2007). HIV symptoms. *Annual Review of Nursing Research, 25,* 259–291.

Rivero-Méndez, M., Holzemer, W., Portillo, C., Solís-Báez, S. S., & Wantland, D. (in review). Symptom experience among men and women living with HIV/AIDS in Puerto Rico.

Sorofman, B., Tripp-Reimer, T., Lauer, G. M., & Martin, M. E. (1990). Symptom self-care. *Holistic Nursing Practice, 4*(2), 45–55.

Tsai, Y. F., Holzemer, W. L., & Leu, H. S. (2005). An evaluation of the effects of a manual on management of HIV/AIDS symptoms. *International Journal of STD & AIDS, 16*(9), 625–629.

Tsai, Y. F., Hsiung, P. C., & Holzemer, W. L. (2002). Symptom management in Taiwanese patients with HIV/AIDS. *Journal of Pain and Symptom Management, 23*(4), 301–309.

Voss, J. G. (2005). Predictors and correlates of fatigue in HIV/AIDS. *Journal of Pain and Symptom Management, 29*(2), 173–184.

Voss, J. G., Dodd, M., Portillo, C., & Holzemer, W. (2006). Theories of fatigue: Application in HIV/AIDS. *Journal of the Association of Nurses in AIDS Care, 17*(1), 37–50.

Voss, J. G., Portillo, C., Holzemer, W., & Dodd, M. (2007). Symptom cluster of fatigue and depression in HIV/AIDS. *Journal of Prevention & Intervention in the Community, 33*(1–2), 19–34.

CHAPTER 9

Theory of Unpleasant Symptoms

Elizabeth R. Lenz and Linda C. Pugh

Symptom management has become increasingly central to nursing practice and, correspondingly, an important focus of nursing science. As nurses assume more of the responsibility for managing the care of patients with both acute and chronic illnesses, their interest in symptom management has fueled additional research that will contribute to the knowledge base of health care. With the notable exception of the symptom management model developed, updated, and revised by faculty and students at the University of California, San Francisco (Dodd et al., 2001; Larson et al., 1994) and the recent work addressing symptom clusters (e.g., Barsevick, Whitmore, Nail, Beck, & Dudley, 2006) much of the theoretical work that has been carried out to elucidate the experience of symptoms and to guide their management has been symptom- or disease-specific. In this chapter we describe the middle range theory of unpleasant symptoms (TOUS): its components, the process by which it was developed, examples and theoretical implications of its application in the nursing literature, and plans for future development.

PURPOSE OF THE THEORY AND HOW IT WAS DEVELOPED

The theory of unpleasant symptoms (TOUS) was designed to integrate existing knowledge about a variety of symptoms. It was based on the premise that there are commonalities across different symptoms experienced by a variety of clinical populations in varied situations. A framework that highlights common elements and dimensions has potential to be useful in both nursing practice and research. The purpose of the theory is to improve understanding of the symptom experience in various contexts and to provide information useful for designing effective means to prevent, ameliorate, or manage unpleasant symptoms and their negative effects. Because it is more general than a theory describing or explaining a specific symptom, the TOUS lacks some of the detail that may be useful in working with a particular symptom in a given clinical population. On the other hand, by highlighting dimensions and considerations that are common to many symptoms, it encourages investigators and clinicians to think about aspects that are not readily apparent and to consider symptoms both alone and in combination. It is heuristic, providing an organizing schema and encouraging thought about the interplay among the many aspects of the symptom experience.

A model such as the TOUS provides a framework within which multiple researchers can work simultaneously, ultimately combining the results of their many programs of research. The TOUS provides common definitions and dimensions for examining symptoms, ultimately enhancing the probability that the results from multiple studies can be combined to produce convincing evidence upon which to base practice.

Because the symptom experience, by definition, occurs at the level of individual perception, the theory is applicable at the level of the individual. However, the TOUS does not consider the individual in isolation. Rather, it positions the individual within the context of his or her family, social and organizational networks, and community by taking into account situational factors in the environment that may influence the symptom experience. It also defines the outcome of the symptom experience in terms of performance, a notion that considers the impact of the symptom experience on the individual's interactions with others and his or her short- and long-term functioning.

The theory of unpleasant symptoms was developed by four nurse researchers who shared interest in the nature and experience of different symptoms (specifically fatigue and dyspnea) and in the processes of concept and theory development. These individuals (Audrey Gift, Renee Milligan, Linda Pugh, and Elizabeth Lenz) had collaborated in dyads or triads on various empirical studies and theoretical articles. They shared geographic proximity, which facilitated collaboration, and by virtue of their common association with one PhD program in nursing, they also shared exposure to the same philosophical and metatheoretical perspectives regarding the development and substance of nursing science. They had access to a philosopher of science colleague, Frederick Suppe, who played an important role in shaping their understanding of middle range theory and who assisted in the theory development process.

This is a theory that was developed inductively from the specific to the general and from concrete observations to theoretical ideas. That is, it had its beginnings at the relatively narrow scope of a single symptom and in the concrete world of practice. Three of the theory's developers had conducted dissertation research regarding a specific symptom: Gift studied dyspnea, and Milligan and Pugh studied fatigue. At the time their initial studies about individual symptoms were carried out, they had no intention of developing a theory. The opportunity to do so evolved over time as they began to realize that their work on individual symptoms represented concept development activity. It became apparent, as they continued to identify and discuss the elements that were common across the symptom experience in both ill and healthy populations, that their thinking was moving to the level of middle range theory.

The initial collaboration took place between Pugh and Milligan, who were both studying fatigue during different phases of the perinatal experience. Pugh (1990) studied correlates of fatigue during labor and delivery. Milligan (1989) had conducted qualitative and quantitative research about fatigue during the postpartum period and was also carrying out concept development and measurement studies (Milligan, Lenz, Parks, Pugh, & Kitzman, 1996). These two researchers, who were also engaged in clinical practice in labor and delivery and postpartum environments, combined their findings about the concept to develop a framework for the study of fatigue during childbearing (Pugh & Milligan, 1993).

Milligan's inductive analysis of fatigue during the postpartum period included clinical observations, interviews with postpartum mothers, and data from a quantitative measure of fatigue. Her work pointed out the importance of differentiating fatigue from related concepts, such as depression, and the desirability of differentiating different types of fatigue. From Pugh's deductive work, which was based on existing models of fatigue, came the identification of physiologic, psychological, and situational factors that influence fatigue during labor, and the recognition that fatigue is a multidimensional phenomenon. These two investigators recognized commonalities in their conceptualizations of and findings about fatigue at different stages in the childbearing process. Pugh and Milligan (1995) tested the framework in a study of pregnant women, examining fatigue longitudinally. Examples of the commonalities include the cumulative nature of the symptom experience and the importance of energy depletion. The framework that emerged from this collaboration incorporated a nursing diagnosis-based definition of fatigue and the results of empirical studies of fatigue from other disciplines, as well as theoretical models developed within nursing to explain fatigue in childbearing situations.

The second collaboration took place when Pugh began to discuss the model of fatigue with Gift (1990, 1991; Gift & Cahill, 1990), who had conducted multiple studies of dyspnea in patients with chronic obstructive pulmonary disease and asthma. They realized that their conceptualizations were similar and discovered a number of commonalities between the two symptoms. They developed a model combining elements of their previous work that was meant to be equally applicable to both dyspnea and fatigue (Gift & Pugh, 1993).

Gift had carried out Wilsonian concept development activities, which clarified the nature and measurement of dyspnea as a subjective phenomenon. She used pain as an analog to develop a model of dyspnea with physiological and psychological components, and variable intensity, duration, and degree of distress experienced. Her conceptualization bore similarities to Pugh and Milligan's framework for studying fatigue: for example, the respective symptom having both acute and chronic manifestations, being influenced by the same categories of factors, and affecting performance or functional ability.

Having developed the multiple-concept dyspnea/fatigue model, which was also potentially applicable to pain, the investigators went on to reason that they could develop a generic theory that was at an even higher level of abstraction and could be extended to encompass additional symptoms. Lenz was familiar with the work of all three researchers and had offered ongoing critique of their work. Collaboratively they decided to develop a middle range theory and began to meet regularly. Discussions revolved around resolving differences in the models for individual symptoms and agreeing on the elements of a more inclusive theory. The resulting TOUS was introduced and described briefly in an article advocating the development of middle range theories to guide nursing practice (Lenz, Suppe, Gift, Pugh, & Milligan, 1995). The call for papers about middle range nursing theory by *Advances in Nursing Science (ANS)* served as an important stimulus to this theory development activity.

The TOUS generated considerable interest in the nursing academic community as indicated by correspondence received by the authors, much of which came from graduate students who sought clinically relevant theories upon which to base their research. Its publication and more general exposure also pointed out some weaknesses of the theory as well as some aspects that were unclear. As a result, the authors continued to work on refining it, and an updated, improved version was subsequently published (Lenz, Pugh, Milligan, Gift, & Suppe, 1997). Again, the prospect of an opportunity to publish the refinements in *ANS* stimulated the revision.

In considering the process by which the TOUS was developed, several observations are pertinent. First, it was not preplanned but occurred spontaneously, stimulated by shared interests and the opportunity for frequent communication. Proximity that allowed face-to-face meetings, a common background in philosophy and theory development acquired during doctoral study, and the ability to take the time required to debate difficult conceptual issues facilitated the collaborative efforts at all stages. Subsequent geographical moves by the authors have slowed continued work on the theory. Second, forward movement on development of the theory has tended to occur in spurts of activity, undertaken in response to external stimuli, primarily publication opportunities and explicit critiques. This seems to underscore the importance of nursing journal editors' willingness to publish the results of theoretical work as well as empirical research findings. It also reaffirms the value of scholarly dialogue and debate of ideas. Third, the development of the theory occurred in an inductive fashion, which contributed to its practice relevance. At every step concept analysis and clarification were grounded in nursing practice and in practice-related research. The theory was not conceived from armchair musings but was based on real-world observations and attempts to study and solve problems encountered in practice. With time the salience of symptoms and their management has only increased.

CONCEPTS OF THE THEORY

The TOUS has three major concepts: the symptom(s), influencing factors, and performance outcomes. The overall structure of the theory, which is portrayed in Figure 9.1, asserts that three interrelated categories of factors (physiologic, psychologic, and situational) influence predisposition to and manifestation of a given symptom or multiple symptoms and the nature of the symptom experience. The symptom experience, in turn, affects the individual's performance, which encompasses cognitive, physical, and social functioning. The performance outcomes can feed back to influence the symptom experience itself as well as to modify the influencing factors. Literature supporting the structure of the theory was cited in the published descriptions of the original theory (Lenz et al., 1995) and the updated version (Lenz et al., 1997), and is incorporated below in the description of the theory components.

Symptoms

Symptoms were the starting point for conceptualizing the theory, and hence should be considered its central concept. Thus far, the TOUS has focused on subjectively perceived symptoms rather than objectively observable signs. However, Kim, McGuire, Tulman, and Barsevick (2005)

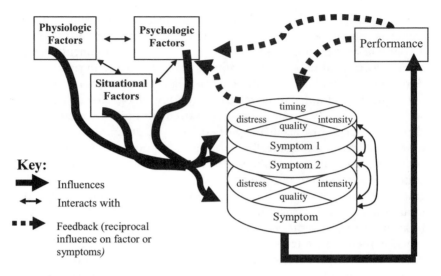

FIGURE 9.1   Unpleasant symptoms.

Reprinted with permission from: Lenz, E. R., Pugh, L. C., Milligan, R., Gift, A., & Suppe, F. (1997). The middle range theory of unpleasant symptoms: An update. *Advances in Nursing Science, 19*(3), 14–27.

argue that the term symptom—and by extension, theories that address them—should be broad enough to include both self-reported symptoms and objective, observed signs. For purposes of the TOUS, symptoms are defined as "the perceived indicators of change in normal function-ing as experienced by patients" (Rhodes & Watson, 1987, p. 242). The perception-based definition assumes awareness by the individual and that the nature of a symptom can be truly known and described only by the individual experiencing it. Therefore, measurement must be subjective. The extent to which objectively observable signs can be explained by the theory has yet to be examined and clearly warrants attention as a pos-sible extension.

The TOUS asserts that symptoms can occur either in isolation—one at a time—or in combination with other symptoms. Although the term is not used in the TOUS and the model does not depict clusters in the usual way, the conceptualization of multiple symptoms potentially occurring concurrently is similar to the notion of symptom clusters. This concept is currently being given considerable attention in the literature regarding cancer and other chronic illnesses (e.g., Armstrong, Cohen, Eriksen, & Hickey, 2004; Barsevick, Dudley, & Beck, 2006; Dodd, Miaskowski, & Lee, 2004; Fox & Lyon, 2006; Kim et al., 2005; Lang et al., 2006;

Miaskowski, Dodd, & Lee, 2004). Symptom clusters are inherent in the definitions and diagnostic criteria for many psychiatric disorders (e.g., Asmundson, Stapleton, & Taylor, 2004; Shelby, Golden-Kreutz, & Anderson, 2005).

In some situations, one symptom may precede and possibly give rise to another. For example, extreme fatigue may precipitate episodes of nausea and vertigo. When more than one symptom is experienced at the same time, or even cumulatively as total symptom burden, the net effect can be powerful (Sarna et al., 2004; Wilmoth, Coleman, Smith, & Davis, 2004). Moderating effects can also occur. That is, when pain is accompanied by one or more other symptoms, such as fatigue and nausea, it tends to be perceived as considerably worse than when it occurs alone. Different levels of pain can also moderate the relationship of fatigue with psychological variables. For example, Francoeur (2005) found several interactions among symptoms in a study of 268 cancer patients with recurrent disease, including the interaction of pain with fever, fatigue, and weight loss in predicting depressive affect.

In the TOUS, symptoms are conceptualized as manifesting multiple variable and measurable dimensions. It is asserted that all symptoms vary in intensity or severity, degree of associated distress, timing, and quality. These dimensions are also related to one another. The *intensity dimension* quantifies the degree, strength, or severity of the symptom and is the most frequently measured aspect of the symptom experience. It is part of the routine assessment of postsurgical patients to ask them to express the intensity or severity of their pain in numerical terms or on a visual analog scale. Intensity is often the simplest characteristic for patients to rate. In pediatric practice, nonnumeric measures of pain are used to capture children's ratings of its intensity (e.g., the faces pain scale).

The *distress dimension* reflects an affective aspect of the symptom experience in that it refers to the degree to which the individual experiencing the symptom is bothered by it. Because of differences in pain threshold levels, for example, individuals exposed to the same intensity of pain-inducing stimuli can experience very different levels of distress. Clearly, the degree of distress experienced with a symptom is related to its intensity; however, it can also be moderated by other considerations. Distress can be influenced by the degree of focused attention that the individual directs toward the symptom. Symptom management strategies designed to lessen distress include diverting attention from the symptom (for example, in the breathing techniques practiced in the Lamaze method of childbirth to divert attention from pain or through introduction of another stimulus that can compete with pain for the individual's attention as suggested in the gate control theory of pain). One of the most important influences on the degree of distress associated with a given symptom is the meaning that the individual attaches to the symptom. For example, a woman who has been treated for infertility may perceive nausea associated with pregnancy as a very welcome symptom and would not be bothered by it, whereas a cancer patient could perceive considerable distress associated with chemotherapy-induced nausea of the same severity because of its potentially negative connotations. Armstrong and colleagues (2004) include meaning as a dimension of the symptom experience that is separate from, and additional to, distress.

The *time dimension* includes the way symptoms vary in duration and frequency. First they vary in duration, the length of time they continue. Duration addresses the importance of the patient's experiential history. It is common to differentiate acute from chronic symptom experiences because they tend to be different in nature and to be treated differently. They also may hold very different meaning for the individual experiencing them. Chronic symptoms may be particularly distress-producing due to their duration; and treatment of symptoms may change with their duration. Strategies that are appropriate for acute pain, for example, are not necessarily useful in treating chronic pain. Secondly, intermittent symptoms vary in the frequency with which they occur; they can also vary in their regularity and periodicity. Nausea that occurs every morning for 3 hours during the first trimester of pregnancy can be described, and hence measured, along several time-related dimensions. The importance of time as a dimension of the symptom experience was emphasized by Henley, Kallas, Klatt, and Swenson (2003), who also underscored the importance of examining intraindividual change over time. They described the impact of time on the meaning the individual attaches to the symptom by virtue of its effect on one's self-evaluation of the symptom experience and emotional response to it.

The final dimension of the symptom experience incorporated in the TOUS is the *quality of* the symptom. This dimension refers to the nature of the symptom or the way in which it is manifested or experienced, that is, what it feels like to have the symptom. By including this dimension, the TOUS acknowledges that in addition to reflecting characteristics that are common across all symptoms, each symptom has unique aspects and characteristics. The descriptors that best characterize each symptom are highly specific. For example, pain is often characterized by the nature of the sensation: stinging, burning, stabbing, pounding, and so forth, and by its location. Changes in the nature of the pain may signal changes in disease progression, hence they are incorporated in many of the widely used symptom-specific measures. Dyspnea can be characterized by the way the shortness of breath feels to the individual: for example, tightness versus suffocation. These descriptors are important because they differ systematically from one disease state—or stage of progression—to another, and so they may provide valuable clues to assessment and effective symptom management.

Describing and measuring the quality of specific symptoms (and symptom clusters) depends on the patient's ability to articulate what he or she is experiencing. Individuals differ in the descriptors that they use and also in their ability to communicate. Qualitative research with a variety of patient populations is often valuable in describing the quality of the symptom experience. Qualitative methods may be used in the early phases of a study to identify descriptors that are then used as the basis for the subsequent development of quantitative measures (e.g., see Lang et al., 2006). The measurement of the symptom(s) would be more descriptive when all four characteristics are included. However, measuring one, two, or three characteristics is valid and informative for health care providers in managing the symptom(s).

Influencing Factors

Three categories of factors that influence the symptom experience (and can, in turn, be influenced by it and by one another) are identified in the TOUS: physiologic factors, psychologic factors, and situational factors. The specific factors that are most relevant in influencing a given symptom may be different from those that are most influential for another. The combination and/or interaction of multiple influencing factors can impact the symptom experience differently from any given influencing factor alone. For example, the combination of a late-stage illness (physiological), depressive mood (psychologic), and lack of social support (situational) is likely to result in a more intense and distressing symptom experience than one of these factors by itself.

Physiologic factors include anatomical/structural, physiological, genetic, and treatment-related variables. Examples of variables in this category include the presence of structural anomalies, existence of pathology or disease states, stage and duration of illness, inflammation due to infection or trauma, fluctuations in hormonal or energy levels, adequacy of hydration and nutrition, level of consciousness, type and duration of treatment, genetic makeup, race/ethnicity, and age. All may influence the occurrence of a symptom and how it is experienced. The interplay among different physiologic influencing factors can be quite complex. For example, breast-feeding mothers' experiences of fatigue are influenced by many physiologic factors, including the duration of labor, type of delivery, level of hydration, time since delivery, maternal age, and the presence of any infection. Symptoms are often the indicators that pathology exists, so clearly there is a reciprocal relationship between physiologic factors and symptoms. Additionally, treatments often give rise to unpleasant symptoms; the classic examples are cancer chemotherapy, radiation, and other medications, many of which produce side effects experienced as unpleasant symptoms (e.g., Wilmoth et al., 2004; Francoeur, 2005).

Psychologic factors represent one of the more complex components of the model. They include both affective and cognitive variables. The individual's affective state or mood (e.g., level of anxiety or depression) at or preceding the time of the symptom experience, even if unrelated to the symptom, and his or her affective response to the illness or the symptom itself (e.g., anger, fear, anxiety) can serve to intensify the symptom. Cognitive variables that may impact the symptom experience include the degree of uncertainty surrounding it, the individual's level of knowledge about the illness or the symptom, and his or her repertoire of cognitive coping skills. As psychobiological research underscores the physiological basis for mood, the psychologic and physiologic factors impacting the symptom experience become difficult to separate.

Situational factors encompass the individual's environment, both social and physical. For instance, the experience of symptoms can vary by culture because there is a learned component to interpreting and expressing symptoms. Other situational factors that can influence the experience of symptoms include those that are associated with the individual's experiential background and access to resources, including the availability of financial, emotional, and instrumental help in dealing with the symptom. Examples are socioeconomic status, marital and family status, availability of social support, and access to health care. Lifestyle behaviors, such as smoking and exercise, can influence the occurrence and intensity of symptoms. The physical environment can also influence symptoms. It includes altitude, temperature, humidity, noise level, light, and presence of pollutants or irritants in the air or water. Some investigators who have used the TOUS in research have categorized treatment-related variables as situational; however, the TOUS authors conceptualized situational variables as external to the individual, so they categorized treatment-related internal changes as physiologic factors.

Performance Outcomes

The outcome concept in the TOUS is performance. It represents the consequences of the symptom experience. Quite simply, the theory asserts that the experience of symptoms can have an impact on the individual's ability to function, with function including motor skills, social behaviors, and cognition. The specification of performance as the key outcome of the model reflects a pragmatic orientation as well as a desire for relatively straightforward measurability. It is also consistent with the genesis of the theory in maternal–infant and adult health nursing practice.

The concept of performance has several possible dimensions: physical activity and impairment; functional role performance, including activities of daily living; cognition, including comprehension, learning, concentration, and problem solving; and social interaction. A given symptom or set of symptoms may generate a number of different performance outcomes that may occur simultaneously but also can be time-ordered. Performance outcomes that are proximal in time to the symptom experience can influence more distal outcomes, particularly if the symptom is sustained in duration. An example would be a heart failure patient who suffers from extreme dyspnea. The symptom interferes with the ability to walk uphill, climb steps, and carry groceries. As a result of these more proximal functional limitations in performance, the more distal performance outcomes might be that an elderly, city-dwelling patient is unable to maintain previous patterns of socializing with friends and shopping independently for food and ultimately would have to move from an apartment or house that requires climbing a hill or climbing stairs. Temporally proximal and distal outcomes can also be conceptualized as primary and secondary outcomes, whereby one outcome gives rise to others.

The TOUS does not explicitly include quality of life (QOL) as an outcome, in part because of the high degree of overlap with functional status in many QOL measures. Evidence that symptoms influence the affective aspects of quality of life (e.g., Fox & Lyon, 2006) and that mood may both impact and be impacted by symptoms (Francoeur, 2005; Gift & McCrone, 1993; Redeker, Lev, & Ruggiero, 2000) suggests the need to consider adding affective outcomes and/or quality of life to the TOUS. Currently the influence of symptoms on affective variables is handled by the feedback loop from the symptom experience to psychologic factors rather than as an explicit outcome.

RELATIONSHIPS AMONG THE CONCEPTS: THE MODEL

The relationships among the major concepts of the TOUS are depicted as lines in Figure 9.1. In the original version of the theory, simplifying assumptions were made, and the relationships between the influencing factors and the symptom experience, and, in turn, between the symptom experience and performance, were depicted as unidirectional. The revised version of the TOUS acknowledges the complexity of the symptom experience by depicting the relationships among the three major components as reciprocal. That is, the influencing factors are assumed to impact the nature of the symptom experience, which, in turn, impacts performance. However, experiencing symptoms can also change the patient's psychological, physiological, or social status. For example, experiencing the symptoms of severe pain and fatigue can negatively impact one's mood state (psychologic influencing factor) (e.g., Francoeur, 2005). Likewise, performance can have a reciprocal relationship to the experience of unpleasant symptoms. For example, the experience of severe pain can restrict an arthritis patient's physical activity, and inactivity may reciprocally increase the intensity of the pain.

The symptom experience can serve as a mediating or moderating variable between influencing factors and performance. A mediating relationship might be exemplified by the finding that Cesarean delivery is associated with higher levels of fatigue than vaginal delivery, and that, in turn, mothers with higher levels of fatigue interact less frequently with their infants than do those who are less fatigued. Fatigue is the mediator that helps explain the link between type of delivery and maternal parenting behavior (Milligan, Parks, & Lenz, 1996; Parks, Lenz, Milligan, & Han, 1999). A scenario in which pain is a moderator would be the relationship of age to the ability to climb stairs following knee replacement surgery. In situations where pain is low and all else being equal, the older the patient, the more limited the ability to climb stairs; however, where pain is high, age might well be unrelated to climbing performance.

The most recent version of the TOUS also asserts that performance can have a feedback effect on the physiologic, psychologic, and situational factors. A breast cancer patient's severe pain (symptom), for example, can impair her desire to interact with others, hence decrease or increase the frequency of her social interaction (performance). Decreased interaction with others in the social network can result not only in decreased network size as others withdraw from the network but also in a reduction in the social support received from her network (situational influencing factors).

The three categories of influencing factors are hypothesized to influence one another and to interact with one another in their relation to the symptom experience. That is, physiologic complications of surgery can interact with a patient's anxiety or depression to create more severe pain than would be experienced had the psychologic factors not been operating as strongly. The positive impact of social support in mitigating the negative impact of physical illness or stress on the severity of symptoms exemplifies the interaction of situational factors with physiologic and psychologic factors. More study is needed about the manner in which they may interact to produce variation in the symptom experience.

As noted above in the discussion of symptom clusters, the TOUS hypothesizes that when patients experience more than one symptom, the symptom experiences are related to one another. The relationship can be an interactive one, even multiplicative. That is, the experience of a given unpleasant symptom, such as pain, is exacerbated or fundamentally changed in other ways when it occurs simultaneously with another symptom, such as nausea. Nipple pain and fatigue, two common symptoms in breast-feeding women during the first postpartum month, can be multiplicative and lead to premature weaning (an unwanted performance outcome). The management of one symptom at a time is clearly easier for the new mother. When she is bombarded with several symptoms, the effect is great.

It is likely that the cumulative effect of multiple symptoms on function is greater than the sum of the individual symptoms; however, this conjecture has not been subjected to thorough and systematic empirical testing and is not necessarily a foregone conclusion. For example, Fox and Lyon (2006) found in a small sample of lung cancer survivors that fatigue and dyspnea were highly correlated. The cluster of the two symptoms explained 29% of the variance in quality of life; however, when the impact of each symptom in the cluster was compared, dyspnea wielded the much greater explanatory power than fatigue. Reishtein (2004) did not find support for the hypothesis that the variance in functional performance that was explained by fatigue, dyspnea, and sleep difficulty taken together was greater than the sum of the contributions of the three symptoms.

USE OF THE THEORY IN NURSING RESEARCH

An increasing number of investigators are using the TOUS as the conceptual framework upon which to base their studies. Other authors have cited it as a middle range theory that effectively highlights aspects of a phenomenon for examination (e.g., Barsevick, Dudley et al., 2006; McCann & Boore, 2000) or is consistent with the findings of a symptom-related study (e.g., Franck et al., 2004; Higgins, 1998). The TOUS has also been used as the basis for instrument development (Kim, Oh, & Lee, 2006; Kim, Oh, Lee, Kim, & Han, 2006) and in a theoretical or concept analysis or in concept development exercises (e.g., Dabbs et al., 2004; Dodd et al., 2001; Henley et al., 2003). Clinical populations in which it has been applied in research include cancer survivors and cancer patients undergoing treatment, patients who have experienced a myocardial infarction or heart failure, patients with mitral valve prolapse syndrome, patients with liver cirrhosis, patients with renal failure who are on hemodialysis, stroke patients, persons with chronic obstructive pulmonary disease (COPD), and pregnant, postpartum, and breast-feeding women. A number of these studies have been carried out in locations outside of the United States (e.g., Korea, Hong Kong, Mainland China). The TOUS authors have received multiple inquiries from master's and doctoral students who have found the theory to be extremely relevant to the phenomena they are interested in examining, and several have expressed the intent to use the TOUS as the theoretical framework for their dissertation research.

A review of the published research based on the TOUS has provided evidence to substantiate many of the conceptualizations and hypothesized relationships in the theory. Some examples of assertions in the TOUS that have been supported empirically are described below.

One of the most frequently validated assertions is that the symptom experience is individualized and highly variable (Higgins, 1998). The TOUS delineation of variable dimensions of symptoms has proven to be very useful and has been validated empirically (e.g., Kapella, Larson, Patel, Covey, & Berry, 2006; Kim, Oh, Lee, Kim, et al., 2006; Liu, 2006). The dimensions most commonly measured have been intensity, distress, frequency, and duration. All of these dimensions have been measured successfully and their importance as predictors of outcomes substantiated. They have been found to vary independently; for example, a symptom that occurs infrequently can be very intense and distressing (Kim, Oh, & Lee, 2006). Quality has been studied less often than the others, but when studied qualitatively, it has yielded descriptors of the symptom experience that may be helpful in differentiating different types or stages of illness and/or have proven useful for incorporation in quantitative measures (e.g., Lang et al., 2006; Liu, 2006; Parshall et al., 2001). As noted above, the meaning of the symptom(s) has been included in some models as an additional dimension of the symptom experience to examine (Armstrong, 2001). In addition, Henley and colleagues (2003) have provided evidence of the complex nature of time in the symptom experience.

The revised version of the TOUS (Lenz et al., 1997) embodied the assertion that multiple symptoms can occur concurrently. The current literature documents that in many illness or stress-related situations multiple symptoms are experienced simultaneously (e.g., Barsevick, Dudley et al., 2006; Scordo, 2005). For example, cancer patients with solid tumors were found to experience an average of 11–13 symptoms concurrently (Armstrong et al., 2004), and Dabbs and colleagues (2003) found as many as 29 symptoms reported by patients who had undergone lung or heart–lung transplantation. Gift, Jablonski, Stommel, and Given (2004) found that fatigue, nausea, weakness, appetite and weight loss, altered taste, and vomiting formed a persistent cluster in elderly lung cancer patients. Lang and colleagues (2006) found that 62% of a sample of people living with chronic hepatitis C infection reported symptom clustering. The TOUS does not depict symptoms as clusters per se but rather as occurring simultaneously, so in that sense it differs from some definitions and depictions of symptom clusters. For example, Kim and colleagues (2005) define symptom clusters as "composed of stable groups of symptoms, are relatively independent of other clusters, and may reveal specific underlying dimensions of symptoms" (p. 270). The assertion that symptoms tend to occur in clusters has been validated in many studies that were based on the TOUS as the conceptual framework (e.g., Dabbs et al., 2003; Franck et al., 2004; Gift et al., 2004; Gift, Stommel, Jablonski, & Given, 2003; Kim, Oh, & Lee, 2006; McCann & Boore, 2000) and is viewed as a critical consideration in conceptualizing the symptom experience (Dodd et al., 2001; Kim et al., 2005). When a number of symptoms are experienced simultaneously, they may not all impact outcomes to the same degree. Instead, one symptom may emerge as the most important predictor, explaining a much higher proportion of the variance in outcomes than any of the others in the cluster (e.g., Reishtein, 2004). Carpenter and colleagues (2004)—similarly to Hutchinson and Wilson (1998)—differentiated primary from secondary symptoms, thus apparently envisioning a sequence of events in which symptoms (e.g., sleep problems) can impact other symptoms (fatigue).

The three categories of influencing factors (physiologic, psychologic, and situational) varied in their importance as predictors or correlates of the symptom experience from one study to another. In some studies a given category of factors was not related to the symptom experience e.g., situational factors were not related to fatigue in McCann and Boore's (2000) study of patients with renal failure who required maintenance hemodialysis. However, such patterns were not consistent, and there is considerable evidence that all three categories are meaningful in explaining the symptom experience (e.g., Gift, 1991; Gift & McCrone, 1993). The inconsistency can be attributed, at least in part, to the specific variables chosen as indicators of the category and other methodological considerations, such as sample size. A given concept (e.g., insomnia) in some studies is set forth as a symptom and in others as a situational factor (see Pugh, Milligan, & Lenz, 2000). Liu (2006) categorized age and gender as situational variables; however, in the TOUS these are included in the physiological factors category. Oh, Kim, Lee, and Kim (2004) categorized dyspnea as a physiological factor impacting the symptom of fatigue, whereas in most studies it is considered to be a symptom. Corwin, Brownstead, Barton, Heckar, and Morin (2005) pointed out the desirability of differentiating stable from variable predictors. Stable predictors (such as psychological traits and many social environmental variables) are difficult to change and hence are less amenable to intervention than variable predictors. The TOUS does not explicitly incorporate this distinction.

All categories of influencing factors have been demonstrated as important correlates or predictors of symptoms; however, the category of influencing factors that was most often documented to be associated with the symptom experience was psychologic factors. A common finding, for example, was the strong association of depression with symptoms such as fatigue and dyspnea (e.g., Corwin et al., 2005; Crane, 2005; Redeker, Lev, & Ruggiero, 2000) and the emergence of psychological factors as more important predictors than physiological (e.g., Kapella et al., 2006). Some issues remain to be clarified regarding the conceptualization and measurement of some of the frequently studied psychologic factors, particularly depression. For example, fatigue is often included as an item on measures of depression. Hutchinson and Wilson (1998) found that the boundaries of the three influencing factor categories and symptom consequences/performance outcomes were blurred and sometimes overlapping. For example, the psychologic factor component of the model (anxiety, memory loss, depression) was difficult to differentiate from the symptoms themselves. They concluded that the components of the TOUS are not necessarily mutually exclusive when applied to Alzheimer's disease patients but are better conceptualized as fluid and possibly interchangeable depending on the context in which they occur.

In the revised version of the TOUS, relationships among the components of the model were hypothesized to be reciprocal and potentially involving complex interactions. This assertion that the interplay among symptoms is often very complex has been substantiated (e.g., Corwin et al., 2005; Dabbs et al., 2000; McCann & Boore, 2000). For example, Lee, Chung, Park, and Chun (2004) found a moderating relationship of situational factors (social support) on the relationship between psychologic factors (mood states) and symptoms in Korean breast cancer patients. In a secondary analysis of data from cancer patients undergoing chemotherapy, Redeker, Lev, and Ruggiero (2000) found that fatigue and insomnia were related but not in the predicted fashion. "Instead of amplifying the effect of the symptoms on performance outcomes as the TOUS suggests, the salience of fatigue and insomnia to quality of life decreased in the presence of the psychological factors, largely due to redundancy among these variables in relation to quality of life" (p. 284). These authors raised important questions about how changes in the relationships among influencing factors, symptoms, and outcomes (in this case quality of life) change over time and over the course of an illness.

The outcome of interest in the TOUS is performance, conceptualized exclusively to include physical, cognitive, and social functioning. This conceptualization has been criticized as too limited (see Dodd et al., 2001; Henly, Kallas, Klat, & Swenson, 2003). The most commonly studied outcome to date has been functional performance or functional health status, measured either by disease-specific or general instruments. Other outcomes have included care-seeking patterns (Jurgens, 2006; Liu, 2006), use of health resources (Scordo, 2005), health concerns (Scordo, 2005), and death (Franck et al., 2004). Virtually all of the studies that included performance outcomes revealed relationships with symptoms. Exceptions are the finding by Michael, Allen, and Macko (2006) that fatigue in a sample of community-dwelling subjects with chronic hemiparetic stroke was not related to ambulatory activity, and Crane's (2005) finding that fatigue was not related to women's participation in physical activity after myocardial infarction.

USE OF THE THEORY IN NURSING PRACTICE

To date there remains little published evidence of the application of the TOUS in clinical practice; however, there have been several studies that have tested clinical interventions. For example, Pugh and Milligan (1995, 1998; Milligan, Flenniken, & Pugh, 1996) conducted several experimental studies to test a positioning intervention based on the TOUS to minimize fatigue in nursing mothers, because fatigue was found to be a major barrier to breast-feeding success. The multifaceted intervention included discussions of diet and exercise, the need for sleep and rest, ways to build the mothers' self esteem, use of social support, comfort measures such as warm compresses, and use of side-lying position while breast-feeding to conserve energy. The intervention, therefore, addressed all three TOUS categories of influential factors. It was found to be effective in that the experimental group of mothers had lower fatigue at 14 days postpartum and sustained breast-feeding for an average of 6 weeks longer than the control group mothers. In several additional studies similar results were found (Pugh, Milligan, & Brown, 2001; Pugh, Milligan, Frick, Spatz, & Bronner, 2002).

A majority of investigators address the practice implications of their research. Virtually all of the studies emphasize the importance of assessing the occurrence of multiple symptoms simultaneously, since the pattern of symptom concurrence has been found across symptoms and clinical populations. They also stress the importance of routinely assessing multiple dimensions of the symptom experience (e.g., Scordo, 2005). For example, Parshall and colleagues' (2001) findings suggest the basis for a multifaceted assessment of dyspnea in heart failure patients, both in ambulatory care settings where these patients are managed on an ongoing basis and in emergency room settings when they seek care for dyspnea that has become particularly distressing. Such assessment can be used to identify ambulatory patients who are at risk for hospital admission and ultimately to guide the design of interventions to decrease dyspnea and decrease hospitalization rates.

Symptom management is one of the most important problems addressed in today's clinical practice. It represents a focus that is squarely within—and perhaps even central to—nursing's practice domain. More specific models at lower levels of abstraction, such as the middle range theory of acute pain management (Good, 1998) or the middle range theory of chronotherapeutic intervention for postsurgical pain management (Auvil-Novak, 1997) can and should be applied in managing individual symptoms such as pain (see Brown, 1996). More inclusive middle range theories also have contributions to make to practice and may provide the advantage of a slightly different perspective than the highly specific (see Lenz, Suppe, Gift, Pugh, & Milligan, 1996). The revised symptom management model (Dodd et al., 2001) is more explicit than the TOUS in addressing symptom management strategies. However, the TOUS also helps highlight certain aspects of the symptom experience and potential strategies for symptom management that are not addressed by more symptom-specific models. For example, the TOUS stresses the importance of a multivariate assessment of the symptom experience itself and of possible influencing factors and provides a rationale and framework for applying a biopsychosocial approach. It suggests that multiple management strategies may need to be applied simultaneously, given the multivariate nature of the factors influencing symptoms. It also underscores the importance of addressing the possibility of several symptom experiences occurring concurrently and, by inference, suggests that some influencing factors may give rise to or impact multiple symptoms. It also emphasizes the importance of considering the effect of several symptoms, occurring together, on the patient's functioning, and encourages assessment of functional patient outcomes.

According to Cooley (2000), the TOUS is valuable because it "proposes a way to integrate information about the complexity and interactive nature of the symptom experience" (p. 146). Hutchinson and Wilson (1998) also stress the importance of the model in encouraging nurses to design interventions in a way that takes into account the interactive nature of symptoms, influencing factors, and consequences, thereby making them client-specific. In its most recent version, the TOUS emphasizes the interplay among influential factors, symptoms, and performance outcomes; thus, it encourages creative thinking about new and different approaches to symptom management. Several clinicians have described it as having intuitive appeal because it is relatively straightforward, easy to understand and apply, and focused on relevant concerns.

CONCLUSION

The theory of unpleasant symptoms, which was grounded in clinical research and practice, is a mid-range theory that holds considerable promise as a basis for additional research and as a guide to nursing practice. Although it is one of the few recent mid-range theories that have undergone revision based on empirical findings (Liehr & Smith, 1999), the TOUS remains a work in progress. The updated version addressed several of the weaknesses of the original; however, we recognize that selected aspects of the theory remain underdeveloped. Subsequent development has been relatively piecemeal, undertaken in response to specific published critiques or applications of the theory. The authors are committed to continued development and publication of updates.

The changes that were made to the theory in the 1997 revision added to the complexity of the model but also made it more consistent with the complex reality that constitutes the symptom experience. The modifications have been validated in several ill (heart failure, cancer, chronic obstructive pulmonary disease, end-stage renal failure) and well (breast-feeding mothers, pregnant and postpartum women) samples. Thus far, the symptoms that have been described in these studies have included pain, dyspnea, nausea and vomiting, insomnia and other sleep problems, hot flashes, and fatigue. More research is needed in additional clinical populations and with additional symptoms. The current research suggests that the symptom dimensions identified in the TOUS are both relevant and measurable; however, additional elaboration is warranted with regard to the conceptualization and measurement of time. For example, the abruptness of onset of a symptom may be important to add. The theory needs to more explicitly address the way the symptom experience unfolds over time (see Henley et al., 2003).

Given the plethora of evidence accruing about symptom clusters, the TOUS needs to be more explicit about them. The inclusion of multiple symptoms in the model introduces a number of areas of complexity that have not yet been addressed in detail, for example, the sequence in which symptoms appear and the extent to which a given symptom tends to influence the appearance and characteristics of others. The notion of primary and secondary symptoms should be included explicitly.

Additional conceptual/theoretical work is needed as well to address several of the issues that have been pointed out by investigators who have used the theory. For example, a question exists as to whether it is relevant for both signs and symptoms. Likewise, its potential applicability to subjects or patients who have perceptual deficits or who are unable to describe the symptom experience (e.g., infants or unconscious patients) has been assumed but has not yet been fully explored.

The complex relationships among the three categories of influencing factors and between these factors and the symptom experience need much fuller elaboration and the categories themselves need continuing clarification. The differentiation between permanent and transitory influencing factors also needs to be considered. Although the potential relevance of all three types of factors has been quite well-supported, there are some inconsistencies that need to be examined. The most influential factors need to be identified and the nature of their complex relationships to the symptom experience explicated. Psychologic influential factors have been found repeatedly to play a key role in exacerbating or mitigating symptoms; however, there is potential for conceptual and empirical overlap between psychological states (anxiety and depression in particular) and the affective or distress component of the symptom experience. The interplay between these two model components needs to be examined.

The performance component of the model needs additional development. Several of the investigations have revealed it to be more complex than originally thought. The notions of primary and secondary outcomes and temporally proximal and distal outcomes need to be incorporated in the model. Although the functional, pragmatic focus of the performance outcome was chosen purposefully, it does de-emphasize other, more inclusive outcomes that may be important consequences of the symptom experience. Quality of life (particularly the affective aspects thereof) is a prime example. Functioning is generally a component of quality of life, but the latter is more inclusive. Its possible place within the TOUS is a topic that needs to be explored conceptually and empirically.

Finally, more attention needs to be paid to symptom assessment and management. As noted above, the TOUS has many practice implications, and recent findings suggest potentially useful interventions; however, these remain to be described in detail and possible patterns discerned.

As was pointed out in the original description of the process that was used to develop the TOUS, it has been and continues to be the product of an exciting group interaction. Multiple practice-grounded observations, a growing body of literature documenting its application, and lively discussions with colleagues and students have led to its continued development. Its richness can only increase as the developers continue to address the input of others who have used the theory in research and practice.

REFERENCES

Armstrong, T. S. (2001). Symptoms experience: A concept analysis. *Oncology Nursing Forum, 30,* 601–606.

Armstrong, T. S., Cohen, M. Z., Eriksen, L. R., & Hickey, J. V. (2004). Symptom clusters in oncology patients and implications for symptom research in people with primary brain tumors. *Journal of Nursing Scholarship, 36*(3), 197–206.

Asmundson, G. J. G., Stapleton, J. A., & Taylor, S. (2004). Are avoidance and numbing distinct PTSD symptom clusters? *Journal of Traumatic Stress, 17*(6), 467–475.

Auvil-Novak, S. E. (1997). A middle-range theory of chronotherapeutic intervention for postsurgical pain. *Nursing Research, 46,* 66–71.

Barsevick, A. M., Dudley, W. N., & Beck, S. L. (2006). Cancer-related fatigue, depressive symptoms, and functional status: A mediation model. *Nursing Research, 55*(5), 366–372.

Barsevick, A. M., Whitmore, K., Nail, L. M., Beck, S. L., & Dudley, W. N. (2006). Symptom cluster research: Conceptual, design, measurement and analysis issues. *Journal of Pain and Symptom Management, 31*(1), 85–95.

Brown, S. J. (1996). Letter to the editor. *Advances in Nursing Science, 18*(4), vi.

Carpenter, J. S., Elam, J. L., Ridner, S. H., Carney, P. H., Cherry, G. J., & Cucullu, H. L. (2004). Sleep, fatigue, and depressive symptoms in breast cancer survivors and matched health women experiencing hot flashes. *Oncology Nursing Forum, 31*(3), 591–598.

Cooley, M. (2000). Symptoms in adults with lung cancer: A systematic research review. *Journal of Pain and Symptom Management, 19,* 137–153.

Corwin, E. J., Brownstead, J., Barton, N., Heckar, S., & Morin, K. (2005). The impact of fatigue on the development of postpartum depression. *Journal of Obstetric, Gynecologic, & Neonatal Nursing, 34*(5) 577–586.

Crane, P. B. (2005). Fatigue and physical activity in older women after myocardial infarction. *Heart & Lung, 34*(1), 30–38.

Dabbs, A. D., Dew, M. A., Stilley, C. S., Manzetti, J., Zullo, T., Kormos, R. L., et al. (2000). *Psychosocial vulnerability, physical symptoms and physical impairment after lung and heart-lung transplantation.* Paper presented at Eastern Nursing Research Society annual meeting, State College, PA.

Dabbs, A. D., Dew, M. A., Stilley, C. S., Manzetti, J., Zullo, T., McCurry, K. R., et al. (2003). Psychosocial vulnerability, physical symptoms and physical impairment after lung and heart-lung transplantation. *The Journal of Heart and Lung Transplantation, 22*(11), 1268–1275.

Dabbs, A. D., Hoffman, L. A., Swigart, V., Happ, M. B., Iacono, A. T., & Dauber, J. H. (2004). Using conceptual triangulation to develop an integrated model of the symptom experience of acute rejection after lung transplantation. *Advances in Nursing Science, 27,* 136–149.

Dodd, M., Jansen, S., Facione, N., Faucett, J., Froelicher, E. S., Humphreys, J., et al. (2001). Advancing the science of symptom management. *Journal of Advanced Nursing, 33*(5) 668–676.

Dodd, M. J., Miaskowski, C., & Lee, K. A. (2004). Occurrence of symptom clusters. *Journal of the National Cancer Institute, 32,* 76–78.

Fox, S. W., & Lyon, D. E. (2006). Symptom clusters and quality of life in survivors of lung cancer. *Oncology Nursing Forum, 33*(5), 931–936.

Franck, L. S., Kools, S., Kennedy, C., Kong, S. K. F., Chen, J-L., & Wong, T. K. S. (2004). The symptom experience of hospitalized Chinese children and adolescents and relationship to pre-hospital factors and behavior problems. *International Journal of Nursing Studies, 41,* 661–669.

Francoeur, R. B. (2005). The relationship of cancer symptom clusters to depressive affect in the initial phase of palliative radiation. *Journal of Pain and Symptom Management, 29*(2), 130–155.

Gift, A. G. (1990). Dyspnea. *Nursing Clinics of North America, 25,* 955–965.

Gift, A. G. (1991). Psychological and physiological aspects of acute dyspnea in asthmatics. *Nursing Research, 40,* 196–199.

Gift, A. G., & Cahill, C. (1990). Psychophysiologic aspects of dyspnea in chronic obstructive pulmonary disease: A pilot study. *Heart & Lung, 19,* 252–257.

Gift, A. G., Jablonski, A., Stommel, M., & Given, C. W. (2004). Symptom clusters in elderly patients with lung cancer. *Oncology Nursing Forum, 31*(2), 203–210.

Gift, A. G., & McCrone, S. H. (1993). Depression in patients with C.O.P.D. *Heart & Lung, 22*(4), 289–297.

Gift, A. G., & Pugh, L. C. (1993). Dyspnea and fatigue. *Nursing Clinics of North America, 28,* 373–384.

Gift, A. G., Stommel, M., Jablonski, A., & Given, W. (2003). A cluster of symptoms over time in patients with lung cancer. *Nursing Research, 52*(6) 393–400.

Good, M. (1998). A middle-range theory of acute pain management: Use in research. *Nursing Outlook, 436,* 120–124.

Henley, S. M., Kallas, K. D., Klatt, C. M., & Swenson, K. K. (2003). The notion of time in symptom experiences. *Nursing Research, 52*(6) 410–417.

Higgins, P. (1998). Patient perceptions of fatigue while undergoing long-term mechanical ventilation: Incidence and associated factors. *Heart & Lung, 27*(3), 177–183.

Hutchinson, S. A., & Wilson, H. S. (1998). The theory of unpleasant symptoms and Alzheimer's disease. *Scholarly Inquiry for Nursing Practice, 22,* 143–158.

Jurgens, C. Y. (2006). Somatic awareness, uncertainty and delay in care-seeking in acute heart failure. *Research in Nursing and Health, 29,* 74–76.

Kapella, M. C., Larson, J. L., Patel, M. K., Covey, M. K., & Berry, J. K. (2006). Subjective fatigue, influencing variables and consequences in chronic obstructive pulmonary disease. *Nursing Research, 55*(1), 10–17.

Kim, H-J., McGuire, D. B., Tulman, L., & Barsevick, A. M. (2005). Symptom clusters: Concept analysis and clinical implications for cancer nursing. *Cancer Nursing, 28*(4), 270–282.

Kim, S-H., Oh, E-G., & Lee, W-H. (2006). Symptom experience, psychological distress, and quality of life in Korean patients with liver cirrhosis: A cross-sectional survey. *International Journal of Nursing Studies, 43,* 1047–1056.

Kim, S-H., Oh, E-G., Lee, W-H., Kim, O-S., & Han, K-H. (2006). Symptom experience in Korean patients with liver cirrhosis. *Journal of Pain and Symptom Management, 31*(4), 325–334.

Lang, C. A., Conrad, S., Garrett, L., Battistutta, D., Cooksley, W. G., Dunne, M., et al. (2006). Symptom prevalence and clustering of symptoms in people living with chronic hepatitis C infection. *Journal of Pain and Symptom Management, 31*(4), 335–344.

Larson, P. J., Carrieri-Kohlman, V., Dodd, M. J., Douglas, M., Fawcett, J., Froelicher, E., et al. (1994). A model for symptom management. *Image: Journal of Nursing Scholarship, 26,* 272–276.

Lee, E-H., Chung, B. Y., Park, H. B., & Chun, K. H. (2004). Relationships of mood disturbance and social support to symptom experience in Korean women with breast cancer. *Journal of Pain and Symptom Management, 27*(5), 425–433.

Lenz, E. R., Pugh, L. C., Milligan, R., Gift, A., & Suppe, F. (1997). The middle-range theory of unpleasant symptoms: An update. *Advances in Nursing Science, 19*(3), 14–27.

Lenz, E. R., Suppe, F., Gift, A. G., Pugh, L. C., & Milligan, R. A. (1995). Collaborative development of middle-range nursing theories: Toward a theory of unpleasant symptoms. *Advances in Nursing Science, 17*(3), 1–13.

Lenz, E. R., Suppe, F., Gift, A. G., Pugh, L. C., & Milligan, R. A. (1996). Letter to the editor: Response to Brown. *Advances in Nursing Science, 18*(4), vi–vii.

Liehr, P., & Smith, M. J. (1999). Middle range theory: Spinning research and practice to create knowledge for the new millennium. *Advances in Nursing Science, 21*(4) 81–91.

Liu, H. E. (2006). Fatigue and associated factors in hemodialysis patients in Taiwan. *Research in Nursing and Health, 29,* 40–50.

McCann, K., & Boore, J. R. P. (2000). Fatigue in persons with renal failure who require maintenance hemodialysis. *Journal of Advanced Nursing, 32,* 1132–1142.

Miaskowski, C., Dodd, M., & Lee, K. (2004). Symptom clusters: The new frontier in symptom management research. *Journal of the National Cancer Institute.* Monographs, no. 32, 17–21.

Michael, K. M., Allen, J. K., & Macko, R. F. (2006). Fatigue after stroke: Relationship to mobility, fitness, ambulatory activity, social support and falls efficacy. *Rehabilitation Nursing, 31*(5), 210–217.

Milligan, R. A. (1989). Maternal fatigue during the first three months of the postpartum period. *Dissertation Abstracts International, 50,* 07B.

Milligan, R. A., Flenniken, P., & Pugh, L. C. (1996). Positioning intervention to minimize fatigue in breastfeeding women. *Applied Nursing Research, 9,* 67–70.

Milligan, R. A., Lenz, F. R., Parks, P. L., Pugh, L. C., & Kitzman, H. (1996). Postpartum fatigue: Clarifying a concept. *Scholarly Inquiry for Nursing Practice, 10,* 279–291.

Milligan, R. A., Parks, P. L., & Lenz, E. R. (1996, June). *Testing the theory of unpleasant symptoms.* Paper presented at the American Nurses' Association Council for Nursing Research Scientific Session, Washington, DC.

Oh, E-G., Kim, C-J., Lee, W-H., & Kim, S. S. (2004). Correlates of fatigue in Koreans with chronic lung disease. *Heart & Lung, 33*(1), 13–20.

Parks, P. L., Lenz, F. R., Milligan, R. A., & Han, H. R. (1999). What happens when fatigue lingers for 18 months after delivery? *Journal of Obstetric, Gynecologic, and Neonatal Nursing, 28*(1), 87–93.

Parshall, M. B., Welsh, J. D., Brockopp, D. Y., Heiser, R. M., Schooler, M. P., & Cassidy, K. B. (2001). Dyspnea duration, distress and intensity in emergency department visits for heart failure. *Heart & Lung, 30*(1), 47–56.

Pugh, L. C. (1990). Psychophysiologic correlates of fatigue during childbearing. *Dissertation Abstracts International, 51,* 01B.

Pugh, L. C., & Milligan, R. A. (1993). A framework for the study of childbearing fatigue. *Advances in Nursing Science, 15*(4), 60–70.

Pugh, L. C., & Milligan, R. A. (1995). Patterns of fatigue during pregnancy. *Applied Nursing Research, 8,* 140–143.

Pugh, L. C., & Milligan, R. A. (1998). Nursing intervention to increase the duration of breastfeeding. *Applied Nursing Research, 11,* 190–194.

Pugh, L. C., Milligan, R. A., & Brown, L. P. (2001). The breastfeeding support team for low-income predominantly minority women: A pilot intervention study. *Health Care for Women International, 22,* 501–515.

Pugh, L. C., Milligan, R. A., Frick, K. D., Spatz, I. D., & Bronner, Y. (2002). Breastfeeding duration and cost effectiveness of a support program for low-income breastfeeding women. *Birth, 29*(2), 95–100.

Pugh, L. C., Milligan, R. A., & Lenz, B. R. (2000). Response to "insomnia, fatigue, anxiety, depression, and quality of life of cancer patients undergoing chemotherapy." *Scholarly Inquiry for Nursing Practice, 14,* 291–294.

Redeker, N. S., Lev, E. L., & Ruggiero, J. (2000). Insomnia, fatigue, anxiety, depression and quality of life of cancer patients undergoing chemotherapy. *Scholarly Inquiry for Nursing Practice: An International Journal, 14*(4), 275–290.

Reishtein, J. L. (2004). Relationship between symptoms and functional performance in COPD. *Research in Nursing and Health, 28,* 39–47.

Rhodes, V., & Watson, P. (1987). Symptom distress—the concept past and present. *Seminars in Oncology Nursing, 3*(4), 242–247.

Sarna, L., Evangelista, L., Tashkin, E., Padilla, G., Holmes, C., Brecht, M. L., et al. (2004). Impact of respiratory symptoms and pulmonary function on quality of life of long-term survivors of non-small cell lung cancer. *Chest, 125,* 439–443.

Scordo, K. A. (2005). Mitral valve prolapse syndrome health concerns, symptoms and treatments. *Western Journal of Nursing Research, 27*(4), 390–405.

Shelby, R. A., Golden-Kreutz, D. M., & Anderson, B. L. (2005). Mismatch of post-traumatic stress disorder (PTSD) symptoms and DOM-IV symptom clusters in a cancer sample: Exploratory factor analysis of the PTSD Checklist-Civilian Version. *Journal of Traumatic Stress, 18*(4), 347–357.

Wilmoth, M. C., Coleman, E. A., Smith, S. C., & Davis, C. (2004). Fatigue, weight gain, and altered sexuality in patients with breast cancer: Exploration of a symptom cluster. *Oncology Nursing Forum, 31*(6), 1069–1077.

Theory of Self-Efficacy

Barbara Resnick

Self-efficacy is defined as an individual's judgment of his or her capabilities to organize and execute courses of action. At the core of self-efficacy theory is the assumption that people can exercise influence over what they do. Through reflective thought, generative use of knowledge and skills to perform a specific behavior, and other tools of self-influence, a person will decide how to behave (Bandura, 1997). To determine self-efficacy an individual must have the opportunity for self-evaluation or the ability to compare individual output to some sort of evaluative criterion. It is this comparative process that enables an individual to judge performance capability and establish self-efficacy expectation.

PURPOSE OF THE THEORY AND
HOW IT WAS DEVELOPED

Self-efficacy theory is based on social cognitive theory and conceptualizes person-behavior-environment interaction as triadic reciprocality, the foundation for reciprocal determinism (Bandura, 1977, 1986). Triadic reciprocality is the interrelationship among person, behavior, and environment; reciprocal determinism is the belief that behavior, cognitive and other personal factors, and environmental influences all operate interactively as determinants of each other. Reciprocality does not mean that the influence of behavioral, personal factors, and environmental influences are equal. Depending on the situation, the influence of one factor may be stronger than another, and these influences may vary over time.

Cognitive thought, which is a critical dimension of the person-behavior-environment interaction, does not arise in a vacuum. Bandura

(1977, 1986, 1995) suggested that individuals' thoughts about themselves are developed and verified through four different processes: (1) direct experience of the effects produced by their actions, (2) vicarious experience, (3) judgments voiced by others, and (4) derivation of further knowledge of what they already know by using rules of inference. Human functioning is viewed as a dynamic interplay of personal, behavioral, and environmental influences.

Initial Theory Development and Research

In 1963, Bandura and Walters wrote *Social Learning and Personality Development*, which expanded on social learning theory to incorporate observational learning and vicarious reinforcement. In the 1970s Bandura incorporated what he considered to be the missing component to that theory, self-efficacy beliefs, and published "Self-Efficacy: Toward a Unifying Theory of Behavior Change" (Bandura, 1977). The work supporting self-efficacy beliefs was based on research testing the assumption that exposure to treatment conditions could result in behavioral change by altering an individual's level and strength of self-efficacy. In the initial study (Bandura, Adams, & Beyer, 1977) 33 subjects with snake phobias were randomly assigned to three different treatment conditions: (1) enactive attainment, which included actually touching the snakes, (2) role modeling, or seeing others touch the snakes, and (3) the control group. Results suggested that self-efficacy was predictive of subsequent behavior, and enactive attainment resulted in stronger and more generalized (to other snakes) self-efficacy expectations.

Expansion of the early research included three additional studies (Bandura, Reese, & Adams, 1982): (1) 10 subjects with snake phobias, (2) 14 subjects with spider phobias, and (3) 12 subjects with spider phobias. Similar to the initial self-efficacy study, enactive attainment and role modeling were effective interventions for strengthening self-efficacy expectations and impacting behavior. The study of 12 subjects with spider phobias also considered the physiological arousal component of self-efficacy. Pulse and blood pressure were measured as indicators of fear arousal when interacting with spiders. After interventions to strengthen self-efficacy expectations (enactive attainment and role modeling), heart rate decreased and blood pressure stabilized.

This early self-efficacy research used an ideal controlled setting in that the individuals with snake phobias were unlikely to seek out opportunities to interact with snakes when away from the laboratory setting. Therefore, there was controlled input of efficacy information. While this ideal situation is not possible in the clinical setting, the theory of self-efficacy has been used to study and predict health behavior change and management in a variety of settings.

I came to use the theory as I reviewed the literature, exploring factors that influenced the willingness of older adults to participate in functional activities and exercise. There was a recurring theme that suggested self-efficacy and outcome expectations mattered to an individual's willingness. It seemed appropriate, therefore, to use the theory to help understand behavior and guide the development of interventions to change behavior.

CONCEPTS OF THE THEORY

Bandura, a social scientist, differentiated between two components of self-efficacy theory: self-efficacy expectations and outcome expectations. These two components are the major ideas of the theory. Self-efficacy expectations are judgments about personal ability to accomplish a given task. Outcome expectations are judgments about what will happen if a given task is successfully accomplished. Self-efficacy and outcome expectations were differentiated because individuals can believe that a certain behavior will result in a specific outcome; however, they may not believe that they are capable of performing the behavior required for the outcome to occur. For example, Mrs. White may believe that rehabilitation will result in her being able to go home independently; however, she may not believe she is capable of ambulating across the room. Therefore, Mrs. White may not participate in the rehabilitation program or be willing to practice ambulation.

Bandura (1977, 1986, 1997) suggests that outcome expectations are based largely on the individual's self-efficacy expectations. The types of outcomes people anticipate generally depend on their judgments of how well they will be able to perform the behavior. Those individuals who consider themselves highly efficacious in accomplishing a given behavior will expect favorable outcomes for that behavior. Expected outcomes are dependent on self-efficacy judgments. Therefore, Bandura postulated that expected outcomes may not add much on their own to the prediction of behavior.

Bandura (1986) does state, however, that there are instances when outcome expectations can be dissociated from self-efficacy expectations. This occurs either when no action will result in a specific outcome or when the outcome is loosely linked to the level or quality of the performance. For example, if Mrs. White knows that *even if she* regains functional independence by participating in rehabilitation she will still be discharged to a skilled nursing facility rather than back home, her behavior is likely to be influenced by her outcome expectations (discharge to the skilled nursing facility). In this situation, no matter what Mrs. White's performance, the outcome is the same; thus outcome expectancy may influence her behavior independent of her self-efficacy beliefs.

Expected outcomes are also partially separable from self-efficacy judgments when extrinsic outcomes are fixed. For example, when a nurse provides care to six patients during an 8-hour shift the nurse receives a certain salary. When the same nurse cares for 10 patients during that shift, she receives the same salary. This could negatively impact performance. It is also possible for an individual to believe he or she is capable of performing a specific behavior but not believe that the outcome of performing that behavior is worthwhile. For example, older adults in rehabilitation may believe that they are capable of performing the exercises and activities involved in the rehabilitation process, but they may not believe that performing the exercises will result in improved functional ability. Some older adults believe that resting rather than exercising will lead to recovery. In this situation outcome expectations may have a direct impact on performance.

Both self-efficacy and outcome expectations play an influential role in the performance of functional activities (Bootsma-van der Wiel et al., 2001; Collins, Lee, Albright, & King, 2004; Cress et al., 2005; Resnick et al., 2005), adoption and maintenance of exercise behavior (O'Connor, Rousseau, & Maki, 2004; Resnick et al., 2005), and recovery of function for disabled older adults in the community (de Blok et al., 2006). Self-efficacy expectations also were associated with functional recovery immediately following a stroke (Robinson-Smith, Johnston, & Allen, 2000), cardiac (Cromwell & Adams, 2006; Gary, 2006; Hiltunen et al., 2005), or orthopedic event such as hip fracture or joint replacement (Harnirattisai, 2003; Harnirattisai & Johnson, 2005; Resnick, Vogel, & Luisi, 2005). Outcome expectations are particularly relevant to older adults. These individuals may have high self-efficacy expectations for exercise, but if they do not believe in the outcomes associated with exercise, for example, improved health, strength, or function, then it is unlikely that there will be adherence to a regular exercise program (Bootsma-van der Wiel et al., 2001; Collins et al., 2004; Cress et al., 2005; Resnick, Orwig, Wehren et al., 2005).

Generally, it is anticipated that self-efficacy will have a positive impact on behavior. It must be recognized, however, that there are times when self-efficacy will have no or a negative effect on performance. Some research has found that there is a negative effect of self-reported personal goals on performance such that higher personal goals can cause poorer performance (Vancouver, Thompson, & Williams, 2001). High self-efficacy expectations can actually be counterproductive. High self-efficacy may lead people to have a false sense of confidence and not put in as much effort as needed to perform optimally (Jones, Harris, Waller, & Coggins, 2005). This may be particularly true of behaviors such as exercise in which adequate resources to perform are needed (i.e., adequate physical strength), and the individual may have limited prior experience on which to draw and appropriately evaluate his or her self-efficacy expectations.

Sources of Self-Efficacy Judgment

Bandura (1986) suggested that judgment about one's self-efficacy is based on four informational sources: (1) enactive attainment, which is the actual performance of a behavior; (2) vicarious experience or visualizing other similar people perform a behavior; (3) verbal persuasion or exhortation; and (4) physiological state or physiological feedback during a behavior, such as pain or fatigue. The cognitive appraisal of these factors results in a perception of a level of confidence in the individual's ability to perform a certain behavior. The positive performance of this behavior reinforces self-efficacy expectations (Bandura, 1995).

Enactive Attainment

Enactive attainment has been described as the most influential source of self-efficacy information (Bandura, 1986; Bandura & Adams, 1977) and is the most common intervention used to strengthen efficacy expectations in older adults (Brassington, Atienza, Perczek, DiLorenzo, & King, 2002; Estabrooks, Fox, Doerksen, Bradshaw, & King, 2005; Gyurcsik, Estabrooks, & Frahm-Templar, 2003; McAuley et al., 2006). There has been repeated empirical verification that actually performing an activity strengthens self-efficacy beliefs. Specifically, the impact of enactive attainment has been demonstrated with regard to snake phobias, smoking cessation, exercise behaviors, performance of functional activities, and weight loss. Enactive attainment generally results in greater strengthening of self-efficacy expectations than do informational sources. However, performance alone does not establish self-efficacy beliefs. Other factors, such as preconceptions of ability, the perceived difficulty of the task, the amount of effort expended, the external aid received, the situational circumstance, and past successes and failures all impact the individual's cognitive appraisal of self-efficacy (Bandura, 1995). An older adult who strongly believes he or she is able to bathe and dress independently because he or she has been doing so for 90 years will not likely alter self-efficacy expectations if he or she wakes up with severe arthritic changes one morning and is consequently unable to put on a shirt. However, repeated failures to perform the activity will impact self-efficacy expectations. The relative stability of strong self-efficacy expectations is important; otherwise an occasional failure or setback could severely impact both self-efficacy expectations and behavior.

Vicarious Experience

Self-efficacy expectations are also influenced by vicarious experiences or seeing other similar people successfully perform the same activity (Bandura, Adams, Hardy, & Howells, 1980). There are some conditions, however, that impact the influence of vicarious experience. If the individual has not been exposed to the behavior of interest or has had little experience with it, vicarious experience is likely to have a greater impact. Additionally, when clear guidelines for performance are not explicated, self-efficacy will be more likely to be impacted by the performance of others. Among older adults with cognitive impairment vicarious experiences are particularly effective in increasing activity (Resnick & Galik, 2006).

Verbal Persuasion

Verbal persuasion involves telling an individual that he or she has the capabilities to master the given behavior. Empirical support for the influence of verbal persuasion has been documented since Bandura's early research of phobias (Bandura & Adams, 1977). Verbal persuasion has proven effective in supporting recovery from chronic illness and in health promotion research. Persuasive health influences lead people with a high sense of self-efficacy to intensify efforts at self-directed change of risky health behavior. Verbal encouragement from a trusted, credible source in the form of counseling and education has been used alone and with performance behavior to strengthen efficacy expectations (Castro, King, & Brassington, 2001; Hiltunen et al., 2005; Moore et al., 2006; Resnick, Simpson et al., 2006). For example, verbal encouragement via telephone calls was successful in increasing physical activity among older adults (Castro et al., 2001).

Physiological Feedback

Individuals rely in part on information from their physiological state in order to judge their abilities. Physiological indicators are especially important in relation to coping with stressors, physical accomplishments, and health functioning. Individuals evaluate their physiological state, or arousal, and if aversive, they may avoid performing the behavior. For example, if the older adult has a fear of falling or getting hurt when walking, a high arousal state associated with the fear can limit performance and decrease the individual's confidence in ability to perform the activity. Likewise if the rehabilitation activities result in fatigue, pain, or shortness of breath, these symptoms may be interpreted as physical inefficacy, and the older adult may not feel capable of performing the activity.

Interventions can be used to alter the interpretation of physiological feedback and help individuals cope with physical sensations, enhancing self-efficacy and resulting in improved performance. Interventions include (a) visualized mastery, which eliminates the emotional reactions to a given situation (Bandura & Adams, 1977), (b) enhancement of physical status (Bandura, 1995), and (c) altering the interpretation of bodily states (McAuley, Jerome, Marquez, Elavsky, & Blissmer, 2003; McAuley, Konopack, Motl, et al., 2006). Interventions that decrease the pain associated with the use of pain medication or ice treatments has been shown to increase participation in rehabilitation and exercise among older adults (Rejeski, Katula, Rejeski, Rowley, & Sipe, 2005; Resnick, 1998, 2002; Resnick, Ory et al., 2006).

RELATIONSHIPS AMONG THE CONCEPTS: THE MODEL

The theory of self-efficacy was derived from social cognitive theory and must be considered within the context of reciprocal determinism. The four sources of experience (direct experience, vicarious experience, judgments by others, derivation of knowledge by inference) that can potentially influence self-efficacy and outcome expectations interact with characteristics of the individual and the environment. Ideally, self-efficacy and outcome expectations are strengthened by these experiences and subsequently moderate behavior. Since self-efficacy and outcome expectations are influenced by performance of a behavior, it is likely that there is a reciprocal relationship between performance and efficacy expectations (see Figure 10.1).

Measurement of Self-Efficacy and Outcome Expectations

Operationalization of self-efficacy constructs is based on Bandura's (1977) early work with snake phobias. Self-efficacy measures were developed as paper and pencil measures that list activities, from least to most difficult, in a specific behavioral domain. In Bandura's (1977) early work, participants were asked to indicate whether they could perform the activity (magnitude of self-efficacy expectations) and then evaluated the level of confidence they had in performing the given activity (strength of self-efficacy).

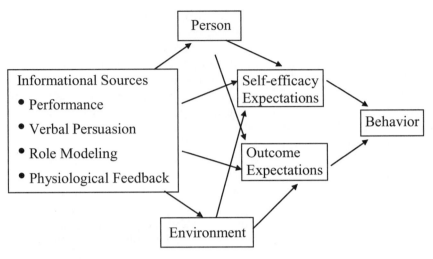

FIGURE 10.1   Self-efficacy.

Traditionally in the development of self-efficacy measures items are derived based on combined quantitative and qualitative research exploring factors that influenced adherence to a specific behavior such as exercise (Resnick & Jenkins, 2000). The self-efficacy for exercise scale, for example, includes nine items, with each item reflecting a commonly recognized challenge associated with exercise for older individuals (Resnick & Jenkins, 2000). Participants then responded by indicating if they have no confidence (0) or are very confident (10) (Table 10.1).

Development of outcome expectation measures has been less well-defined, although the process of establishing appropriate items is the same as it is for self-efficacy expectations. For example, the Outcome Expectations for Exercise (OEE) Scale was developed specifically to measure outcome expectations for exercise for the older adult (Resnick, Zimmerman, Orwig, Furstenberg, & Magaziner, 2001). The items for the OEE were written based on findings from qualitative research (Resnick & Spellbring, 2000) in which older individuals expressed the benefits they derived from exercise. Five of the items reflect physical benefits and four focused on mental health benefits. Individuals either agree or disagree with the statements provided.

USE OF THE THEORY IN NURSING RESEARCH

The theory of self-efficacy has been used in nursing research focusing on clinical aspects of care, education, nursing competency, and profes-

TABLE 10.1   How Confident Are You Right Now That You Could Exercise Three Times per Week for 20 Minutes if . . .

	Not Confident								Very Confident		
1. the weather was bothering you	0	1	2	3	4	5	6	7	8	9	10
2. you were bored by the program or activity	0	1	2	3	4	5	6	7	8	9	10

sionalism. Over the past 10 years there have been approximately 1,500 articles in nursing journals that focus on the measurement and use of self-efficacy expectations and/or outcome expectations to predict behavior.

These articles address education of nurses and caregivers, as well as management of chronic illnesses, health promotion, and disease prevention. The majority of this work has been geared toward behavior change-type interventions such as smoking cessation and increasing physical activity. The majority of these studies have been done within the United States, though there is an increasing literature supporting the use of this theory among Asians as well as other cultural groups. The majority of the work has been descriptive and correlational in nature, although there is a large base of research that has tested interventions implemented to strengthen self-efficacy and, less commonly, outcome expectations across a wide range of behaviors. What is most important with regard to the use of the theory of self-efficacy in nursing research is that the researcher maintains the behavioral specificity by developing a specific fit between the behavior that is being considered and efficacy and outcome expectations. If the behavior of interest is walking for 20 minutes every day, the self-efficacy measure should focus on the challenges related to this specific behavior (time, fatigue, pain, or fear of falling).

Self-Efficacy Studies Related to Managing Chronic Illness

Over the past 10 years there have been 71 studies in the nursing literature that focus on self-efficacy related to management of chronic illness. This work started in the area of management of cardiac disease (Taylor, Bandura, Ewart, Miller, & DeBusk, 1985), and Gortner and colleagues were some of the first nurses to initiate self-efficacy intervention research (Gortner, Rankin, & Wolfe, 1988). Jenkins's work built off that of Gortner et al., and she tested a self-efficacy intervention on recovery of 156 patients following cardiac surgery (Gortner & Jenkins, 1990). The use of self-efficacy theory to help individuals manage chronic illness continues to be prevalent in patients with congestive heart failure (Granger,

Moser, Germino, Harrell, & Ekman, 2006; Han, Lee, Park, Park, & Cheol, 2005; Johansson, Dahlström, & Bromström, 2006) and has extended to include those with stroke (Michael, Allen, & Macko, 2006), renal disease (Curtin, Mapes, Schatell, & Burrows-Hudson, 2005), diabetes (Hörnsten, Norberg, & Lundman, 2002; Lorig, Ritter, & Jacquez, 2005), and Parkinson's disease (Caap-Ahlgren & Dehlin, 2004). In addition, the self-efficacy work in chronic illness has focused on self-management of the symptoms associated with chronic problems such as pain (Arnstein, 2004; Boyle et al., 2004; Wells-Federman, Arnstein, & Caudill, 2002).

As with other areas of self-efficacy research, the majority of this work is correlational, although there are an increasing number of intervention studies testing self-efficacy-based interventions that add greatly to the literature. Siu, Chan, Poon, Chui, & Chan (2007) tested the impact of a self-management program on self-efficacy expectations in 148 Chinese individuals. Participants were matched on duration of illness and gender and then randomly allocated to experimental and comparison groups. The experimental group participated in the self-management program, while the comparison group joined a tai chi interest class in a mass-activity format. One week following the program the treatment group participants demonstrated significantly higher self-efficacy in managing their illness, used more cognitive methods to manage pain and symptoms, and felt more energetic than the subjects in the comparison group. Similarly a nurse-led pain management program for 154 patients with chronic pain resulted in increased self-efficacy, decreased pain intensity and pain-related disability, and fewer depressive symptoms among patients with chronic pain.

Several studies have considered self-efficacy expectations in adults with diabetes. Sousa, Zauszniewski, Musil, McDonald, & Milligan (2004) provided support theoretically for the use of self-efficacy theory in patients with diabetes. Specifically, the Sousa research team tested a conceptual framework for diabetes self-care management and found that individuals with greater diabetes knowledge had greater self-care agency and self-efficacy. Those with a higher score in social support had greater self-care agency and better diabetes self-care management, and those with greater self-efficacy had better diabetes self-care management. Multiple interventions have been developed using the theory to help patients with diabetes management. Sturt, Whitlock, and Hearnshaw (2006) recently described development and initial testing of a self-efficacy-based intervention, called the self-efficacy goal achievement intervention. It is comprised of patient goal-setting consultations with practice nurses using the Diabetes Management Self-Efficacy Scale. Pilot testing showed a reduction in participants' glycosylated hemoglobin of 0.93% between baseline and 3 months postintervention, an increase in patient self-efficacy, and some decline in patient diabetes treatment satisfaction. Heisler and Piette (2005) provide another example of an innovative nurse-initiated self-efficacy-based intervention in which role models, or peer supports, were used to improve diabetes management. Their study tested the feasibility and acceptability of using an interactive voice response (IVR)-based platform to facilitate peer support among older adults with diabetes. Of the 40 participants, 70% found the calls helpful in managing diabetes symptoms, 73% reported that their partner helped them improve their self-care, and 70% stated that they helped their partner do things to stay healthy. There were significant improvements in participants' reported diabetes self-care self-efficacy between baseline and follow-up assessments ($P < .01$).

The use of self-efficacy in diabetes management has been extended to include multiple ethnic and cultural groups. Specifically, self-efficacy has effectively been used with Turkish individuals (Kara, van der Bijl, Shortridge-Baggett, Asti, & Erguney, 2006), Australian (McDowell, Courtney, Edwards, & Shortridge-Baggett, 2005; Rapley, Passmore, & Phillips, 2003), and Chinese individuals (Shiu & Wong, 2002). More commonly self-efficacy measures and interventions have been used with African American populations (Montague, Nichols, & Dutta, 2005; Samuel-Hodge, DeVellis, Ammerman, Keyserling, & Elasy, 2002) and Hispanic groups (Lorig, Ritter, & Gonzalez, 2003; Lorig, Ritter, & Jacquez, 2005; Morgan, Buscemi, & Fajardo, 2004). The use of self-efficacy in diabetes management also crosses the life span and begins with use among women to control gestational diabetes (Homko, Sivan, & Reece, 2002) and includes the use of the theory among children (Faro, Ingersool, Fiore, & Ippolito, 2005) and older adults (Wolf, 2006).

Self-Efficacy for Exercise

There were approximately 200 studies over the past 10 years in the nursing literature that have focused on self-efficacy expectations and exercise behavior. Self-efficacy expectations have generally been positively associated with exercise (Jones et al., 2005; Vancouver et al., 2001), especially in correlational studies. Self-efficacy was significantly associated with the adoption and maintenance of exercise behavior (Hiltunen et al., 2005; McAuley et al., 2006; Moore et al., 2006). Expected outcomes in the form of perceived benefits from exercise were likewise associated with exercise behavior among older adults (Resnick, Vogel, & Luisi, 2005; Wilcox, Castro, & King, 2006).

Using the theory of self-efficacy, interventions have been developed and tested to increase exercise behavior in healthy community-dwelling

adults (Resnick, Palmer, Jenkins, & Spellbring, 2000) as well as those
who have sustained a hip fracture or orthopedic event (Resnick, 1998;
Resnick, Orwig et al., 2006), or among those who have cardiac disease
(Cromwell & Adams, 2006; Gary, 2006; Hiltunen et al., 2005), in cancer
survivors (Bennett, Lyons, Winters-Stone, Nail, & Scherer, 2007), in patients with chronic obstructive pulmonary disease (de Blok et al., 2006),
and in diabetics (Chau, Shiu, Ma, & Au, 2005). De Blok et al. (2006), for
example, tested a counseling intervention and noted that among 21 patients with chronic obstructive pulmonary disease (COPD) those exposed
to the treatment showed an increase of 1,430 steps/day (+69% from
baseline), whereas the control group showed an increase of 455 steps/day
(+19%) ($p = 0.11$ for group $\times$ time interaction). Resnick, Orwig et al.
(2006) tested a comprehensive exercise program, the Exercise Plus Program, for older adults post hip fracture that incorporated all sources of
self-efficacy information (mastery, verbal persuasion, self-modeling, and
physiological feedback) and likewise noted that those in the treatment
group showed an increase in time-step in physical activity and increased
number of steps when compared to those who received routine care.

   Although there is a consistent relationship between self-efficacy and
outcome expectations and exercise behavior when considered in cross-
sectional samples, it should be recognized that self-efficacy and outcome
expectations do not always increase when individuals are exposed to self-
efficacy-based interventions for exercise. In the study by Resnick, Orwig
et al. (2006) there were trends indicating that individuals in the treatment groups had a greater increase in their self-efficacy and outcome
expectations when compared to controls, but these differences were not
statistically significant. This may, in part, be due to measurement issues in
that the individuals participating volunteered for this exercise intervention study and therefore generally had strong self-efficacy and outcome
expectations at baseline. It is also possible that the intervention was not
strong enough to result in a change in self-efficacy and outcome expectations. Specifically, it is possible that changes might have been noted if the
intervention had started earlier (i.e., in the first 60 days postfracture). In
addition, the study addressed self-efficacy expectations with regard to
challenges associated with exercise, not confidence in the performance of
the actual exercises prescribed (e.g., walking for 20 minutes). The inclusion of such a measure might have shown a different outcome.

   The lack of a statistically significant improvement in self-efficacy and
outcome expectations has, however, been previously reported. McAuley
et al. (2006) suggested that a decline in self-efficacy following exposure
to an exercise intervention can also occur when there is a decrease in
exposure to exercise classes (or in this case the trainer in the home setting), when exposed to a new exercise program, when there is a change in

clinical condition or ability, or when the exercise program is progressively more challenging. It is therefore critical to consider these aspects when implementing exercise intervention studies.

Self-Efficacy for Health Promotion

In addition to using self-efficacy to increase exercise activities, self-efficacy theory has directed research in nursing with regard to a variety of health promotion activities. These studies focus on (a) weight loss (Beckman, Hawley, & Bishop, 2006; Burke, Dunbar-Jacob, Orchard, & Sereika, 2005; Walker, Pullen, Hertzog, Boeckner, & Hageman, 2006); (b) smoking cessation (Andrews, Felton, Ellen Wewers, Waller, & Tingen, 2007; Chen & Yeh, 2006; Sheahan & Free, 2005); (c) cancer prevention, specifically related to breast cancer (Crombie et al., 2005; Kelley, 2004); (d) safe sexual activity (Dancy & Berbaum, 2005; Dilorio, Dudley, Soet, Watkins, & Maibach, 2000); and (e) education related to pre- and post-operative care for cardiac surgeries (Parent & Fortin, 2000) and ortho-pedic surgeries (Moon & Backer, 2000). The theory has likewise driven research in the area of maternal–child nursing related to childbirth activities, breast-feeding (Wilhelm, Stepans, Hertzog, Rodenhorst, & Gardner, 2006), maternal self-efficacy related to care of toddlers (Hall, Clauson, Carty, Janssen, & Saunders, 2006), and care of children with asthma (Winkelstein et al., 2006).

In addition to a clinical focus, self-efficacy-based research has also guided the exploration of education techniques for nursing. Studies of undergraduates have focused on self-efficacy expectations related to academic performance (Pauli, 2005) and clinical skills (Schoening, Sittner, & Todd, 2006; Smith-Miller, 2006), and the impact of self-efficacy expectations for nurse practitioner students (Chang, Mu, & Tsay, 2006; Theroux & Pearce, 2006).

This report covers a wide array of topics and yet is only a small representation of the last decade of nursing research that used self-efficacy theory. Clearly, the theory is used extensively to guide nursing research, and the research has contributed to guidance for nursing practice.

USE OF THE THEORY IN NURSING PRACTICE

Translation of research findings into practice is not often done in a timely fashion. This is particularly true of research findings that focus on behavior change. There is, however, evidence to demonstrate that the theory of self-efficacy can help direct nursing care. The theory has been particularly helpful with regard to motivating individuals to participate in health-promoting activities such as regular exercise, smoking cessation, weight loss, and going for recommended cancer screenings. For example, Resnick and her research teams (Resnick, 1998, 2002; Resnick, Vogel, & Luisi, 2005; Resnick, Simpson et al., 2006; Resnick, Magaziner, Orwig, & Zimmerman, 2002) have used self-efficacy theory as a foundation for programs that encourage exercise and physical activity in older adults. The seven step approach to developing and implementing an exercise program for community-dwelling older adults incorporates the theory of self-efficacy. The seven steps include (1) education, (2) exercise prescreening, (3) setting goals, (4) exposure to exercise, (5) role models, (6) verbal encouragement, and (7) verbal reinforcement/rewards, all of which are designed to strengthen self-efficacy and outcome expectations. Each of the steps will be briefly discussed.

Education about exercise can be done both formally and informally, incorporating written materials appropriate for the individual. For older patients routine health care visits offer opportunities for education, as do periods of time during hospitalization. It is important that education be delivered with sensitivity to the unpleasant sensations associated with exercise, offering interventions to decrease unpleasantness. For instance, anticipating pain and fatigue, or identifying that the older adult fears getting hurt during exercise, the nurse can provide specific interventions to manage these problems. Exercise prescreening, the second step, is done using a simple prescreening form (Resnick, Ory et al., 2006), with the intent of assuring older individuals that it is safe for them to exercise at a moderate level. Next, it is useful to help patients identify appropriate short- and long-term exercise goals. The goals should be very specific. An example of a short-term goal might be walking three times per week for 10 minutes. The long-term goal might include being able to walk without an assistive device, going on a trip, or being able to get on the floor and play with a grandchild. The next steps focus on motivating the patient to actually begin exercising. Attempts should be made to get the individual to engage in the first exercise session. This exposure will help emphasize the benefits. Identifying role models such as a neighbor, friend, relative, or celebrity who exercise can be helpful, especially to get the individual to initiate the appropriate behavior. To be most effective the role models should be similar to the individual in terms of characteristics such as age and overall health status. Verbal encouragement to continue the exercise behavior, and positive reinforcement for any attempt at exercise, is an ongoing necessity for the program. When a patient comes back for a health care visit, the nurse must remember to ask about exercise activity, review how progress toward goals is occurring, and be enthusiastic with the patient regarding any progress. In many cases the reward can be support, excitement, and a hug for work well done.

The theory of self-efficacy also guides recommended steps for the development and implementation of restorative care nursing programs (Fleishell & Resnick, 1998). A five-step approach is recommended as a practical way to implement a successful restorative care nursing program and includes the following steps: (1) establishing an appropriate philosophy of care; (2) evaluating the resident; (3) motivating the resident to engage in functional activities; (4) getting to work, recognition, reinforcement, and reward; and (5) documentation, re-evaluation, and demonstrating outcomes. Steps 3 and 4, both of which focus on motivating the residents to participate in functional activities, are specifically geared toward strengthening self-efficacy and outcome expectations. Techniques such as verbal encouragement, performance accomplishment, role modeling, and decreasing the unpleasant sensations associated with performance are addressed. Similarly, self-efficacy theory has been used to guide the development of cardiac rehabilitation programs (Hiltunen et al., 2005). For patients to achieve the greatest benefit from such programs, nurses must help them modify unhealthy behaviors. The theory of self-efficacy provides systematic guidance, which allows the nurse to interpret, modify, and predict the patient's behaviors. Changes in lifestyle are commonly needed for individuals who must learn to live with chronic illness. The ease with which such changes occur is affected by self-efficacy and outcome expectations. Self-efficacy theory has been especially useful in helping patients to manage chronic disease and to adopt healthy lifestyles.

CONCLUSION

The studies that nurse researchers have done using the theory of self-efficacy provide support for the importance of self-efficacy and outcome expectations with regard to behavior change. The studies also provide support for the effectiveness of specific interventions that have been tested to strengthen both self-efficacy and outcome expectations and thereby improve behavior. It is important to note, however, that studies have also demonstrated that self-efficacy and outcome expectations may not be the only predictors of behavior. Other variables, such as tension/anxiety, barriers to behavior, and other psychosocial experiences impact behavior. Bandura (1986) recognized that expectations alone would not result in behavior change if there were no incentive to perform or if there were inadequate resources or external constraints. Certainly an individual may believe he or she can participate in a rehabilitation program but may not have the resources (i.e., transportation or money) to do so. In addition, when considered over time it is possible that self-efficacy and outcome expectations will not get stronger. Rather, the individual may recognize that it is not as easy to perform a given behavior, and self-efficacy and outcome expectations may actually weaken.

Self-efficacy theory is situation-specific. It is difficult, therefore, to generalize an individual's self-efficacy from one type of behavior to another. If an individual has high self-efficacy with regard to diet management, this may or may not generalize to persistence in an exercise program. Future nursing research needs to focus on the degree to which specific self-efficacy behaviors can be generalized. To what degree is self-efficacy a dimension of individual humanness, distinct for each person but consistent across a range of related behaviors for one person?

Measurement of self-efficacy and outcome expectations requires the development of situation-specific scales with a series of activities listed in order of increasing difficulty or by a contextual arrangement in non-psychomotor skills such as dietary modification (Bandura, 1997). It is important to carefully construct these scales and establish evidence of reliability and validity. These scales, which are behavior-specific, can be used as the foundation for assessing an individual's self-care abilities in a particular area. Interventions can then be developed that are relevant for that individual.

A persistent problem with the use of the theory of self-efficacy in nursing research has been the lack of consideration of outcome expectations. In particular, with regard to exercise in older adults, outcome expectations have been noted to be better predictors of exercise behavior than self-efficacy expectations (Resnick, Vogel, & Luisi, 2005; Wilcox et al., 2006). The influence of self-efficacy expectations beyond incentive to initiate behavior also needs to be considered. More important, how does self-efficacy influence behavior over time? Clearly, social cognitive theory and the theory of self-efficacy have helped guide nursing research related to behavior change. Ongoing studies are needed to continue to evaluate the impact of both self-efficacy and outcome expectations on behavior change, as well as develop and test interventions that strengthen these expectations.

REFERENCES

Andrews, J. O., Felton, G., Ellen Wewers, M., Waller, J., & Tingen, M. (2007). The effect of a multi-component smoking cessation intervention in African American women residing in public housing. *Research in Nursing and Health, 30*(1), 45–60.

Arnstein, P. (2004). Chronic neuropathic pain: Issues in patient education. *Pain Management Nursing, 5*(4), 34–41.

Bandura, A. (1977). Self-efficacy: Toward a unifying theory of behavioral change. *Psychological Review, 84*, 191–215.

Bandura, A. (1986). *Social foundations of thought and action.* Englewood Cliffs, NJ: Prentice Hall.

Bandura, A. (1995). *Self-efficacy in changing societies.* New York: Cambridge University Press.

Bandura, A. (1997). *Self-efficacy: The exercise of control.* New York: W. H. Freeman.

Bandura, A., & Adams, N. (1977). Analysis of self-efficacy theory of behavioral change. *Cognitive Therapy and Research, 1,* 287–308.

Bandura, A., Adams, N., & Beyer, J. (1977). Cognitive processes mediating behavioral change. *Journal of Personality and Social Psychology, 35*(3), 125–149.

Bandura, A., Adams, N., Hardy, A., & Howells, G. (1980). Tests of the generality of self-efficacy theory. *Cognitive Therapy and Research, 4,* 39–66.

Bandura, A., Reese, L., & Adams, N. (1982). Microanalysis of action and fear arousal as a function of differential levels of perceived self-efficacy. *Journal of Personality and Social Psychology, 43,* 5–21.

Bandura, A., & Walters, R. (1963). *Social learning and personality development.* New York: Holt, Rinehart and Winston.

Beckman, H., Hawley, S., & Bishop, T. (2006). Application of theory-based health behavior change techniques to the prevention of obesity in children. *Journal of Pediatric Nursing, 21*(4), 266–275.

Bennett, J. A., Lyons, K. S., Winters-Stone, K., Nail, L. M., & Scherer, J. (2007). Motivational interviewing to increase physical activity in long-term cancer survivors: A randomized controlled trial. *Nursing Research, 56*(1), 18–27.

Bootsma-van der Wiel, A., Gussekloo, J., DeCraen, A., Van Exel, E., Knook, D., Lagaay, A., et al. (2001). Disability in the oldest old: "Can Do" or "Do Do"? *Journal of the American Geriatric Society, 49,* 909–914.

Boyle, M., Murgo, M., Adamson, H., Gill, J., Elliott, D., & Crawford, M. (2004). The effect of a chronic pain on health related quality of life amongst intensive care survivors. *Australian Critical Care, 17*(3), 104–106, 108–113.

Brassington, G. S., Atienza, A., Perczek, R. E., DiLorenzo, T. M., & King, A. C. (2002). Intervention-related cognitive versus social mediators of exercise adherence in the elderly. *American Journal of Preventive Medicine, 23*(2 suppl), 80–86.

Burke, L. E., Dunbar-Jacob, J., Orchard, T. J., & Sereika, S. M. (2005). Improving adherence to a cholesterol-lowering diet: A behavioral intervention study. *Patient Education & Counseling, 57*(1), 134–142.

Caap-Ahlgren, M., & Dehlin, O. (2004). Sense of coherence is a sensitive measure of changes in subjects with Parkinson's disease during 1 year. *Scandinavian Journal of Caring Sciences, 18*(2), 154–159.

Castro, C. M., King, A. C., & Brassington, G. S. (2001). Telephone versus mail interventions for maintenance of physical activity in older adults. *Health Psychology, 20*(6), 438–444.

Chang, W. C., Mu, P. F., & Tsay, S. L. (2006). The experience of role transition in acute care nurse practitioners in Taiwan under the collaborative practice model. *Journal of Nursing Research, 14*(2), 83–89.

Chau, Y. S., Shiu, A. T., Ma, S. F., & Au, T. Y. (2005). A nurse-led walking exercise program for Hong Kong Chinese diabetic patients: Implications for facilitating self-efficacy beliefs. *Journal of Clinical Nursing, 14*(10), 1257–1259.

Chen, H. H., & Yeh, M. L. (2006). Developing and evaluating a smoking cessation program combined with an Internet-assisted instruction program for adolescents with smoking. *Patient Education and Counseling, 61*(3), 411–418.

Collins, R., Lee, R. E., Albright, C. L., & King, A. C. (2004). Ready to be physically active? The effects of a course preparing low-income multiethnic women to be more physically active. *Health Education & Behavior, 31*(1), 47–64.

Cress, M. B., Buchner, D. M., Prohaska, T., Rimmer, J., Brown, M., Macera, C., et al. (2005). Best practices for physical activity programs and behavior counseling in older adult populations. *Journal of Aging & Physical Activity, 13*(1), 61–74.

Crombie, K., Hancock, K., Chang, E., Vardanega, L., Wonghongkul, T., Chanakok, A., et al. (2005). Breast screening education at Australian and Thai worksites: A comparison of program effectiveness. *Contemporary Nurse: A Journal for the Australian Nursing Profession, 19*(1–2), 181–196.

Cromwell, S. L., & Adams, M. M. (2006). Exercise, self efficacy, and exercise behavior in hypertensive older African-Americans. *Journal of National Black Nurses' Association, 17*(1), 17–21.

Curtin, R. B., Mapes, D., Schatell, D., & Burrows-Hudson, S. (2005). Self-management in patients with end stage renal disease: Exploring domains and dimensions. *Nephrology Nursing Journal, 32*(4), 389–395.

Dancy, B. L., & Berbaum, M. L. (2005). Condom use predictors for low-income African American women. *Western Journal of Nursing Research, 27*(1), 28–44; discussion 45–49.

de Blok, B. M., de Greef, M. H., ten Hacken, N. H., Sprenger, S. R., Postema, K., & Wempe, J. B. (2006). The effects of a lifestyle physical activity counseling program with feedback of a pedometer during pulmonary rehabilitation in patients with COPD: A pilot study. *Patient Education and Counseling, 61*(1), 48–55.

Dilorio, C., Dudley, W., Soet, J., Watkins, J., & Maibach, E. (2000). A social cognitive-based model for condom use among college students. *Nursing Research, 49,* 208–214.

Estabrooks, P. A., Fox, E. H., Doerksen, S. E., Bradshaw, M. H., & King, A. C. (2005). Participatory research to promote physical activity at congregate-meal sites. *Journal of Aging and Physical Activity 13*(2), 121–144.

Faro, B., Ingersoll, G., Fiore, H., & Ippolito, K. S. (2005). Improving students' diabetes management through school-based diabetes care. *Journal of Pediatric Healthcare, 19*(5), 301–308.

Fleishell, A., & Resnick, B. (1998). *Stayin alive: Minimizing loss and maximizing potential: Manual for restorative care nursing programs.* Laurel, MD: Joanne Wilson's Gerontological Nursing Ventures.

Gary, R. (2006). Exercise self-efficacy in older women with diastolic heart failure: Results of a walking program and education intervention. *Journal of Gerontological Nursing, 32*(7), 31–41.

Gortner, S., & Jenkins, L. (1990). Self-efficacy and activity level following cardiac surgery. *Journal of Advanced Nursing, 15,* 1132–1138.

Gortner, S., Rankin, S., & Wolfe, M. (1988). Elders' recovery from cardiac surgery. *Progress in Cardiovascular Nursing, 3*(2), 54–61.

Granger, B. B., Moser, D., Germino, B., Harrell, J., & Ekman, I. (2006). Caring for patients with chronic heart failure: The trajectory model. *European Journal of Cardiovascular Nursing, 5*(3), 222–227.

Gyurcsik, N., Estabrooks, P., & Frahm-Templar, M. (2003). Exercise-related goals and self-efficacy as correlates of aquatic exercise in individuals with arthritis. *Arthritis and Rheumatology, 49*(3), 306–313.

Hall, W. A., Clauson, M., Carty, E. M., Janssen, P. A., & Saunders, R. A. (2006). Effects on parents of an intervention to resolve infant behavioral sleep problems. *Pediatric Nursing, 32*(3), 243–250.

Han, K. S., Lee, S. J., Park, E. S., Park, Y., & Cheol, K. H. (2005). Structural model for quality of life in patients with chronic cardiovascular disease in Korea. *Nursing Research, 54*(2), 85–96.

Harnirattisai, T. (2003). *Exercise, physical activity and physical performance in Thai elders after knee replacement surgery: A behavioral change intervention study.* Unpublished doctoral dissertation, University of Missouri-Columbia.

Harnirattisai, T., & Johnson, R. (2005). Effectiveness of a behavioral change intervention in Thai elders after knee replacement. *Nursing Research, 54*(2), 97–107.

Heisler, M., & Piette, J. D. (2005). "I help you, and you help me": Facilitated telephone peer support among patients with diabetes. *Diabetes Educator, 31*(6), 869–879.

Hiltunen, E. F., Winder, P. A., Rait, M. A., Buselli, E. F., Carroll, D. L., & Rankin, S. H. (2005). Implementation of efficacy enhancement nursing interventions with cardiac elders. *Rehabilitation Nursing 30*(6), 221–229.

Homko, C. J., Sivan, E., & Reece, E. A. (2002). The impact of self-monitoring of blood glucose on self-efficacy and pregnancy outcomes in women with diet-controlled gestational diabetes. *Diabetes Educator, 28*(3), 435–443.

Hörnsten, Å., Norberg, A., & Lundman, B. (2002). Psychosocial maturity among people with diabetes mellitus. *Journal of Clinical Nursing, 11*(6), 777–784.

Johansson, P., Dahlström, U., & Bromström, A. (2006). Consequences and predictors of depression in patients with chronic heart failure: Implications for nursing care and future research. *Progress in Cardiovascular Nursing, 21*(4), 202–211.

Jones, F., Harris, P., Waller, H., & Coggins, A. (2005). Adherence to an exercise prescription scheme: The role of expectations, self-efficacy stage of change and psychological well-being. *British Journal of Health Psychology, 10,* 359–378.

Kara, M., van der Bijl, J. J., Shortridge-Baggett, L. M., Asti, T., & Erguney, S. (2006). Cross-cultural adaptation of the Diabetes Management Self-Efficacy Scale for patients with type 2 diabetes mellitus: Scale development. *International Journal of Nursing Studies, 43*(5), 611–621.

Kelley, M. A. (2004). Culturally appropriate breast health educational intervention program for African-American women. *Journal of National Black Nurses' Association, 15*(1), 36–47.

Lorig, K. R., Ritter, P. L., & Gonzalez, V. M. (2003). Hispanic chronic disease self-management: A randomized community-based outcome trial. *Nursing Research, 52*(6), 361–369.

Lorig, K. R., Ritter, P. L., & Jacquez, A. (2005). Outcomes of border health Spanish/English chronic disease self-management programs. *Diabetes Educator, 31*(3), 401–409.

McAuley, E., Jerome, G. J., Marquez, D. X., Elavsky, S., & Blissmer, B. (2003). Exercise self-efficacy in older adults: Social, affective, and behavioral influences. *Annals of Behavioral Medicine, 25*(1), 1–7.

McAuley, E., Konopack, J. F., Motl, R. W., Morris, K. S., Doerksen, S. E., & Rosengren, K. R. (2006). Physical activity and quality of life in older adults: Influence of health status and self-efficacy. *Annals of Behavioral Medicine, 31,* 99–103.

McDowell, J., Courtney, M., Edwards, H., & Shortridge-Baggett, L. (2005). Validation of the Australian/English version of the Diabetes Management Self-Efficacy Scale. *International Journal of Nursing Practice, 11*(4), 177–184.

Michael, K. M., Allen, J. K., & Macko, R. F. (2006). Fatigue after stroke: Relationship to mobility, fitness, ambulatory activity, social support, and falls efficacy. *Rehabilitation Nursing, 31*(5), 210–217.

Montague, M. C., Nichols, S. A., & Dutta, A. P. (2005). Self-management in African American women with diabetes. *Diabetes Educator, 31*(5), 700–711.

Moon, L., & Backer, J. (2000). Relationships among self-efficacy, outcome expectancy, and postoperative behaviors in total joint replacement patients. *Orthopedic Nursing, 19*(2), 77–85.

Moore, S. M., Charvat, J. M., Gordon, N. H., Pashkow, F., Ribisl, P., Roberts, B. L., et al. (2006). Effects of a CHANGE intervention to increase exercise maintenance following cardiac events. *Annals of Behavioral Medicine, 31*, 53–62.

Morgan, B. S., Buscemi, C. P., & Fajardo, V. P. (2004). Assessing instruments in a Cuban American population with type 2 diabetes mellitus. *Journal of Transcultural Nursing, 15*(2), 139–146.

O'Connor, B. P., Rousseau, F. L., & Maki, S. A. (2004). Physical exercise and experienced bodily changes: The emergence of benefits and limits on benefits. *International Journal of Aging and Human Development, 59*(3), 177–203.

Parent, N., & Fortin, F. (2000). A randomized, controlled trial of vicarious experience through peer support for male first time cardiac surgery patients: Impact on anxiety, self-efficacy expectation, and self-reported activity. *Heart & Lung, 29*, 389–400.

Pauli, P. (2005). Using games to demonstrate competency. *Journal of Nurses Staff Development, 21*(6), 272–276.

Rapley, P., Passmore, A., & Phillips, M. (2003). Review of the psychometric properties of the Diabetes Self-Efficacy Scale: Australian longitudinal study. *Nursing Health Science, 5*(4), 289–297.

Rejeski, W. J., Katula, J., Rejeski, A., Rowley, J., & Sipe, M. (2005). Strength training in older adults: Does desire determine confidence? *Journal of Gerontology B Psychological Sciences and Social Science, 60*(6), P335–P337.

Resnick, B. (1998). Functional performance of older adults in a nursing home setting. *Clinical Nursing Research, 7*, 230–246.

Resnick, B. (2002). Testing the impact of the WALC intervention on exercise adherence in older adults. *Journal of Gerontological Nursing, 28*(6), 40–49.

Resnick, B., & Galik, E. (2006). Essentials in diagnosis of dementia. *Clinical Advisor Supplement*, 9–14.

Resnick, B., & Jenkins, L. (2000). Testing the reliability and validity of the self-efficacy for exercise scale. *Nursing Research, 49*(3), 154–159.

Resnick, B., Magaziner, J., Orwig, D., & Zimmerman, S. (2002). Evaluating the components of the Exercise Plus Program: Rationale, theory and implementation. *Health Education Research, 17*(5), 648–658.

Resnick, B., Orwig, D., Wehren, L., Zimmerman, S., Simpson, M., & Magaziner, J. (2005). The Exercise Plus Program for older women post hip fracture: Participant perspectives. *The Gerontologist, 45*(4), 539–544.

Resnick, B., Orwig, D., Zimmerman, S., Hawkes, W., Golden, J., Werner-Bronzert, M., et al. (2006). Testing of the SEE and OEE post-hip fracture. *Western Journal of Nursing Research, 28*(5), 586–601.

Resnick, B., Ory, M., Rogers, M., Page, P., Lyle, R. M., Coday, S., et al. (2006). Screening for and prescribing exercise for older adults. *Geriatrics and Aging, 9*(3), 174–182.

Resnick, B., Palmer, M. H., Jenkins, L. S., & Spellbring, A. M. (2000). Path analysis of efficacy expectations and exercise behavior in older adults. *Journal of Advanced Nursing, 31*(6), 1309–1315.

Resnick, B., Simpson, M., Bercovitz, A., Galik, E., Gruber-Baldini, A., & Zimmerman, S. (2006). Pilot testing of the restorative care program: Impact on residents. *Journal of Gerontological Nursing, 2*, 11–14.

Resnick, B., & Spellbring, A. M. (2000). Understanding what motivates older adults to exercise. *Journal of Gerontologic Nursing, 26*(3), 34–42.

Resnick, B., Vogel, A., & Luisi, D. (2005). Motivating minority older adults to exercise. *Cultural Diversity and Ethnic Minority Psychology, 12*(1), 17–29.

Resnick, B., Zimmerman, S., Orwig, D., Furstenberg, A. L., & Magaziner, J. (2001). Model testing for reliability and validity of the outcomes, expectations for exercise scale. *Nursing Research, 50,* 293–299.

Robinson-Smith, G., Johnston, M. V., & Allen, J. (2000) Self-care self-efficacy, quality of life and depression after stroke. *Archives of Physical Medicine & Rehabilitation, 81*(4), 460–464.

Samuel-Hodge, C. D., DeVellis, R. F., Ammerman, A., Keyserling, T. C., & Elasy, T. A. (2002). Reliability and validity of a measure of perceived diabetes and dietary competence in African American women with type 2 diabetes. *Diabetes Educator, 28*(6), 979–988.

Schoening, A. M., Sittner, B. J., & Todd, M. J. (2006). Simulated clinical experience: Nursing students' perceptions and the educators' role. *Nurse Educator, 31*(6), 253–258.

Sheahan, S. L., & Free, T. A. (2005). Counseling parents to quit smoking. *Pediatric Nursing, 31*(2), 98–102, 105–109.

Shiu, A. T., & Wong, R. Y. (2002). Fears and worries associated with hypoglycemia and diabetes complications: Perceptions and experience of Hong Kong Chinese clients. *Journal of Advanced Nursing, 39*(2), 155–163.

Siu, A. M. H., Chan, C. C. H., Poon, P. K. K., Chui, D. Y. Y., & Chan, S. C. C. (2007). Evaluation of the chronic disease self-management program in a Chinese population. *Patient Education & Counseling, 65*(1), 42–50.

Smith-Miller, C. (2006). Graduate nurses' comfort and knowledge level regarding tracheostomy care. *Journal of Nurses Staff Development, 22*(5), 222–229; quiz 230–231.

Sousa, V. D., Zauszniewski, J. A., Musil, C. M., McDonald, P. E., & Milligan, S. E. (2004). Testing a conceptual framework for diabetes self-care management. *Research and Theory in Nursing Practice, 18*(4), 293–316.

Sturt, J., Whitlock, S., & Hearnshaw, H. (2006). Complex intervention development for diabetes self-management. *Journal of Advanced Nursing, 54*(3), 293–303.

Taylor, C. B., Bandura, A., Ewart, C. K., Miller, N. H., & DeBusk, R. F. (1985). Exercise testing to enhance wives' confidence in their husbands' cardiac capability soon after clinically uncomplicated acute myocardial infarction. *The American Journal of Cardiology, 55*(6), 635–638.

Theroux, R., & Pearce, C. (2006). Graduate students' experiences with standardized patients as adjuncts for teaching pelvic examinations. *Journal of the American Academy of Nurse Practitioners, 18*(9), 429–435.

Vancouver, J. B., Thompson, C. M., & Williams, A. A. (2001). The changing signs in the relationships among self-efficacy, personal goals and performance. *Journal of Applied Psychology, 86*(4), 605–620.

Walker, S. N., Pullen, C. H., Hertzog, M., Boeckner, L., & Hageman, P. A. (2006). Determinants of older rural women's activity and eating . . . including commentary by Wilbur, J., Zenk, S. N., with response by Walker, Pullen, Boeckner, and Hageman. *Western Journal of Nursing Research, 28*(4), 449–474.

Wells-Federman, C., Arnstein, P., & Caudill, M. (2002). Nurse-led pain management program: Effect on self-efficacy, pain intensity, pain-related disability, and depressive symptoms in chronic pain patients. *Pain Management Nursing, 3*(4), 131–140.

Wilcox, S., Castro, C. M., & King, A. C. (2006). Outcome expectations and physical activity participation in two samples of older women. *Journal of Health Psychology, 11*(1), 65–77.

Wilhelm, S. L., Stepans, M. B. F., Hertzog, M., Rodenhorst, T. K. C., & Gardner, P. (2006). Motivational interviewing to promote sustained breastfeeding. *JOGNN: Journal of Obstetric, Gynecologic, & Neonatal Nursing, 35*(3), 340–348.

Winkelstein, M. L., Quartey, R., Pham, L., Lewis-Boyer, L., Lewis, C., Hill, K., et al. (2006). Asthma education for rural school nurses: Resources, barriers, and outcomes. *Journal of Scholarship in Nursing, 22*(3), 170–177.

Wolf, J. (2006). The benefits of diabetes self-management education of the elderly veteran in the home care setting. *Home Healthcare Nurse, 24*(10), 645–651.

CHAPTER 11

Story Theory

Patricia R. Liehr and Mary Jane Smith

Our belief in the healing potential of story-sharing, and our recognition of the importance of building theory at the intersection of practice and research have been essential to the development of story theory. The theory was first published in 1999 (Smith & Liehr) with the name "attentively embracing story." Since that time, after discussion with colleagues and students, most of whom questioned the complexity of the name, we thoughtfully simplified the name to "story theory," which has always been the essence of the theory. The central otology and epistemology of the theory remains as Reed (1999) described it nearly a decade ago. The ontology affirms that "story is an inner human resource for making meaning," and the epistemology is based in the understanding that "middle range theory bonds research and practice in a method of knowledge development" (p. 205).

PURPOSE OF THE THEORY AND
HOW IT WAS DEVELOPED

Stories are a fundamental dimension of the human experience. They bind humans to other humans and times to other times (Taylor, 1996). Stories express who people are, where they've been, and where they are going. The purpose of story theory is to describe and explain story as the context for a nurse–person health-promoting process. The theory was developed to provide a story-centered structure for guiding nursing practice and research. The core nursing process for practice and research is intentional dialogue occurring in a nurse–person relationship. In this

205

relationship the nurse gathers a story about a health situation that matters to the person.

The authors have had a long-term relationship that started in an educational program and cultivated discussion of common values about nursing practice and research. Smith began studying rest in 1975 with her dissertation research (Smith, 1975). Later, she conceptualized rest as "easing with the flow of rhythmic change in the environment" (Smith, 1986, p. 23). Liehr's (1992) dissertation examined the blood pressure effects of talking about the usual day and listening to a story. These early works were harbingers of what was to come in collaboration.

Years passed and we both pursued our own work. A serendipitous meeting at a nursing conference led to discussion of the importance of story for promoting health and human development. In talking about our individual work, we were struck by the commonalities that surfaced when we gathered stories. It became clear that story was a context for guiding practice and research. This clarity demanded articulation of a theory as a basis for further work. It was important that the theory be at the middle range level of abstraction to ensure applicability. The theory was developed in an enthusiastic discourse that fits the description by Belenky, Clinchy, Goldberger, and Tarule (1996) "as a place where people work at the very edges of their abilities, constantly pushing each other's thinking into new territory, giving names to things that have gone unnamed, dreaming of better ways, describing common ground and finding ways to realize shared dreams" (p. 13).

We began trying to name the theory to reflect our experience with patients and research participants. We had an image of the way story-sharing mattered to people when we listened with full attention. It took time to engage in the creative process of naming the theory. After several months and many names, we had the name that we believed accurately captured what we were describing. Once the theory was named, each of us began to view practice and research situations through the lens of attentively embracing story. As we used this lens to consider practice and research and discussed the theory with colleagues and students, we reflected on the theory name. We came to recognize that all people do not attentively embrace their story even when given the opportunity for story-sharing with someone who truly cares to listen. Readiness for embracing story and experiencing ease varies from individual to individual. The attentively embracing part of the theory name came from our early work with pregnant teens and persons in cardiac rehabilitation (Smith & Liehr, 2003). People who embraced their story of pregnancy or broken heart were people who moved on to purposeful living.

The original name limited expression of the complexity that is naturally inherent in the emergent human health story. We changed the name between 2003 and 2006. Although the process of attentive embracing is incorporated into the theory's meaning, the words were removed from the theory name. The current name, story theory, is more precise, parsimonious, and at the middle range level of discourse while still reflecting the basic nature and the complex process described in the theory. The name change is consistent with the original intent of theory applicability to any situation where a nurse engages a person to intentionally dialogue about what matters most to them about their complicating health challenge.

In our earliest writing on middle range theory (Smith & Liehr, 1999) we emphasized the importance of naming the theory in a way that describes the central core shaping the structure of the theory. What we did not discuss was that the theory name, like any other element or dimension of a theory, is a work in progress. When authors of a theory find that an element or dimension, such as a designated name, is not consistent with the core meaning of the theory, a change is in order. It is essential that the name be appropriate to the theory and offer a unique identity that clearly represents the theory.

We describe story as a narrative happening of connecting with self-in-relation through intentional dialogue to create ease. Ease emerges in the midst of accepting the whole story as one's own . . . a process of attentive embracing.

Foundation Literature and Assumptions

Story theory is at the middle range level of abstraction, holding assumptions congruent with unitary and neomodernist perspectives (Parse, 1981; Reed, 1995; Rogers, 1994). In these nonreductionistic views, human beings are transforming and transcending in mutual process with their environment. The mutual, ever-changing motion of creating meaning is essential to the unitary perspective. Developmental personal history and human potential for health and healing are essential to the neomodernist perspective.

The human story is a health story in the broadest sense. It is a recounting of one's current life situation to clarify present meaning in relation to the past with an eye toward the future, all in the present moment. The idea of story is not new to nursing. Several extant nursing theories explicitly or implicitly incorporate dimensions of story (Boykin & Schoenhofer, 2001; Newman, 1999; Parse, 1981; Peplau, 1991; Watson, 1997). The nursing literature frequently addresses the importance of the nurse's story (Benner, 1984; Chinn & Kramer, 1999; Ford & Turner, 2001), and Banks-Wallace (2002) emphasizes the place of story for researchers seeking to understand African American culture, which is embedded in an oral tradition. In her discussion about story as a vehicle for research, Banks-Wallace (2002) also notes the therapeutic value of storytelling.

Sandelowski has evaluated both the research (1991) and practice (1994) merits of the human story. Burkhardt and Nagai-Jacobson (2002) call attention to the power of story: "In the process of telling and hearing stories, persons often come to new insights and deeper understandings of themselves because stories include not only events in our lives, but also the meanings and interpretations that define the significance of the events for particular lives" (p. 296). McAdams (1993) describes processes occurring when interpreted meaning supports healing: "Stories help us organize our thoughts, providing a narrative for human intentions and interpersonal events that is readily remembered and told. In some instances, stories may also mend us when we are broken, heal us when we are sick" (p. 31). Arthur Frank (1997) refers to stories as ways to repair the damage caused by illness so that one's life path is reconstructed in the context of illness; he refers to "redrawing maps and finding new destinations" (p. 53).

Recent literature has called attention to "narrative" in health care (Charon, 2006; Charon & Montello, 2002). Charon and Montello (2002) address the role of narrative in medical ethics and interchangeably use the terms "narrative" and "story." Charon (2006) distinguishes the terms and simultaneously ties them together. "The word *narrate* itself combines roots meaning "to count" and "to tell" . . . narrative contains, almost like a repository or reliquary, aspects of human knowledge and experience that can, once stored—and *storied*—be drawn on again and again" (p. 60). Bruner (2002) reminded readers that both "telling" and "knowing in some particular way" are implicit in roots of "to narrate," and these roots are twisted together in complex connection.

For the purposes of our work, we refer to narrative within the context of story . . . story is a narrative happening. In this definition, story incorporates narration of events-as-remembered and infuses unique personal perspectives that shape meaning and guide choices in-the-moment. The current plethora of writings about narrative confirm our beliefs about the significance of story and remind us that this core dimension of nursing practice is now being recognized by other disciplines. Attention to story is a growing phenomenon. The multidisciplinary perspectives have contributed to more precise understanding and inspired continued effort to articulate the meaning of story for nursing practice. Nightingale (1946) called for a rejection of mindless chattering and a devotion to listening to the patient: "He feels what a convenience it would be, if there were any single person to whom he could speak simply and openly . . . to whom he could express his wishes and directions" (p. 96). Nurses have long known the importance of listening and they have known how to listen so that they could understand what matters most. Story theory articulates the implicit wisdom of practicing nurses . . . enabling guidance for practice and a framework for research. The assumptions that underlie story theory create a values-laden niche where the theory emerges.

The assumptions of the theory are that persons (1) change as they interrelate with their world in a vast array of flowing connected dimensions, (2) live an expanded present where past and future events are transformed in the here and now, and (3) experience meaning as a resonating awareness in the creative unfolding of human potential. The first assumption grounds sensitivity to the complexity of entangled health story dimensions to highlight persons moving with, through, and beyond their unfolding story. The second assumption invites a focus on the storyteller's present health experience with the listener's understanding that the storyteller's unique perspective incorporates the past and future in the here and now. The third assumption supports the human propensity to create meaning through awareness of thoughts, feelings, behavior, bodily experience, and other human expressions, all in the rhythm of the unfolding health story.

CONCEPTS OF THE THEORY

Story theory is composed of three interrelated concepts: (1) intentional dialogue, (2) connecting with self-in-relation, and (3) creating ease. According to the theory, story is a narrative happening of connecting with self-in-relation through intentional dialogue to create ease. Ease emerges in the midst of accepting the whole story as one's own . . . a process of attentive embracing.

Intentional Dialogue

Intentional dialogue is purposeful engagement with another to summon the story of a complicating health challenge. There is intention to engage in dialogue about the unique life experience of one's pain, confusion, joy, broken relationships, satisfaction, or suffering as a catalyst to seek a message and begin a process of change. Telling one's story happens in a trusting relationship with another where the nurse walks with the storyteller along a path, journeying a little further along to uncover what is happening, and paying attention to the unfolding movement of story, where both the storyteller and the nurse come to know better who they are (Campbell, 1988; Keen & Valley-Fox, 1989). Intentional dialogue energizes the experience of being alive by touching that which matters most of all to the storyteller. Throughout the flow of the story, the nurse holds fast to what has real meaning for the person who is recollecting what is past in the here and now, and accepting self as truly alive in the present moment of hopes, dreams, and expectations. In giving full attention to the other, the nurse "conveys to the speaker that his contribution is worth listening to, that as a person he is respected enough to receive the undivided attention of another" (Rogers, 1951, p. 34).

There are two processes of intentional dialogue: true presence and querying emergence. True presence is the nurse's nonjudgmental rhythmical focusing/refocusing of energy on the other, which is open to what was, is, and can be. It is "bringing one's humanness to the moment while simultaneously giving self over to the other who is exploring the meaning of the situation" (Liehr, 1989, p. 7). True presence is crucial to walking with the other who is sharing story. It is the substance of the nurse's activity during story sharing. Attending to the emergence of the unfolding health story assumes true presence and focuses on seeking clarification of the patterns that connect the beginning, middle, and end of a story. The nurse lives true presence by staying in while staying out. There is an all-at-once staying close to the story rhythm from the perspective of the storyteller while simultaneously distancing to discern patterns of connectedness. If the story is told over many encounters, it helps the nurse to make notes about story progress, possible patterns, and hunches about meaning.

Querying the emergence of the health story is clarification of vague story directions. Both the nurse and the storyteller attend to the story of the complicating health challenge. The nurse concentrates and tries to understand the story from the other's perspective. Nothing can be assumed about the story; only the storyteller knows the details. The story is never finished. There is always more to the story, including parts that the individual may not want to tell. The nurse in true presence stays with the longing to tell and the desire to tell only so much at a time.

Connecting With Self-in-Relation

Connecting with self-in-relation is the active process of recognizing self as related with others in a story plot. Hall and Allan (1994) identified self-in-relation as a central concept in their model for nursing practice and focused on the meaning of the concept for nurse–client interaction, noting that the "self is created in relation to others" (p. 112). Surrey (1991), who has developed a theory of self-in-relation, proposes it as the primary developmental process for women. The conceptualizations of Hall, Allan, and Surrey fit with our ideas in some places and misfit in others, but their ideas confirm a common ground of valuing self-in-relation as a dimension of human development and caring processes.

In story theory, connecting with self-in-relation is composed of personal history and reflective awareness. Personal history is the unique narrative uncovered when individuals reflect on where they have come from, where they are now, and where they are going in life. Venturing into the story is following the path of life as recollected. In the recollection, the nurse invites an awareness of self-in-relation to the complex context of a unique life. In following the story path, the nurse encourages reckoning with a personal history by traveling to the past to arrive at the story beginning, moving through the middle, and into the future all in the present, thus going into the depths of the story to find unique meanings that often lie hidden in the ambiguity of puzzling dilemmas. Self is affirmed in recognition and acceptance of nuances, faults and strengths, as well as understanding of how one has lived and how one envisions future hopes and dreams.

Reflective awareness, which is the opposite of taking life for granted, is being in touch with bodily experience, thoughts, and feelings. It relates to being in touch with one's view of and place in the world and, more concretely, in the moment (Kabat-Zinn, 1994). Reflective awareness enables thoughtful observation of self so that bodily experience, thoughts, and feelings are recognized for what they are as separate and distinct entities rather than personal defining qualities. For instance, when people in pain recognize that their pain is separate and distinct from who they are, they simultaneously recognize that they are more than their pain; that the pain is not a personal life-defining entity; and that they can be with the pain rather than being defined by it. With this mindful way of being in the moment, "there is a profound shift in one's relationship to thoughts and emotions, the result being greater clarity, perspective, objectivity and ultimately, equanimity" (Shapiro, Carlson, Astin, & Freedman, 2006, p. 379).

As the nurse guides reflective awareness on bodily experiences, thoughts, and feelings in a given moment of story, the storyteller becomes present to what is known and unknown, allowing unrecognized meaning to surface. Maslow (1967) describes the desire to know and the simultaneous fear of knowing. He states, "It is certainly demonstrable that we need the truth and we love to seek it. And yet it is just as easy to demonstrate that we are also simultaneously afraid to know the truth" (p. 167). Meaning changes when the unknown comes to light as known in an expanded present moment where there is coherence and integration. In telling the story, the person is telling the story to the nurse who is attentively present and at the same time telling the story to self. Reflective awareness on the personal history of story enlivens one's connection with self-in-relation to others and the world. It establishes an environment for creating ease.

Creating Ease

Creating ease is an energizing release experienced as the story comes together in movement toward resolving. It happens in the context of a person's search for ease and the nurse's intention to enable ease. The two dimensions of creating ease are remembering disjointed story moments and flow in the midst of anchoring. Remembering disjointed story moments is connecting events in time through the realization, acceptance, and understanding that come as health story fragments sort and converge as a meaningful whole. Polanyi (1958) discusses understanding as "a grasping of disjointed parts into a comprehensive whole" (p. 28). In the nurse–person dialogue, there is a remembering of disconnected moments as the nurse moves with the person through the story. Patterns surface as individuals shed a momentary light on the meaning of important experiences. Often, the nurse does not divert attention to the highlighted experiences when they are first introduced but tucks them into the background while staying with the foreground story. With focused presence over time, the nurse enables the other to illuminate issues, values, ideas, and context, uncovering coherent patterns of meaning in the tapestry of life experience. Disjointed moments are woven together as the storyteller remembers the health story in the presence of a caring nurse.

Flow is an experience of dynamic harmony, and anchoring is an experience of comprehending meaning. As patterns are discerned, named, and made explicit, anchoring and flowing occur all at the same time. Meaning surfaces while anchoring in a moment of pattern clarity, allowing a sense of flow and calmness. "Flow is the way people describe their state of mind when consciousness is harmoniously ordered and they want to pursue whatever they are doing for its own sake" (Csikszentmihalyi, 1990, p. 6). Csikszentmihalyi describes the harmony that ensues when one anchors to meanings, which capture purposeful unity and focus on life direction. He provides descriptions of individuals who used changing health situations to achieve clarity of purpose, noting that "a person who knows how to find flow from life is able to enjoy even situations that seem only to allow despair" (Csikszentmihalyi, 1990, p. 193). The defining feature of flow is "intense experiential involvement in moment-to-moment activity" (Csikszentmihalyi, 2005, p. 600).

Justice (1998), in describing pain, states that "when I keep mindful of the connections I have with a larger wholeness and order, I can often lift myself out of my pain or relieve it" (p. 108). He advocates paying attention to both sides of life to enable a sense of a larger wholeness or order. A whole story encompasses a life of gladness and melancholy, restriction and freedom, fear and security, and discrepancy and coherence. No story is one-sided. The person experiencing loss is also experiencing gain and the one who is lonely often has uplifting interactions with others. As the disjointed story moments come together as a whole, there is a simultaneous anchoring and flow through recognizing meaning and attentively embracing who one is in this moment of a life story. When story-sharing becomes a vehicle for healing, "embracing story" happens. Embracing story energizes release from the confines of a disjointed story where story moments are scattered making it difficult to discern a plot. Ease is resonating energy, enabling vision even for only a moment—a powerful moment creating possibilities for human development.

RELATIONSHIPS AMONG THE CONCEPTS:
THE MODEL

The theory comes to life in practice and research through traditional dimensions of story. Franklin (1994) asserts that stories are composed of complicating, developmental, and resolving processes. When gathering health story data, the complicating process focuses on a health challenge that arises when there is a change in the person's life; the developmental process is composed of the story-plot that links to the health challenge and suffuses it with meaning; and the resolving process is a shift in view that enables progressing with new understanding. The relationships among the concepts of the theory are depicted in Figure 11.1. This model is different from the first model of the theory (Smith & Liehr, 1999), which attempted to show the dynamic nature of the theory but failed to capture the all-at-once nature of intentional dialogue, connecting with self-in-relation and creating ease.

The current model attempts to depict a common flow of energy between nurse and person where story emerges. In this shared flux of energy all the concepts of story come together. The model incorporates story processes (complicating health challenge, developing story-plot, movement toward resolving) that provide a base for gathering story in research and practice. Story-plot is the organizing theme that brings events of the story together in a meaningful whole (Polkinghorne, 1988). It is proposed that developing story-plot about a complicating health challenge facilitates movement toward resolving.

Story is a narrative happening of connecting with self-in-relation through intentional dialogue to create ease. Ease emerges in the midst of accepting the whole story as one's own . . . a process of attentive embracing. Implicit in the description is the suggestion that story process begins with intentional dialogue to support connecting with oneself in relationship with others and with one's world with the possibility of experiencing ease. There is no doubt that the relationship among the concepts appears on the

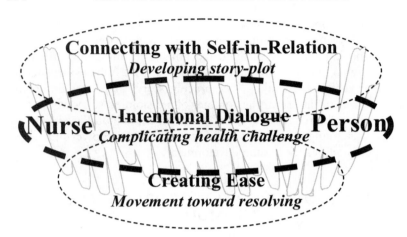

FIGURE 11.1   Story.

printed page as linear. However, the intent is that these concepts are in a dynamic interrelationship, a quality that is difficult to depict in a model. For example, moments of ease surface when the nurse first engages the person in a caring way to identify what really matters. Even a brief encounter with a caring nurse enables a connection before story parts come together as a whole . . . before embracing story occurs. Needless to say, the complexity of human interaction defies linearity. As nurse scientists we are called to fit language to the relationships among the concepts as best we can, recognizing that the simplicity necessary for models conflicts with the complexity recognized in most nursing phenomena.

Theory-Guided Story Gathering

The theory proposes common processes for gathering a story, whether the nurse is doing research or practice. These common processes are: complicating health challenge, developing story-plot, and movement toward resolving.

Complicating Health Challenge

A complicating health challenge is any circumstance where life change or pattern disruption generates uneasiness in everyday living. The health challenge may be an obvious illness-related phenomenon, such as the diagnosis of a serious illness, or it may be a naturally occurring developmental event like sending a youngest child off to college. It may be discomfort brought on by bullying or by the demand for lifestyle change. Whatever the health challenge, story-gathering begins when the nurse asks about "what matters most" to the storyteller. Attentive presence to "what matters" is a way of "being with," which places the storyteller at the center of attention. It carries the storyteller into the moment so that the present moment can be explored as mystery. Movement into the moment calls for connecting with the clear and centered intention to listen and hear the story with the storyteller leading the direction.

Developing Story-Plot

The nurse invites a reflection on the past, focusing on issues that have importance for the complicating health challenge in the present moment. These issues are the beginnings of the developing story-plot and are critical to understanding self-in-relation. We have described story-plot as "the unfolding story qualities, critical moments, and turning points that contribute to the health challenge" (Liehr & Smith, 2007, p. 121) and "issues that are critical to understanding the story and . . . the unfolding story qualities" (Smith & Liehr, 2005, p. 276). For instance, issues of changing life circumstances, cited by the storyteller when talking about a complicating health challenge, will generally be recognized as story-plot turning points. At the empirical level, story-plot may be documented as high points, low points, and turning points synthesized in the description of the complicating health challenge. High points include times when things are going well, low points are times when things are not going so well, and turning points can be important decisions or twists in the story all in the expanded present of the unfolding health story. Csikszentmihalyi (1997) believes that "the only path to finding out what life is about is a patient, slow attempt to make sense of the realities of the past and the possibilities of the future as they can be understood in the present" (p. 4). This path is a synthesis of high points, low points and turning points that characterize critical moments of the story.

Sometimes, the high points, low points, and turning points that create the story-plot can be uncovered by taking pen to paper and drawing relationship structures such as a family tree, which notes important relationships and serves as a base for understanding connecting with self-in-relation. The authors have described the use of a story path (Liehr & Smith, 2000) as a relationship structure that links present, past, and future of an unfolding story-plot. Another promising approach to story-gathering is photovoice, where people are encouraged to document a particular experience through photographs, which are then used as a foundation for story sharing about the experience. Carlson, Engebretson, and Chamberlain (2006) described the use of photovoice to collect stories about things that generated pride and things that needed to be changed in a lower-income African American urban community. Possible vehicles for story-gathering are limited only by the imagination of the nurse-scholar. The underlying principle to keep in mind when identifying a story-gathering structure is the intent of the story-gathering work and the potential of the structure to mirror the intent and enable a sense of the past and future expressed in the current moment of intentional dialogue about a complicating health challenge.

Movement Toward Resolving

Resolving happens in keeping the storyteller immersed in the "now" health experience. Finding a center of stillness and letting go of busyness and distractions energizes mindful attention to the story and propels movement toward resolving. Kunz (1985) contends that "centering quiets both the mind and emotions and thereby helps develop the power of focusing and intent" (p. 299). The experience of flow happens when the person is fully engaged in overcoming a challenge "that is just about manageable" (Csikszentmihalyi, 1997, p. 30). In a centered-present focus, one is free to take on the complicating health challenge and to view it in a manageable way. Oftentimes this shift to a manageable view energizes a sense of ease as a person attentively embraces the fullness of life emerging in the moment. It is an opportunity to change thinking and feeling and to move on differently.

Over the years, we have learned that movement toward resolving emerges along a spectrum including subtle recognition as well as all-out embracing the now-moment. Resolution does not close when the storytelling ends; it occurs in its own time. On some occasions, subtle recognition is a huge step along the path of human development, opening doors and pointing directions, enabling next steps.

USE OF THE THEORY IN NURSING RESEARCH

Since story theory was first published nearly a decade ago, we have explored ways to measure what is learned from practice stories and we have debated the best qualitative approach as well as the value of a quantitative approach for analyzing story data when guided by the theory. We have learned that there is neither a simple destination for the exploration nor an answer to the debate. To some extent, we ourselves, our students, our colleagues, and anyone who uses story theory to guide research is pushing the edge of understanding about how nursing practice stories collected through research can best be gathered and analyzed to access their inherent wisdom. Several examples of published research will be presented, highlighting the place that story theory has had in the research process. In these examples, the reader will find that the theory has been used to guide a story-centered care intervention and it has been used to guide story-gathering for research with both quantitative and qualitative analyses. Regardless of the place of story theory in a study design, health story gathered for the purpose of scholarly inquiry requires an analysis strategy based on a research question. It is the wording of the question that guides the method of analysis. Therefore, for each example, the research question will be made explicit. Finally, a recently introduced story inquiry analysis method will be described.

Research on a Story-Centered Care Intervention

In an effort to assess the power of story-gathering guided by story theory, Liehr and colleagues (2006) tested story-centered care for people with stage one hypertension. In this instance, story-centered care was an intervention randomly assigned to people who were receiving structured exercise and nutritional counseling after being diagnosed with stage one hypertension. The research question was: What is the difference in 24-hour ambulatory blood pressure (BP) when story-centered care is added to structured exercise and nutrition counseling for people with stage one hypertension? None of the participants was medicated for hypertension; rather, prior to entering the study, they had been instructed by their health care providers to adjust their diet and increase exercise. The major outcome variable, 24-hour ambulatory BP, was measured twice before and twice after the intervention over a 6-month period. Participants who received story-centered care in addition to the structured exercise and nutrition counseling had statistically significant lower systolic BP while awake than those who received only the exercise and nutrition intervention ($p < .05$). During story-centered care, advanced practice nurses engaged participants in four 1-hour dialogue sessions about the health challenge of integrating lifestyle change into their everyday patterns. This study was conducted with a small number of participants ($N = 24$), but the significant findings suggest that story-centered care guided by story theory shows promise for enhancing the effect of structured exercise and nutrition counseling for people with stage one hypertension.

Gathering and Analyzing Story Data

The story path approach has been effectively used to collect research data. When using this approach, the researcher generally begins with a line on a blank piece of paper and labels the line "the story of . . . ." to orient the research participant to the dialogue. The story will always be about a health challenge. Most often, the researcher begins with the present

. . . asking participants to identify where they are right now, today, on their life/health journey. Then, attention turns to the past and finally to the future. Researchers have found that the time-oriented dimension of this approach is more important than the actual line on a piece of paper. Sometimes participants engage with the researcher to "populate" the line with meaningful health challenge high points, low points, and turning points, and sometimes the line is seemingly dismissed by the participant as the present-past-future story unfolds. When this approach for gathering stories was first described (Liehr & Smith, 2000), its utility for collecting practice evidence was emphasized. As a research approach, story path enables collection of stories about a particular health challenge with the consistent structure of present-past-future focus. To this point, research-ers who have used the story path approach have collected focused stories in 20–40 minutes, and they have collected larger numbers of stories than might be traditional for qualitative studies. Therefore, researchers have sampled a broad range of participants before being assured of redundancy in the stories of health challenge. In addition, there are a greater number of shorter stories for analysis.

Analyses appropriate for story data include both qualitative and quantitative approaches. The use of a quantitative indicator may raise questions about the fit between the analysis strategy and the paradigmatic and theoretical underpinnings. A quantitative analysis that captures story progression offers congruence, as does relationship analysis where word-use is analyzed in association with health outcome indicators to expand understanding of a health challenge. Pennebaker and Stone (2003) refer to word-use analysis as a tool for accessing a window into personality. If one accepts this vision of word-use, a relationship analysis has potential to tie together personality–health qualities in an informative way. When word-use in a story about a health challenge is quantified, quantification is not intended to represent a measure of the story but rather a chronicle of story moments over time or an amplified understanding of a story–health outcome connection.

Research Using the Story-Path Approach for Data Gathering

Hain (2008) studied 63 people undergoing hemodialysis and she analyzed story data using a quantitative approach. One research question was: "What is the relationship between word-use in stories of lifestyle change and cognitive function for older adults undergoing hemodialysis?" She con-sidered word count, big words, words per sentence, and cognitive process words in her analysis. Story path was used to collect the stories about liv-ing with the challenge of lifestyle change. Cognitive function was measured with the modified mini-mental state (3MS) exam, which measures global cognitive function including orientation, attention, recall, and language.

Word-use was analyzed with Linguistic Inquiry and Word Count (LIWC), a software program developed by Pennebaker, Francis, and Booth (2001). The LIWC program is a word-based computerized text analysis software that discerns linguistic elements (word count and sentence punctuation); affective, cognitive, sensory, and social words; and words that reflect relativity and personal concerns. Seventy-two dimensions of language use comprise the LIWC structure for narrative evaluation. The structure has had psychometric testing, and reliability and validity estimates are reported by Pennebaker and King (1999).

Preparation of the nurse–participant transcripts for analysis included deletion of the nurse's words, correction of spelling errors, and removal of utterances that did not constitute recognizable words. After cleaning the data in this way, each transcript was saved as a text file. The LIWC program computes the percentage of words used for each word category and linguistic element. Hain's research questions the relationship between LIWC outcome indicators and cognitive function. The story data were considered in relation to the cognitive data, with the intent that word use in stories of lifestyle change would enhance understanding of cognitive function. Hain found statistically significant relationships between global cognitive function and the linguistic elements of words per sentence ($r = .41$; $p < .01$) and use of big words ($r = .37$, $p < .01$). In her discussion of the findings she suggests that these linguistic elements could be indicators readily detected by nurses who work with hemodialysis patients, allowing referral for cognitive assessments, which could contribute to better quality of care and improved adherence to lifestyle prescriptions (Hain, 2008).

Williams studied 40 caregivers of oncology patients and analyzed story data using a qualitative approach. The research question was: What are the sources of energy used by caregivers of bone and marrow transplant patients to meet their caregiving challenge? Story path was used to collect data (Williams, 2007). Data were analyzed with a descriptive exploratory qualitative approach using a model of informal caregiving dynamics previously created by Williams. Details about the findings of this study can be found in Chapter 14, where Williams introduces a midrange theory of caregiving dynamics.

Story Inquiry Research Method

Stories are the substance of qualitative research, and traditional approaches can be used when analyzing stories gathered with the guidance of story theory. For instance, phenomenological analysis is an example of an established way to analyze story data when the research question addresses the human experience (Giorgi, 1985; Smith & Liehr, 1999; Van Manen, 1990). Narrative inquiry may be another way to analyze story data. Clandinin and Connelly (2000) propose narrative inquiry for analysis when the researcher wishes to understand experience emerging in a social context over time. Their simple definition of narrative inquiry is "stories lived and told" (p. 20).

In 2007, we proposed a story inquiry research method closely tied to story theory to be used when analyzing stories collected for the purpose of addressing a complicating health challenge (Liehr & Smith, 2007). When using the story inquiry method, the researcher will naturally pose a research question related to a complicating health challenge. For example, what is the health challenge of being overweight? There are five processes in this inquiry method: (1) gather stories about a complicating health challenge using a meaningful consistent structure to encourage story-sharing; (2) begin deciphering the complicating health challenge with a focus on what "matters most" for the person sharing the story; (3) describe the developing story plot, noting critical moments (high points, low points, turning points) that carry the unfolding story forward; (4) identify movement toward resolving, recognizing that there will be a range in the "resolving" activity, and (5) synthesize findings to address the research question. We have just begun to apply the story inquiry method as proposed in these processes and, as usual, we are working out the kinks in the process. However, the method shows promise for contributing to development of nursing knowledge with direct applicability to nursing practice.

USE OF THE THEORY IN NURSING PRACTICE

The question leading the story when the foremost intention is caring-healing is "what matters" to the client about the complicating health challenge. In eliciting the story, the nurse leads the client along, clarifying meaningful connections about what is happening in everyday living in the context of the client's complicating health challenge. Sharing the health challenge story brings developing story-plot and movement toward resolving to the surface. The resulting story about "what matters" to the client provides distinct information about how one person lived the presenting health challenge.

Health Stories Collected During Nursing Practice

Health stories collected through application of story theory during nursing practice include those about exploring a new territory of calmness (Smith & Liehr, 1999); setting aside life burdens (Liehr & Smith, 2000); shifting vision (Smith & Liehr, 2003); drinking-driving (Smith & Liehr, 2005), and expressing disagreement through behavioral messages (Ito,

Takahashi, & Liehr, 2007). Summers (2002) used the theory as a foundation for mutual timing, a concept she believes is critical for effective health care encounters. Hain (2007) described querying "what matters most" in her work with hemodialysis patients. Jolly and colleagues (2007) used story theory when coming to know the meaning of "voice" for vulnerable adolescents in an urban practice setting. In Chapter 3, there is a story about yearning to be recognized from a woman who suffers migraines and a story about catastrophic cultural immersion from practice with hurricane survivors. In each of these instances, story theory was the lens for viewing nursing practice interactions, and most of the stories were gathered using the story-path method.

Stories are so integral to nursing practice that they are often gathered by nurses and used to guide health care decision making without a second thought about their potential for knowledge development. In 2005, Smith and Liehr introduced an approach for analyzing practice stories guided by story theory. Seven phases of inquiry were proposed to direct practicing nurses wishing to use stories as practice evidence contributing to knowledge development. The phases of inquiry are (1) gather a story about a complicating health challenge, (2) compose a reconstructed story, (3) connect existing literature to the health challenge, (4) refine the name of the complicating health challenge, (5) describe the developing story plot, (6) identify movement toward resolving, and (7) collect additional stories about the complicating health challenge (Smith & Liehr, 2005).

As the discipline of nursing moves toward educating greater and greater numbers of nurses with practice doctorates, it is important to honor the wisdom found in practice stories; to consider the potential of practice stories for advancing nursing practice scholarship; and to identify systematic approaches for using practice stories for nursing knowledge development. Story theory provides one systematic approach for viewing practice stories, where the stories create the foundation for knowledge development.

CONCLUSION

Collaborative work on story theory began in 1996, and the theory was first published in 1999. In the 12 years since we first began thinking through the meaning of story sharing for health, we have accomplished a great deal and have moved a short distance from where we began. Development and publication of the theory led to further consideration and description of use in practice (Liehr & Smith, 2000; Smith & Liehr, 2005). We believe that story is central to nursing practice and to nursing practice scholarship and we are committed to providing a structure enabling ready access to the wisdom of practice stories. Story theory provides a substantive guide for story-gathering in research and practice. Story processes focused on the complicating health challenge, developing story plot, and movement toward resolving have an inherent potential for growing nursing knowledge and guiding nursing practice.

Both quantitative and qualitative analyses have been applied to story data. We believe that several methods are appropriate for the qualitative analysis of story data, and we have recently proposed story inquiry method (Liehr & Smith, 2007), which is relevant when the researcher is pursuing understanding of a complicating health challenge. Linguistic analysis, using software programs such as LIWC, shows promise for quantitative analysis. Each time we share another dimension of our thinking on story theory with the nursing community, we learn more about the theory and formulate next directions. Middle range theory development is scholarship in progress with practice and research. As these thoughts are shared, new questions are realized, and so the story goes.

REFERENCES

Banks-Wallace, J. (2002). Talk the talk: Storytelling and analysis rooted in African-American oral tradition. *Qualitative Health Research, 12*(3), 410–426.

Belenky, M. F., Clinchy, B. M., Goldberger, N., & Tarule, J. M. (1996). *Women's ways of knowing: The development of self, voice, and mind.* New York: Basic Books.

Benner, P. (1984). *From novice to expert.* Menlo Park, CA: Addison-Wesley.

Boykin, A., & Schoenhofer, S. (2001). The role of nursing leadership in creating caring environments in health care delivery systems. *Nursing Administration Quarterly, 25*(3), 1–7.

Bruner, J. (2002). *Making stories: Law, literature, life.* New York: Farrar, Straus & Giroux.

Burkhardt, M. A., & Nagai-Jacobson, M. G. (2002). *Spirituality: Living our connectedness.* Albany, NY: Delmar.

Campbell, J. (1988). *The power of myth.* New York: Doubleday.

Carlson, E. D., Engebretson, J., & Chamberlain, R. M. (2006). Photovoice as a social process of critical consciousness. *Qualitative Health Research, 16*(6), 836–852.

Charon, R. (2006). *Narrative medicine: Honoring the stories of illness.* New York: Oxford University Press.

Charon, R., & Montello, M. (Eds.). (2002). *Stories matter: The role of narrative in medical ethics.* New York: Routledge.

Chinn, P. L., & Kramer, M. K. (1999). *Theory and nursing integrated knowledge development.* New York: Mosby.

Clandinin, D. J., & Connelly, F. M. (2000). *Narrative inquiry: Experience and story in qualitative research.* San Francisco: Jossey-Bass.

Csikszentmihalyi, M. (1990). *Flow: The psychology of optimal experience.* New York: Harper & Row.

Csikszentmihalyi, M. (1997). *Finding flow.* New York: Basic Books.

Csikszentmihalyi, M. (2005). Flow. In A. J. Elliot & C. S. Dweck (Eds.), *Handbook of competence and motivation* (pp. 598–608). New York: Guilford.

Ford, K., & Turner, D. (2001). Stories seldom told: Pediatric nurses' experiences of caring for hospitalized children with special needs and their families. *Journal of Advanced Nursing, 33,* 288–295.

Frank, A. W. (1997). *The wounded storyteller: Body, illness, and ethics.* Chicago: University of Chicago Press.

Franklin, J. (1994). *Writing for story.* Middlesex, England: Penguin.

Giorgi, A. (1985). *Phenomenology and psychological research.* Pittsburgh, PA: Duquesne University Press.

Hain, D. (2007). What matters most? Promoting adherence by understanding health challenges faced by hemodialysis patients. *American Kidney Fund: Professional Advocate, 7*(1), 3.

Hain, E. (2008). Cognitive function and adherence of older adults undergoing hemodialysis. *Nephrology Nursing Journal, 35*(1), 23–30.

Hall, B. A., & Allan, J. D. (1994). Self in relation: A prolegomenon for holistic nursing. *Nursing Outlook, 15,* 110–116.

Ito, M., Takahashi, R., & Liehr, P. (2007). Heeding the behavioral message of elders with dementia in day care. *Holistic Nursing Practice, 21*(1), 12–18.

Jolly, K., Weiss, J. A., & Liehr, P. (2007). Understanding adolescent voice as a guide for nursing practice and research. *Issues in Comprehensive Pediatric Practice, 30*(3), 3–13.

Justice, B. (1998). *A different kind of health: Finding well-being despite illness.* Houston, TX: Peak.

Kabat-Zinn, J. (1994). *Wherever you go, there you are.* New York: Hyperion.

Keen, S., & Valley-Fox, A. (1989). *Your mythic journey.* Los Angeles: Jeremy P. Tarcher.

Kunz, D. (1985). Compassion, rootedness and detachment: Their role in healing. In D. Kunz (Ed.), *Spiritual aspects of the healing arts* (pp. 289–305). Wheaton, IL: The Theosophical Publishing House.

Liehr, P. (1989). A loving center: The core of true presence. *Nursing Science Quarterly, 2,* 7–8.

Liehr, P. (1992). Uncovering a hidden language: The effects of listening and talking on blood pressure and heart rate. *Archives of Psychiatric Nursing, 6,* 306–311.

Liehr, P., Meininger, J. C., Vogler, R., Chan, W., Frazier, L., Smalling, S., et al. (2006). Adding story-centered care to standard lifestyle intervention for people with Stage 1 hypertension. *Applied Nursing Research, 19,* 16–21.

Liehr, P., & Smith, M. J. (2000). Using story theory to guide nursing practice. *International Journal of Human Caring, 4,* 13–18.

Liehr, P., & Smith, M. J. (2007). Story inquiry: A method for research. *Archives of Psychiatric Nursing, 21*(2), 120–121.

Maslow, A. H. (1967). Neurosis as a failure of personal growth. *Humanitas, 8,* 153–169.

McAdams, D. P. (1993). *The stories we live by.* New York: Guilford.

Newman, M. A. (1999). The rhythm of relating in a paradigm of wholeness. *Image: Journal of Nursing Scholarship, 31,* 227–230.

Nightingale, F. (1946). *Notes on nursing: What it is and what it is not.* Philadelphia: J. B. Lippincott.

Parse, R. R. (1981). *Man-living-health: A theory of nursing.* New York: Wiley.

Pennebaker, J. W., Francis, M. E., & Booth, R. J. (2001). *Linguistic inquiry and word count: LWIC2001.* Mahwah, NJ: Erlbaum.

Pennebaker, J. W., & King, L. A. (1999). Linguistic styles: Language use as an individual difference. *Journal of Personality and Social Psychology, 77,* 1296–1312.

Pennebaker, J. W., & Stone, L. (2003). Words of wisdom: Language use over the life span. *Journal of Personality and Social Psychology, 85*(2), 291–301.

Peplau, H. (1991). *Interpersonal relations in nursing.* New York: Springer Publishing.

Polanyi, M. (1958). *The study of man.* Chicago: University of Chicago Press.

Polkinghorne, D. E. (1988). *Narrative knowing and the human sciences.* Albany: State University of New York Press.

Reed, P. A. (1995). Treatise on nursing knowledge development for the 21st century: Beyond postmodernism. *Advances in Nursing Science, 17,* 70–84.

Reed, P. A. (1999). Response to "Attentively embracing story: A middle-range theory with practice and research implications." *Scholarly Inquiry for Nursing Practice: An International Journal, 13,* 205–209.

Rogers, C. R. (1951). *Client-centered therapy.* Boston: Houghton Mifflin.

Rogers, M. E. (1994). The science of unitary human beings: Current perspectives. *Nursing Science Quarterly, 7,* 33–35.

Sandelowski, M. (1991). Telling stories: Narrative approaches in qualitative research. *Image: Journal of Nursing Scholarship, 23,* 161–166.

Sandelowski, M. (1994). We are the stories we tell. *Journal of Holistic Nursing, 12,* 23–33.

Shapiro, S. L., Carlson, L. E., Astin, J. A., & Freedman, B. (2006). Mechanisms of mindfulness. *Journal of Clinical Psychology, 62*(3), 373–386.

Smith, M. J. (1975). Changes in judgment of duration with different patterns of auditory information for individuals confined to bed. *Nursing Research, 24,* 93–98.

Smith, M. J. (1986). Human-environment process: A test of Rogers' principle of integrality. *Advances in Nursing Sciences, 9,* 21–28.

Smith, M. J., & Liehr, P. (1999). Attentively embracing story: A middle-range theory with practice and research implications. *Scholarly Inquiry for Nursing Practice: An International Journal, 13,* 187–204.

Smith, M. J., & Liehr, P. (2003). The theory of attentively embracing story. In M. J. Smith & P. R. Liehr (Eds.), *Middle range theory for nursing* (pp. 167–187). New York: Springer Publishing.

Smith, M. J., & Liehr, P. (2005). Story theory: Advancing nursing practice scholarship. *Holistic Nursing Practice, 19*(6), 272–276.

Summers, L. (2002). Mutual timing: An essential component of provider/patient communication. *Journal of the Academy of Nurse Practitioners, 14,* 19–25.

Surrey, J. L. (1991). The self-in-relation: A theory of women's development. In J. Jordan, A. G. Kaplan, B. Miller, I. P. Stiver, & J. L. Surrey (Eds.), *Women's growth in connection: Writings from the Stone Center* (pp. 51–66). New York: Guilford.

Taylor, D. (1996). *The healing power of stories.* New York: Doubleday.

Van Manen, M. (1990). *Researching lived experience.* Albany: State University of New York Press.

Watson, J. (1997). The theory of human caring: Retrospective and prospective. *Nursing Science Quarterly, 10,* 49–52.

Williams, L. (2007). Whatever it takes: Informal caregiving dynamics in blood and marrow transplantation. *Oncology Nursing Forum, 34*(2), 379–387.

CHAPTER 12

Theory of Family Stress and Adaptation

Geri LoBiondo-Wood

Defining family for the purpose of nursing research and practice is a complex endeavor. Attempts to visualize and identify what family is gives rise to many pictures, all with their own nuances and character. Yet it is important to conceptualize family in a substantive way. In the last half of the 20th century, nurse family researchers have endeavored to explain through theory and research how some families, even amid misfortune, chaos, and tragedies, seemingly are able to cope and in some cases flourish. Explanation of family dynamics and what allows a family to grow and function across developmental levels and through normal and situational crises has led to the growth and the complexity of family theories and associated research.

A major area of work in family research has become known as family stress theory. The purpose of this chapter is to present a family stress framework known as the Double ABCX Model of Family Adaptation (McCubbin & Patterson, 1982, 1983a, 1983b). This middle range theory's purpose, major concepts and their relationship, and use in practice and research will be described.

PURPOSE OF THE THEORY AND HOW IT WAS DEVELOPED

To understand the Double ABCX Model, it is important to understand family stress theory. Family stress theory was originally developed by Hill (1949, 1958), who, after World War II, studied families' responses to war,

war separation, and eventual reunion. Hill's original ABCX family crisis model detailed three components that produced a crisis: a stressor event, family's existing resources, and the family's perception of the stressor. How these three factors interacted indicated the crisis-proneness of the family. An important point to understand in the history of family stress theory is that the original work was based on the traditional nuclear family of mother, father, and children.

The Double ABCX Model (Figure 12.1) conceptualized by McCubbin and Patterson (1982, 1983a, 1983b) is an expansion of Hill's original model, which has its roots in sociology. To Hill's original model, postcrisis concepts were added that predict family adaptation over time. The Double ABCX model has been used extensively to study family stressors such as chronic illness in children, cancer, and elder care. In order to emphasize adaptation as the key outcome of the Double ABCX Model, the extended model was renamed the Family Adjustment and Adaptation Response (FAAR) Model (Patterson, 1988, 1989).

As the body of family stress research grew and the variability of families was recognized, additional extensions were added to the model that focused on the key role that family types, strengths, and capabilities played in the understanding of family behavior. The extensions led to the development of another version of the family stress model called the T-Double ABCX Model of Family Adjustment and Adaptation. This

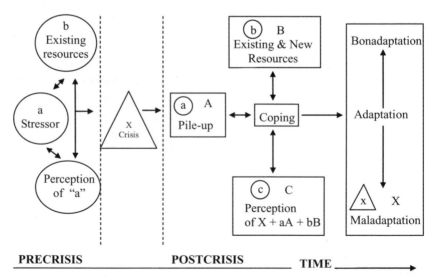

FIGURE 12.1   Family stress and adaptation.

model underscored the importance of family patterns of functioning for adjustment and adaptation (McCubbin & McCubbin, 1987).

The most recent conceptualization of the model was put forth to emphasize resiliency and includes Hill's ABCX Model, the Double ABCX Model, and the FAAR model (McCubbin & McCubbin, 1988, 1993a, 1996). All of these conceptualizations add important pieces to the puzzle of what the family is and how it functions and adapts in periods of tranquility as well as upheaval. The process of adaptation is active and includes the family's immediate environment and community relationships. McCubbin and McCubbin (1996) have outlined five overarching assumptions that underpin the middle range theory:

1. Families over the course of life face hardships and changes as a natural and predictable aspect of family life.
2. Families develop basic competencies, patterns of functioning, and capabilities to foster the growth and development of family members and the family unit, and to protect the family from major disruptions in the face of transitions and changes.
3. Families develop basic and unique competencies, patterns of functioning, and capabilities designed to protect the family from unexpected or non-normative stressors and strains and to foster the family's recovery following a family crisis or major transition or change.
4. Families draw from and contribute to the network of relationships and resources in the community, including its ethnicity and cultural heritage, particularly during periods of family stress and crises.
5. Families faced with crisis situations demanding changes in the family's functioning work to restore order, harmony, and balance even in the midst of change.

The focus of this chapter will be on the Double ABCX Model of Family Adaptation (McCubbin & McCubbin, 1996). As noted in the description of historical roots, this middle range theory was the first expansion of Hill's original work. The use of the Double ABCX Model alone versus the use of its extensions is a source of discussion (McCubbin & McCubbin, 1996). The original Double ABCX Model is straightforward in the definition of concepts and has many tested measures for research and clinical purposes, but it is possible to argue that ignoring the extensions may well be ignoring the highly complex and diverse processes and types of families seen in practice. An important consideration when choosing among the models and the model's extensions for research purposes is to follow the rule, as always, of carefully thinking through the problem that the research intends to explore and selecting a framework consistent with the problem being investigated.

For me, the choice was made after I had spent time with children who had received a transplant or who were waiting for a transplant. I was especially aware of the transplant experience as it affected the families of these children. There was little literature on the family impact of having a child receive a transplant. Therefore, interventions and caring strategies that could be used to educate and support families throughout this long-term process were lacking. In order to systematically develop this area I began to think about designing a research program. The first step was to explore the short- and long-term family impact of having a child who received a transplant so that later work could include development of research-based interventions for children and their families.

Research not only needs a clear question, it also needs a clear theoretical base that is consistent with the problem. This need took me to the literature about family theories. Qualities used to guide the search for a theory included (a) the theory had to fit or complement nursing, (b) it had to address the individual in the family as well as the family unit, (c) it had to conceptualize the family as a unit of interacting individuals, (d) it had to be multifactorial in nature, (e) it had to address strengths as well as weaknesses, and (f) it had to address the adaptability of families. The search was narrowed to a family stress and coping approach, and within this area the McCubbin Double ABCX Model was found.

This framework was well developed, had been tested in instances both of health and illness, took into account family strengths and weaknesses, and both individual (mother and father) and family adaptability could be assessed. Multiple-tested instruments were available that were consistent with the model. The Double ABCX model met the established criteria and offered a testable structure to guide research.

CONCEPTS OF THE THEORY

Key concepts of the Double ABCX Model are depicted in Figure 12.1. Each concept contributes either positively or negatively to the family's ability to adjust and adapt. The concepts are presented and discussed from the perspective of the theory.

Stressor (A)

The stressor was originally defined by Hill (1958) as a stressor event and later extended by McCubbin and Patterson (1983a, 1983b) as the "life event or transition impacting the family unit that produces, or has the potential of producing, change in the family social system" (McCubbin & Patterson, 1983b, p. 8). The stressor or demand has the potential to affect some or all of the aspects of a family's life. The change can occur in any aspect of the family's life, for example, in roles, functions, or goals. Though not depicted in the model, discussion of stressors is often accompanied by discussion of hardships, which are the demands placed on the family. These demands must be met as a result of the stressor event.

Existing Resources (B)

All families have some level of resources. The concept of existing resources is the family's use of community as well as intrafamilial resources. For instance, the parents' level of education and socioeconomic status serve as major resources. Within the framework the stressor is viewed as interacting with the family's use of resources, which act as a buffer for resisting crisis. Resources can be economic or social and can include hardiness and religious beliefs. The resources in the family may be adequate or inadequate, depending on the nature of the stressor event, level of family development, or the family's level of functioning.

Perception of the Stressor (C)

The perception of the stressor is defined by Hill (1958) and McCubbin and Patterson (1983a, 1983b) as the meaning the family assigns to the crisis event and the total circumstances that lead to the crisis. How well a family is able to clarify all aspects of the problem contributes to the family's problem-solving ability. Along with the cultural views of the family, it is the family's subjective interpretation of the effect of the stressor event that is most important. The concept of perception focuses on whether the family views the stressor as manageable or unmanageable. If the stressor is seen as unmanageable it has the potential to initiate family disintegration. In the model, stress is distinguished from a stressor. Whereas a stressor is an event, stress is a state of demand that arises from an actual or perceived demand with the capability of creating instability in family functioning (McCubbin & Patterson, 1983a, 1983b). Stress varies and can affect the family both psychologically and physiologically.

Crisis (X)

The crisis is a demand for change that reflects the sum of the family's disorganization, turmoil, and disruption triggered by an event (Burr, 1973). Within the model the crisis is regarded as the family's inability to maintain stability due to the continuous struggle in the situation. The stressor (a), interacting with the resources (b), and the family perception of the stressor or how the family defines the stressor (c), produces the crisis (x) (Hill, 1949, 1958). If a family has the ability to meet the demands of a stressor event then a crisis may be averted.

Pile-Up (aA Factor)

Pile-up is the effect of managing changes, strains, and stressors over time. The stressors families deal with change and accumulate, affecting each member. This concept was added in the extension of Hill's model to the Double ABCX Model. The idea of pile-up was based on longitudinal research in families where a father/husband was held prisoner or was missing in action during the Vietnam War (McCubbin & Patterson, 1983a, 1983b). The findings of this research suggested that families facing a stressor event experience phases of adjustment and adaptation exemplified by a range of complex interacting processes depicted by the theory.

The Double ABCX Model of Adaptation and Adjustment was conceptualized from the perspective that families rarely are managing a single event or stressor, but, in fact, manage a pile-up of stressors and strains over time. The demands may arise as a result of an individual in the family, the family system, and/or from the community in which the family resides. The demands are caused by an initial stressor and the resultant pressures of the stressor. McCubbin and Patterson (1983a, 1983b) suggest that five types of stressors contribute to a pile-up:

1. The initial crisis with the resultant need for role change and readjustments;
2. Normative transitions that occur concomitantly with the stressor event;
3. Prior strains or earlier strains that a family may not have fully resolved that emerge at the time of a new crisis;
4. Disapproval from family members as one attempts to cope with the crisis by changing behavior;
5. Ambiguity related to structure, roles, and functions of the family.

Existing and New Resources (bB)

Existing, new, and expanded resources allow the family to adapt and meet demands and needs. Usual mechanisms of support are the existing resources. A family in the face of a crisis will call on existing resources to prevent an event from creating further crisis. Expanded family resources are resources strengthened or developed in response to the crisis or as a result of the pile-up of stressors. In a longitudinal study of families with children with cerebral palsy, McCubbin and Patterson (1982) identified four types of resources that strengthened or developed in response to the crisis situation:

1. Self-reliance—personal resources of individual family members, such as self-esteem;
2. Family integration—internal workings of the family that assist members, such as communication patterns;
3. Social support—family members' knowledge that they are cared for, loved, valued, and belong to a network of mutual understanding and responsibility;
4. Collective group support (including group action)—networks of family, friends, and community beyond the immediate family group, who provide support.

Family Perception of the Stressor (cC)

The family's view, definition, and significance given to the stressor and its resultant hardships, the pile-up of stressors, and the meaning the family attaches to the total situation define the family's perception of the stressor. A family that aims to comprehend the meaning of the situation can minimize the psychological toll related to the crisis. In addition, comprehending the meaning can facilitate being more able to cope, use and develop resources, and adapt. The family's perception of the crisis is a key element and becomes a central factor of family coping.

Coping

Coping is an active process encompassing the use of existing and new resources that help to strengthen the family unit, reduce the impact of the stressors, and enhance the family's perception of the crisis and resultant behavioral responses. In the Double ABCX framework, coping with the crisis is related to adaptation. Coping has both behavioral and cognitive elements.

Parents' coping strategies are an important management resource during a family crisis. Coping allows the family to eliminate, reduce, or avoid stressors and strain, manage the situation, and implement changes where necessary to maintain the family system. Coping then becomes a bridging concept in which the family's efforts are directed to decrease situation stressors and increase family movement toward adaptation and adjustment.

Adaptation (xX)

Adaptation, the outcome concept in this middle range theory, means that the family has accommodated, compromised, and, through inner workings, regulated and given meaning to a crisis. Family adaptation is considered at the levels of individual, family system, and community. Each of these levels has demands and capabilities. Adaptation is realized when there is a balance between one of the levels with another. Family coherence, which is the ability of the family to balance the elements depicted in the model of the theory, is a core component of adaptation. Adaptation exists as a continuum from bonadaptation to maladaptation. Bonadaptation is positive and occurs when the family has achieved a balance minimizing discrepancy between resources and demands. With bonadaptation the family has used coping strategies to accept and understand the meaning of the crisis. This understanding gives the family a sense of balance and coherence. Maladaptation is the negative end of the continuum and is typified by family imbalance. The family that presents as maladaptive exhibits physical or psychological ill health and deterioration in family integrity and family functioning.

RELATIONSHIPS AMONG THE CONCEPTS: THE MODEL

The process that the theory's model depicts is viewed as an interactive process of system-environment fit over time (see Figure 12.1). Based on research (McCubbin, Dahl, Lester, & Ross, 1977; McCubbin, Hunter, & Metres, 1974), the recognition that the family is not stagnant, and that crises have long-term implications, the Double ABCX Model was extended to include three stages of adaptation. These stages are resistance, restructuring, and consolidation. They were used to reconceptualize and extend the Double ABCX Model into the Family Adjustment and Adaptation Response (FAAR) Model. The processes in the model emphasize the importance of the element of time for the family and suggest that families do not move in a linear manner from crisis to adaptation. For an extensive discussion of the FAAR model and other additions to the Double ABCX Model, the reader is referred to the many works that have been published by the Center for Excellence in Family Studies at the University of Wisconsin–Madison and the publication *Family assessment: Resiliency, coping and adaptation.* (McCubbin, Thompson, & McCubbin, 1996).

Double ABCX Model: Strengths and Limitations

The Double ABCX Model has both strengths and limitations. Among the model's strengths is the fact that it is a tested middle range theory that focuses on the family as a whole and allows for measurement of multiple family qualities. As the view of family has changed and expanded so has the model to reflect growth in conceptual assessment. All concepts of the theory have been operationally defined with instruments that have been tested widely for their psychometric properties, and all have more than one measure that can be used to test it.

On the negative side, it has been noted that the model has a large number of concepts, and that with all its extensions the concepts are sometimes not distinguished well from each other. For example, it has been noted that family resources overlap with family problem solving and coping (Rungreangkulkij & Gilliss, 2000). Earlier, Walker (1985), while emphasizing the importance of the framework, pointed out that individual resources are interchangeable with family resources even though they are conceptually distinct; she further suggested that an event-specific stressor may not be an adequate conceptualization because it is too narrowly focused. The crisis event, if viewed more broadly as a situation, allows for a more expanded view of the concept of crisis. McCubbin and McCubbin (1996) have stated that the crisis is not necessarily event specific but an imbalance that can be the result of a normative or developmental situation or of a traumatic situation that called the family members into action.

Therefore, if one views family and the work of the family as a process, one cannot say that it is one event that leads to a crisis but rather several components of a situation and how a family adjusts. In the later iterations of the model the crisis event has been minimized and the picture of the family and its resiliency in response to a situation has become a stronger focus. Because of the number of concepts in the model's extension and because of overlapping of some of the concepts, it is important for researchers to clearly identify and define the concepts being addressed in their research questions. It is also important to clearly specify the parts of the theory being studied and which iteration of the theory is being used.

Clarity about the concept being tested will enable appropriate selection of measures. As more concepts are added to a study, the complexity of analysis increases, and the importance of being conceptually clear escalates. Rungreangkulkij and Gilliss (2000) alert researchers to the challenge of multicolinearity and the use of complex statistical analysis when using the model to guide research.

USE OF THE THEORY IN NURSING RESEARCH

The Double ABCX Model has sometimes been studied as a whole. For instance, McCubbin (1988) used the model to study family stress, resources, and family types in families with chronically ill children. Mc-Cubbin later compared single-parent and two-parent families with handicapped children using the Typology Model, an expansion of the Double ABCX Model.

McCubbin (1988) found no significant differences between single-parent and two-parent families in the accumulation of stressors and demands, resource strains, family types, family cohesion, family resources of esteem/communication, mastery/health, extended social support, and child health indices of physical health status. Single-parent families had significantly lower financial cooperation and situational optimism. This study matched families on the child's handicap severity and the parent's age and gender.

More often than not studies select and study specific concepts from the model rather than the whole model. Leske (2003) used the resiliency extension of the model to guide her study that compared family stressors, family strengths, family coping, family well-being, and family adaptation after trauma such as motor vehicle crashes, gunshot wounds (GSW), and coronary-artery by-pass surgery (CABG). The instruments used, except for the measure of patient injury factors the APACHE III and the Family Adaptation Scale (Antonovsky & Sourani, 1988), were specifically developed for use when studying concepts in the model. The results indicated that family members of patients with different types of critical injury or CABG surgery seemed to be more alike than different in terms of responses to measures of hardiness, well-being, and adaptation. Yet, family members of patients who were injured from a GSW reported significantly higher levels of prior stress than the other two groups. The findings of this study are interesting because they seem to support the underlying theory, yet they should be taken with caution as the sample size was small and the design was cross-sectional.

In another example of research using a limited set of the theory's concepts, Board and Ryan-Wenger (2003) and Board and Ryan-Wenger (2002) used the extended McCubbin and McCubbin Resiliency Model of Family Stress (1993b) framework and focused on measuring prospectively the differences in family perception of stress between parents who had a child in the Pediatric Intensive Care Unit (PICU), parents with a child in a general care unit (GCU), and parents with a non-hospitalized ill child. The researchers measured indicators of family adaptation including parental stress, stress symptoms, family functioning, and family pile-up of life events. The researchers who conducted these studies address some of the issues related to doing family research, such as difficulty with recruiting fathers and the challenge of selecting a representative set of concepts for measurement. Suddaby, Flattery, and Luna (1997) used the Double ABCX Model but focused on measuring stress and coping among families awaiting their child's cardiac transplant. This study found parents' use of coping mechanisms decreased over a 3-month pretransplant period, yet overall stress remained at a moderate level and did not change significantly.

The Research of LoBiondo-Wood and Colleagues

The specific example of several studies from one research program that focused on children undergoing liver transplantation and their families will be described as framed within the Double ABCX Model. When an individual requires solid organ transplantation the processes involved in obtaining and maintaining the recipient's new organ affect the family as a whole. The stages before and after the transplant require adjustment and adaptation. Each stage of the process, for both the recipient and the family, has costs in terms of physical and psychological factors, time, money, and stress. LoBiondo-Wood and Williams and colleagues conducted several studies that used the Double ABCX Model (McCubbin & Patterson, 1983a, 1983b) as its guiding framework. Only the postcrisis concepts were measured in both the pretransplantation and posttransplantation periods. Data documenting these postcrisis findings will be reported, and the precrisis concepts noted in the model will be discussed as related to the research (Figure 12.1).

Stressors (A). By the time the parents of a child who needs a liver transplant make the decision with their care providers to seek a transplant evaluation and pursue transplantation, the child often has experienced multiple bouts of illness and/or surgery. The parents have had varying amounts of time to adjust to the idea that their child has a chronic and potentially fatal disease.

Existing Resources (B). The existing resources for the family include use of community resources, parents' education level, medical resources, and socioeconomic status. Availability of support from the extended family for a family entering the transplantation process is important.

Perception of the Stressor (C). The meaning that the family gives to the child's illness and the help received from caregivers contributes to the family's definition of the stressor as manageable or unmanageable.

Crisis (X). The time until transplant and the impending needs and challenges that the family faces when seeking a transplant on behalf of their child constitutes the crisis.

Pile-Up (aA). For the family with a child with end-stage liver disease, the parents awaiting a transplant, and the parents who have a child who has received a transplant, stressors can be found at any point. The first type of stressor is inherent to the diagnosis and medical care needed in the face of recurring illnesses that accompany liver disease. Parents are told of long waiting lists and of the necessity of keeping the child as well as possible before the transplant; yet the parents also know that the sicker child receives a transplant first. Parents have to work with multiple caregivers and may have to take their child to a different health care setting.

Parents whose child is in the pretransplantation period may feel abandoned and forgotten. Other stressors include the family life changes and events that occur irrespective of the central stressor, such as child and parental developmental needs and job-related stressors. Stressors also pile up related to financial burdens, loss of control, and the potential need to involve the public with fund raising. Long-term stressors include the uncertainty of the child's long-term prognosis and the painful affect that burdens parents of chronically ill children (Benning & Smith, 1994; Uzark, 1992).

Family Existing and New Resources (bB). For families seeking and obtaining a transplant for their child, the network of resources and social support may vary over time. Potential support sources are family, health caregivers, friends, and community. Because of the long-term nature of the situation, the family, in order to adapt and adjust, must assimilate new resources and supports that will help the family and the child before and after transplantation. During hospitalization, a strong network among the families and the health care team persists and can either serve as a source of support or reinforce stressors, such as would occur if one of the recipients in the network dies or needs retransplantation. Once the child is discharged and returns home old networks as well as newer ones must be maintained.

Perception of the Stressor (cC). The process of seeking transplantation places multiple new stressors on an already stressed system, consequently reframing and redefining the situation. A family might perceive the diagnosis of a chronic and possibly fatal disease as a relief because it provides a label for the problem and a potential solution. The diagnosis also may be a threat because of the implications that the label brings with it. After transplantation parents voice concerns about whether their child will live and lead a normal life in light of the reality that liver transplantation does not cure the child's liver disease but rather trades the original disease for a new liver that requires lifelong specific health care (LoBiondo-Wood, Bernier-Henn, & Williams, 1992).

Coping. Coping requires the family to actively manage a variety of factors and situations at each stage of the transplant process. Coping is viewed as an active process of engaging management strategies, which may be psychological or behavioral. The movement to adjustment and adaptation is predicated on the assumption that the family has developed adaptive coping strategies.

Adaptation (xX). The view of adaptation is based on McCubbin and Patterson's (1983a, 1983b) belief that adaptation is the continuum of outcomes toward which the family's efforts are directed. The process of adaptation is interactive over time. Though not using the Double ABCX Model, Mishel and Murdaugh (1987) found in a study of family adjustment 1 year following adult heart transplantation that family members initially thought that the patient would return to normal after the transplant. However, they found that adjustments were continually being made and the family member's belief of a return to normal was gradually eroded. In the process of reconceptualization and adjustment, the families became aware of the need to redefine the term *normal*.

In a series of studies LoBiondo-Wood and colleagues (LoBiondo-Wood, Bernier-Henn, & Williams, 1992; LoBiondo-Wood, Williams, Kouzekanani, & McGhee, 2000; LoBiondo-Wood, Williams, & McGhee, 2004) found that families seeking transplantation for their child live through an experience depicted by the Double ABCX Model. Adaptation was not viewed as ending but as continuing over time. Before the transplant and after a successful transplant, the child and the parents have to cope, use resources, and deal with the stressors of the long-term situation. The pile-up of stressors at each stage of the process may lead to bonadaptation or maladaptation, depending on the family's ability to use new and old strategies.

In this research, after the concepts for study were selected, measurement instruments were chosen. The concepts of the double ABCX Model and the measurement instruments are outlined in Table 12.1. In the pretransplantation period the researchers found that higher family stressors, fewer coping skills, and higher perceptions of stress were related to more unhealthy family adaptation (LoBiondo-Wood, Williams, Kouzekanani, & McGhee, 2000). In the prospective study (LoBiondo-Wood, Williams, & McGhee, 2004), from the mothers' perspective, families seemed to be able to adapt and maintain balance over time moving toward health while in the midst of adapting to the child's needs.

USE OF THE THEORY IN NURSING PRACTICE

Although technology has improved health care for individuals and families, the number of families with chronically ill members has increased. The concepts of the Double ABCX Model focus on specific aspects of the illness trajectory that families experience. Therefore, the theory can be useful in assessing, planning, and implementing practice interventions.

The theory calls nurses to understand the processes and stages of the illness and to understand how families adjust and adapt to a crisis situation. Development of a short- and long-term plan for the individual and family can be based on the concepts of stressors, existing resources, and perception of stressors, crisis, and pile-up. As a plan is developed it

TABLE 12.1   Instruments to Measure the Concepts of the Double ABCX Model

Concept		Measure	Number of Items	Reliability
aA	Pile-up	Family Inventory of Life Events & Changes (FILE)	71	.78
bB	Existing and new resources	Family Inventory of Resource Management (FIRM)	69	.80
	Coping	Coping Health Inventory for Parents (CHIP)	45	.89
cC	Perception of the stressor	Family Coping Coherence Index (FCCI)	4	.66
xX	Adaptation	Family Adaptation Device (FAD)	60	.87

Source: LoBiondo-Wood, G., Williams, L., Kouzekanani, K., & McGhee, C. (2000). Family adaptation to a child's transplantation: Pretransplant phase. *Progress in Transplantation, 10*, 81–87.

is important to assess how the family dynamics contribute to stress and adaptation.

Each family member has unique strengths and vulnerabilities. Factoring each of these into a nursing practice plan is essential. The plan should incorporate strategies to enable family members to learn from each other, capitalize on each other's strengths, and be assistive when times of new illness-related crises arise. Coping has been referred to as a bridging concept; therefore assessing types of coping strategies available and planning to supplement coping strategies is inherent to the plan. The practitioner caring for the individual and family experiencing a chronic illness is required to establish a long-term relationship built upon knowing the individual and the family. The long-term relationship rests on a foundation of trust ensuing as the nurse, the individual, and the family get to know each other over time.

CONCLUSION

The Double ABCX model and its multiple extensions has provided a wealth of instruments for testing family response to chronic illness. The model, extensions, and conceptual distinctions may seem cumbersome, but when the model is broken down and the concepts that are consistent with a problem are delineated, the measurement and testing of hypotheses can be accomplished. The aim of using any model is to move its inherent ideas from testing to practice. To accomplish this end with the theory of Family Stress and Adaptation, prediction models need to be tested to determine which concepts, in what order, best explain family adaptation.

Although a vast amount of theoretical and empirical work has been done since Hill introduced the model, there is still room for questions and development. The fit of ethnicity and culture needs further attention when testing the Double ABCX Model. Intervention studies that foster adaptation and adjustment are still necessary. How the instruments are analyzed in constructing a family picture with the vast variety of family types needs to be assessed. Instrument reliability and validity reports generally describe mothers' and fathers' scores separately rather than conceptualizing family scores or considering unique qualities of current family structures.

In actuality, parents may be a male and a female, two individuals of the same gender, or two individuals from different generations within the family who coparent a child. This reality must be considered. Complex family structures require nurse researchers to clearly demonstrate how the family constellation is defined, how it can be addressed with the theory, and how the data will be interpreted. The realities of family research should not lead one to avoid the area but to embrace its multiple challenges and dynamic approaches.

REFERENCES

Antonovsky, S. P., & Sourani, T. (1988). Family sense of coherence and family adaptation. *Journal of Marriage Family, 50,* 79–92.

Benning, C. R., & Smith, A. (1994). Psychological needs of family members of liver transplant patients. *Clinical Nurse Specialist, 8,* 280–288.

Board, R., & Ryan-Wenger, N. (2002). Long term effects of pediatric intensive care unit hospitalization on families with young children. *Heart & Lung, 31*(1), 53–66.

Board, R., & Ryan-Wenger, N. (2003). Stressors and stress symptoms of mothers with children in the PICU. *Journal of Pediatric Nursing, 18,* 195–202.

Burr, W. F. (1973). *Theory construction and the sociology of the family.* New York: Wiley.

Hill, R. (1949). *Families under stress: Adjustment to the crises of war, separation, and reunion.* New York: Harper.

Hill, R. (1958). Generic features of families under stress. *Social Casework, 49,* 139–150.

Leske, J. S. (2003). Comparison of family stresses, strengths, and outcomes after trauma and surgery. *AACN Clinical Issues, 14,* 33–41.

LoBiondo-Wood, G., Bernier-Henn, M., & Williams, L. (1992). Impact of the child's liver transplant on the family: Maternal perspective. *Pediatric Nursing, 18,* 461–466.

LoBiondo-Wood, G., Williams, L., Kouzekanani, K., & McGhee, C. (2000). Family adaptation to a child's transplantation: Pretransplant phase. *Progress in Transplantation, 10*, 81–87.

LoBiondo-Wood, G., Williams, L., & McGhee, C. (2004). Liver transplantation in children: Maternal and family stress, coping and adaptation. *Journal of the Society of Pediatric Nursing, 9*(2) 59–66.

McCubbin, H. I., Dahl, B. B., Lester, G., & Ross, B. (1977). The returned prisoner of war and his children: Evidence for the origin of second generational effects of captivity. *International Journal of Sociology of the Family, 7*, 25–36.

McCubbin, H. I., Hunter, E., & Metres, P. (1974). The adjustment of families of service men missing in action and prisoners of war: An overview. In *Proceedings of the Army Current Trends Behavioral Science Conference*. Washington, DC: Department of the Army.

McCubbin, H. I., & McCubbin, M. A. (1987). Family stress theory and assessment: The T-double ABCX model of family adjustment and adaptation. In H. I. McCubbin & A. I. Thompson (Eds.), *Family assessment for research and practice* (pp. 3–34). Madison: University of Wisconsin–Madison.

McCubbin, H. I., & McCubbin, M. A. (1988). Typologies of resilient families: Emerging roles of social class and ethnicity. *Family Relations, 37*, 247–254.

McCubbin, H. I., & Patterson, J. M. (1982). Family adaptation to crises. In H. I. McCubbin, A. Cauble, & J. Patterson (Eds.), *Family stress, coping and social support* (pp. 26–47). Springfield, IL: Charles C. Thomas.

McCubbin, H. I., & Patterson, J. M. (1983a). Family stress and adaptation to crises: A double ABCX model of family behavior. In D. Olson *Si* B. Miller (Eds.), *Family studies review yearbook* (Vol. 1, pp. 87–106). Beverly Hills, CA: Sage.

McCubbin, H. I., & Patterson, J. M. (1983b). The family stress process: The double ABCX model of adjustment and adaptation. *Marriage and Family Review, 6*, 7–37.

McCubbin, H. I., Thompson, A. L., & McCubbin, M. A. (1996). *Family assessment: Resiliency, coping and adaptation*. Madison: University of Wisconsin Press.

McCubbin, M. A. (1988). Family stress, resources, and family types: Chronic illness in children. *Family Relations, 37*, 367–377.

McCubbin, M., & McCubbin, H. I. (1993a). Families coping with illness: The resiliency model of family stress, adjustment, and adaptation. In C. B. Danielson, B. Hamel-Bissell, & P. Winstead-Fry (Eds.), *Families, health and illness: Perspectives on coping and intervention* (pp. 21–63). St. Louis: Yearbook.

McCubbin, M. A., & McCubbin, H. I. (1993b). Family coping with health crises: The resiliency model of family stress and adaptation. In C. Danielson, B. Hamel-Bissell, & P. Winstead-Fry (Eds.), *Families, health and illness* (pp. 21–63). New York: Mosby.

McCubbin, M. A., & McCubbin, H. I. (1996). Resiliency in families: A conceptual model of family adjustment and adaptation in response to stress and crises. In *Family assessment: Resiliency, coping and adaptation* (pp. 1–64). Madison: University of Wisconsin Press.

Mishel, M. H., & Murdaugh, C. L. (1987). Family adjustment to heart transplantation: Redesigning the dream. *Nursing Research, 36*(6), 332–338.

Patterson, J. M. (1988). Families experiencing stress. The family adjustment and adaptation response model. *Family System Medicine, 6*(2), 202–237.

Patterson, J. M. (1989). Illness beliefs as a factor in patient-spouse adaptation to coronary artery disease. *Family Systems Medicine, 7*(4), 428–442.

Rungreangkulkij, S., & Gilliss, C. L. (2000). Conceptual approaches to studying family caregiving for persons with severe mental illness. *Journal of Family Nursing, 6*, 341–366.

Suddaby, E. C., Flattery, M. P., & Luna, M. (1997). Stress and coping among parents of children awaiting cardiac transplantation. *Journal of Transplant Coordination, 7,* 36–40.

Uzark, K. C. (1992). Caring for families of pediatric transplant recipients: Psychosocial implications. *Critical Care Clinics of North America, 4,* 255–261.

Walker, A. (1985). Reconceptualizing family stress. *Journal of Marriage & Family, 47*(4), 827.

CHAPTER 13

Theory of Cultural Marginality

Heeseung Choi

As transportation and communication technology advances, there is a complementary increase in contacts between culturally distinct populations. The number of immigrants has continued to grow; as of 2005, about 12.4% of the U.S. population was foreign-born immigrants (U.S. Census Bureau, 2005). Although society is becoming more and more ethnically and culturally diverse, the lack of mutual understanding between health care providers and clients from different cultural backgrounds remains a barrier to progress in health care services for immigrants. The theory of cultural marginality was developed to increase understanding of the unique experiences of individuals who are straddling distinct cultures and to offer direction for providing culturally relevant care.

PURPOSE OF THE THEORY AND HOW IT WAS DEVELOPED

While working with immigrant adolescents and living in the United States as an immigrant, I noticed unique circumstances that immigrant adolescents encountered due to the immigration process and the impact of the process on their mental health development. A review of related theories and research on immigrant adolescents' mental health issues provided the foundation for developing a program of research that began with Korean American adolescents. In a community-based study, I discovered that Korean American adolescents demonstrated significantly lower levels of self-esteem, coping, and mastery in addition to higher levels of depression and

243

somatic symptoms than American adolescents (Choi, Stafford, Meininger, Roberts, & Smith, 2002). The response pattern was more prominent among foreign-born Koreans than U.S.-born Koreans. In a subsequent school-based study, compared to Whites, Asian, and Hispanic American adolescents experienced higher levels of social stress as well as somatic symptoms and depression (Choi, Meininger, & Roberts, 2006). Among White, African, Hispanic, and Asian Americans, Asian American adolescents reported the lowest scores on self-esteem, coping, and family cohesiveness, and the highest score in family conflicts (Choi et al., 2006). These findings led to pondering reasons for the adolescents' vulnerability and to exploring the stress originating from the immigration process as a significant risk factor for mental distress. The next step in building my program of research required an extensive literature review searching for theories that contributed to understanding how distress was associated with immigration for Asian American adolescents.

Theories contributing to the development of the theory of cultural marginality were acculturation, acculturative stress, and marginality. Acculturation was first defined by the Social Science Research Council (SSRC) as "phenomena which result when groups of individuals having different cultures come into continuous first-hand contact, with subsequent changes in the original cultural patterns of either or both groups" (Redfield, Linton, & Herskovits, 1936, p. 149). Theories addressing acculturation have undergone many changes over time, expressed originally through unidimensional models to current expression as multidimensional and orthogonal models (Berry, Poortinga, Segall, & Dasen, 1992; Keefe & Padilla, 1987; Oetting & Beauvais, 1990–1991; Vega, Gil, & Wagner, 1998). The unidimensional bipolar model suggested that individuals inevitably lost their culture of origin as they became acculturated into a new culture (Redfield et al., 1936). Individuals were believed to have only two options: either they acculturated or they remained in their old culture. On the other hand, the multidimensional model focuses on the complex nature of acculturation and selective, or uneven, acculturation across domains of social life (Berry et al., 1992; Keefe & Padilla, 1987; Vega et al., 1998). The orthogonal model proposes biculturality and assumes that acculturating individuals could maintain two different cultural identities simultaneously (Oetting & Beauvais, 1990–1991). An individual may identify him- or herself as a member of both cultural groups, not necessarily choosing either cultural group. These two models opened a new era for theories of acculturation.

One of the popular approaches to acculturation is the fourfold theory of acculturation (Berry, 1995; Berry & Kim, 1988; Berry et al., 1992). The fourfold theory explains strategies that acculturating individuals use. Depending on the chosen culture of reference, strategies are categorized as assimilation, separation, integration, and marginalization. In assimilation, individuals give up their cultural identity and are absorbed into the dominant, or new, culture. Separation, by contrast, is withdrawal from the dominant culture to reside within the old culture. Integration is regarded as the ideal response and refers to "making the best of both worlds" (Berry et al., 1992, p. 279). In marginalization, individuals lose their cultural and psychological contacts with both cultures. Theories of acculturation are broad-ranging and complex, incorporating social, economic, and political components, as well as values, attitudes, self-identity, and behavior change components (Berry & Kim, 1988; Berry et al., 1992).

Acculturative stress, a second theory that contributed to cultural marginality, was developed to highlight the link between acculturation and mental health outcomes. Acculturative stress was defined by Vega et al. (1998) as "a by-product of acculturation that is specific to personal exposure to social situations and environments that challenge individuals to make adjustments in their social behavior or the way they think about themselves" (p. 125). Individuals experience acculturative stress during the acculturating process or as a result of discrimination or being different (Chavez, Moran, Reid, & Lopez, 1997). Acculturative stress has been associated with declining mental health status in acculturating immigrants (Gil, Wagner, & Vega, 2000; Hovey & Magana, 2002; Noh & Kaspar, 2003). The intensity of the relationship between acculturative stress and mental health outcomes is determined by a number of moderating factors including the nature of the dominant culture and the characteristics of the acculturating individuals and groups (Berry & Kim, 1988; Berry et al., 1992).

The third theory to contribute to the development of the theory of cultural marginality was the theory of marginality. The theory of marginality was first proposed by Park in 1928 (Park, 1928). Park introduced the "marginal man" concept with special attention to social context (Park 1928, p. 893). He described the mind of the marginal man as experiencing conflicts of the divided self, the old and new self, a lack of integrity, spiritual instability, restlessness, malaise, and moral turmoil between at least two cultural life-worlds. The theory was expanded by Stonequist (1935) who further explored the nature, variations, social situations, and life cycle of the marginal man. By Stonequist's (1935) definition life cycles consist of an introductory period of preparation, a crisis period, and an adjustment period that may provide opportunities and impetus for social and psychological growth. The theory of marginality has been applied to a wide range of situations, such as middle managers' experiences in the social hierarchy of the workplace (Ziller, 1973), student nurse's experiences (Andersson, 1995), and menopause experiences (Im & Lipson, 1997). In nursing, Hall, Stevens, and Meleis (1994) defined marginality as the condition of persons being peripheralized from mainstream society or the center of the society based on their identities, status, and experiences.

Marginalization and marginality were viewed from a sociopolitical perspective in relation to racial, gender, political, or economic oppression and were scrutinized along with inequities in economic, political, and social power and resources (Hall, 1999; Hall, Stevens, & Meleis, 1994).

The broad perspective that characterizes the theories of acculturation, acculturative stress, and marginality has led to criticisms that cite vagueness and a lack of empirical support (Del Pilar & Udasco, 2004; Rudmin, 2003) as major weaknesses. Del Pilar and Udasco (2004) claimed that marginality contains so many different layers of experiences that it is impossible to explain it in a unified way. Keeping in mind the strengths as well as the limitations and criticisms of the previous theories, I began defining cultural marginality. The first definition of cultural marginality was "situations and feelings of passive betweeness when people exist between two different cultures and do not yet perceive themselves as centrally belonging to either one" (Choi, 2001, p. 198). With continued contemplation of this definition, thoughtful ongoing review of literature, and research with immigrant adolescents, the theory of cultural marginality was developed. Schwartz-Barcott and Kim (2000) emphasized the importance of an empirical component in the process of theory development. To validate the theory of cultural marginality with empirical data, I conducted a qualitative study exploring Korean American adolescents and their parents' perceptions of being in between two different cultures. Twenty Korean American adolescents between the ages 11 and 14 years and 21 parents were interviewed.

The qualitative study revealed that the main sources of stress for Korean American adolescents were managing a balanced peer relationship, discrimination, pressure to excel academically and to be successful, and lack of in-depth parent–child relationships. Difficulties that parents experienced were feeling uneasy and insecure about parenting children in American culture, lack of sense of belonging, being ambivalent toward children's ethnic identity, and inability to advocate for children. Parents also reported struggling with lack of in-depth parent–child relationships. As a result of these experiences, parents often felt inadequate, guilty, and regretful. The findings were integrated into the conceptual structure of the theory. This process provides a strong empirical foundation for the theory of cultural marginality. I will introduce relevant quotes as I discuss the main concepts of the theory.

CONCEPTS OF THE THEORY

The major concepts of the theory of cultural marginality are across-culture conflict recognition, marginal living, and easing cultural tension.

As an individual recognizes conflicts between cultures, he or she engages in marginal living and initiates adjustment responses to ease cultural tension. Therefore, cultural marginality is marginal living while recognizing across-culture conflicts and striving to ease cultural tension. An important dimension of cultural marginality, in addition to the major concepts, is contextual/personal influences that create the foundation for a person's experience of cultural marginality. Each of the major concepts of the theory will be discussed as will contextual/personal influences. In describing the major concepts of the theory, quotes shared by parents and adolescents in my most recent qualitative study will be described.

Marginal Living

Marginal living, a major concept of the theory, is defined as passive betweeness in the pushing/pulling tension between two cultures while forging new relationships in the midst of old and living with simultaneous conflict/promise. In the theory of cultural marginality, marginal living is viewed as a process of being in between two cultures with emphasis on being in transition rather than being on the periphery of one culture.

Passive betweeness is the essential quality of marginal living. Park (1928) described the marginal experience as a situation that "condemned him to live in two worlds, in neither of which he ever quite belonged" (p. 893). Nobody chooses to be on the edge of two different cultures or to be in between. It is especially true for children who usually have no option when moving from one country to another (Guarnaccia & Lopez, 1998). They simply follow their parents' choice of new country for a better life. Even adults who decide to live in a new country really do not want to be in an "in between" position. It is a passive choice. Some people who have experienced marginality recalled the time as "a period when they stand with both feet in different boots" (Andersson, 1995, p. 131). The experience has been described as "trapped," "being betwixt and between," and "being located within a structure of double ambivalence" (Bennett, 1993, p. 113; Weisberger, 1992, p. 429). The following quotes capture the quality of passive betweeness. A mother said:

> I, myself, have to live a life of the crippled in this country. . . . I feel like I am floating in the air. I don't know if I will be able to stand on my feet before I die. I worry whether my children will grow up well. . . . I know for sure that I came here for my children, but I was in agony because I thought I made a wrong decision. . . . I am so worried about how to live my life as a mother.

An adolescent said:

> I go crazy over . . . Korean pride and World Cup. But my friends are
> like, "Outside, you are Korean, but inside, you are White." So I feel
> like I'm part of them. Sometimes I'm like that and sometimes I'm not.

When people move to a new country or a different culture, they inevitably must become engaged in new relationships (Rogler, 1994). Coming into new relationships does not happen in a single day, and it is not as simple as taking off old clothes and changing into new ones. One of the qualities of marginal living is forging new relationships in the midst of old relationships. This quality is often more prominent among adolescents since forming new allegiances with peers and confirming their identities and values within the peer group are critical developmental tasks. Adolescents, who are eager to forge new relationships in the midst of old relationships, often encounter contradiction and conflicts. While moving forward to engage in new relationships, adolescents are concerned about losing connection with their old relationships. As adolescents actively forge new relationships while parents dwell in the past, the parent–child relationship gets untied. The majority of Korean American adolescents and their parents reported struggling with lack of in-depth parent–child relationships. The following quote describes the experience of an adolescent who began to engage in new relationships in a new world:

> We (mom and herself) will grow apart since we will be living in two
> different cultures, using different languages. I think she's already having a hard time. . . . I wish you had a program to help her overcome
> such barriers so we may stay close.

Adolescents who are living in between face pushing/pulling tension between two cultures. Parents encourage their children to mingle with new friends, to pursue further opportunities, so that they will be successful in the new society. This phenomenon is prominent especially among families who came to this country for better education and opportunities. Parents, however, feel threatened and become anxious about losing control over their children as their children blend into the new culture. The following quote illustrates the quality of pushing/pulling tension from the perspective of the father of a 12-year-old boy:

> Many of their parents have double standards for them. They want
> their children to be successful in America as American citizens, yet they
> want them to remain Koreans at the same time. And that gives children
> an ambiguous message, which confuses them. . . . If you keep giving
> such contradicting messages to children especially at a sensitive stage

when they start questioning their parents' authority, they will surely get confused and it might lead to creating other problems. I think that is the real problem.

The new society or dominant culture also shows similar contradicting attitudes toward immigrants. The dominant culture welcomes immigrants warmly with its slogan, country of immigrants, and a promise to provide them abundant opportunities and resources. However, in reality, what immigrants often face is overt and covert discrimination. Discrimination was repeatedly reported by both Korean American adolescents and their parents during the interviews. They reported that Korean American adolescents encountered teachers' insensitive attitudes toward different cultures, experienced limited opportunities, got unfair grades and punishment. Korean American adolescents also reported that they had been teased or bullied because of their accent and physical appearance.

There is a demand for immigrants to make choices between contradicting norms, expectations, roles, and values. They often find themselves struggling in simultaneous conflict/promise. Conflict/promise is a quality of marginal living rooted in identity confusion, anxiety, ambivalence, feelings of alienation, loss, helplessness, worthlessness, a feeling of uncertainty, and apprehension about the future (Andersson, 1995; Berry et al., 1992; Fuertes & Westbrook, 1996; Scribner, 1995; Weisberger, 1992). However, conflict does not always create negative outcomes. Depending on how the individual perceives and manages conflict, it may offer possibility for change. In a previous article on the concept of cultural marginality (Choi, 2001), conflict and promise were categorized as two distinct attributes; however, subsequent research has indicated that promise is integral to conflict. Thus, for the theory of cultural marginality, conflict/promise is conceptualized as a single quality of marginal living. Hall and colleagues (Hall, 1999, p. 100; Hall et al., 1994) identified resilience and a "hope-positive view of the future" as well as vulnerabilities when marginalized people struggled to acquire their own survival strategies to protect themselves and enhance well-being. Therefore, marginal living is both a conflict and promise, a crisis and turning point, thus providing impetus for growth.

During the interviews, Korean American parents expressed hopes for their children's future even in the midst of feelings of alienation, powerlessness, worthlessness, and a feeling of uncertainty. They expected their children to blend in the mainstream society and move up the social ladder by obtaining high educational status. The hopes often led children to feel pressured to excel academically and to be successful. Integral to this experience of marginal living is the recognition of across-culture conflict, a second concept of the theory of cultural marginality.

Across-Culture Conflict Recognition

Across-culture conflict recognition is a beginning understanding of differences between two contradicting cultural values, customs, behaviors, and norms. Just as people feel and react to perceived temperature, not measured temperature, people feel and react to their recognition of differences while in between cultures. Conflict emerges as individuals face distinct value systems with accompanying expectations and are forced to make difficult choices. Korean American adolescents reported encountering two distinct cultural values and expectations between peers and their parents and between Korean and American friends.

Acknowledging across-culture conflict recognition as a concept of the theory of cultural marginality has significant implications for research and practice since it allows for individual differences in perception, responses, and mental health outcomes associated with cultural marginality. This is consistent with the theorizing of Lazarus (1997) who identified cognitive appraisal of cultural environment as one of the significant determinants of mental health outcomes. An adolescent said:

> You know how parents raise their kids based on how they were raised . . . well, if I compare my style with regular White friends, it's completely different. They are always out and my parents think you play too much or you do this too much but if you compare me with them, that's not really true. Well, I know it's best for me what they say but sometimes it's like that's how we live here in America.

Easing Cultural Tension

Easing cultural tension is a naturally occurring adjustment response intended to resolve across-culture conflict. Adjustment responses proposed in the theory of cultural marginality are adapted from Weisberger's work on marginality among German Jews (1992). Four responses, assimilation, reconstructed return, poise, and integration, are processes for easing cultural tension. The responses are not mutually exclusive; rather, they are mixed empirically (Weisberger, 1992) and will be referred to as response patterns to connote their contextual, situational, dynamic nature.

The first response pattern is assimilation. It is a process whereby individuals are absorbed into the dominant or new culture (Berry, 1995; Berry & Kim, 1988; Berry et al., 1992). This is usually the first response pattern exhibited by new immigrants, particularly when the dominant, or new culture, is unfavorable to the newcomers. Immigrants strive hard to acquire new language and customs and to mingle with people of the new society. It is a useful strategy for survival in the new culture; however, it may create self-denial, self-hatred, and feelings of guilt (Weisberger, 1992).

After encountering the new culture, individuals may return to their own culture, exhibiting the pattern of reconstructed return. They may choose to return as a result of resistance, obstacles, and conflicts with a new culture or as a result of reminiscence and longing for one's own culture. When they return, they do so with a new perspective toward their own culture as well as to the new culture since they cannot be free from the influences of the new culture (Anderson & Levy, 2003; Weisberger, 1992). Thus, every return is a reconstructed return. A typical characteristic of people who return to or remain in their culture is an overidentification with their own culture. Weisberger (1992, p. 442) describes the characteristics among the returning German Jews as "more Jewish than Jewish." The following quote is from a mother of a 14-year-old daughter. Her daughter has been referred by her teacher to a school counselor for her misbehavior at school:

> Even if she was born here (United States) and has never been to Korea, she always hangs out with Korean friends, particularly Korean kids who recently moved from Korea. She likes to have Korean clothes, accessories, phone, and stuff. . . . I think it is because her longing for Korea and Korean culture.

Poise is a response pattern characterized by a tentative fit on the margin regardless of emotional conflict and struggle. Individuals who respond with poise may become free from obligation or attachment to a certain culture, but they have to be "homeless in a cultural sense" (Weisberger, 1992, p. 440). Even when responding with a pattern of poise, individuals will continue to experience emotional conflicts, and a period of personal crisis continues. Accumulated effects of crisis may include stress and poor mental health outcomes such as personality changes, substance abuse, depression, and even suicidal ideation (Hovey & Magana, 2002; Park, 1928; Vega et al., 1998; Williams & Berry, 1991).

Integration is an adjustment response pattern where an individual creates a third culture by merging and integrating the old and new cultures. Through integration, individuals surpass cultural boundaries, contexts, and identities, and acquire superior social functioning, gaining access to multiple cultural worlds (Park, 1928; Guarnaccia & Lopez, 1998; Weisberger, 1992) and easing cultural tension. They will experience a sense of cultural home, sense of belonging, integration of identity, and psychological and cognitive growth (Bennett, 1993; Vivero & Jenkins, 1999). For them, the possibility of returning to the cultural tension of marginal living is minimized. When faced with another circumstance of cultural tension, it is likely that they will respond successfully. The level of ease experienced during the process will influence mental health and well-being of the individual. A 14-year-old boy who used to struggle to fit in with peers due to language and cultural barriers now becomes comfortable with both American and Korean cultures and feels confident:

> I feel very special in a positive way. There are my friends who think I'm cool. They rather look UP to me. . . . I explain to my friends what Korean culture is. Like New Year's Day, they called me to go with them and watch fireworks. I was like, "I can't" and I explained to them what 'Duk-gook' (Korean traditional food) is and 'Sae-bae'. Like I have to bow down and I get money. And they are like, "Can we come to your house and do 'Sae-bae' so we get money too?" I explained to them and they want to know more about it. One of my friends can actually count from 1 to like 25. They actually go to Web site so they can learn, so they can talk to me. And I actually gave them Korean music, and he's like, can you type the lyrics in English? So they are more into Koreanness. They are more interested.

One adjustment response pattern may have more constructive impact on an individual's mental health than the others; however, there is no ideal or most useful pattern that works for everyone nor is there one pattern that works for one person all of the time. For instance, integration may be a feasible adjustment response pattern for immigrant adolescents but not for immigrant elderly. For the elderly, remaining in contact with the old culture and returning to old culture ways may make them more comfortable. So, the pattern of reconstructed return may be most useful for them. For health care providers working with immigrant populations, it is important to assess unique experiences and perceptions rather than categorize individuals based on their adjustment response pattern. However, knowledge about the response patterns individuals use to ease cultural tension may enable understanding of the complex processes that are central to the struggle that many immigrants face.

Contextual/Personal Influences

Recognizing across-culture conflict, undergoing marginal living, and easing cultural tension occurs in relation to contextual/personal influences. Scholars of acculturation theory recognized nature or types of the dominant society and characteristics of acculturating individuals as significant factors in the acculturation process (Berry & Kim, 1988; Williams & Berry, 1991). In this theory of cultural marginality, the factors influencing the process of across-culture conflict recognition, marginal living, and easing cultural tensions are defined as contextual/personal influences.

Contextual/personal influences identified in literature reviews and shared in interviews with Korean Americans are the nature of the dominant society, such as openness or tolerance to diversity, available social and health care resources for immigrants, racial and/or ethnic composition of school and neighborhood, support from teachers and peers, significant others' attitudes toward the dominant culture, knowledge about the dominant society, age at immigration, length of stay in the United States, educational backgrounds, socioeconomic status, language proficiency, ethnic identity, preimmigration experiences, reasons for immigration, loyalty to own culture, resilience or ability to endure the hardship, openness, parent–child relationships, and coping strategies (Berry, 1995; Berry & Kim, 1988; Berry et al., 1992; Trueba, 2002).

These influences govern not only the individuals who are in the midst of cultural marginality but also the dominant culture that is a source of interaction for immigrant people. Existing theories describing acculturation have been criticized for ignoring the influences of the acculturating individuals or groups to the dominant culture (Rudmin, 2003). The theories viewed acculturating individuals only as passive recipients. When two cultures clash, the interaction is reciprocal although the strength of the influence may not be comparable. Contextual/personal influences make the interaction between two cultures and the effect of one culture on another a mutual process.

RELATIONSHIPS AMONG THE CONCEPTS:
THE MODEL

Figure 13.1 depicts the relationships among the major concepts of the theory. Marginal living begins with the recognition of across-culture conflict. As individuals encounter marginal living, they strive to ease cultural tension through adjustment response patterns. The four response patterns are assimilation, return, poise, and integration. Although not an explicit concept in the theory, the importance of contextual/personal influences is recognized by its inclusion as a foundation for the theory of cultural marginality.

USE OF THE THEORY IN NURSING RESEARCH

The theory of cultural marginality is being introduced for the first time in this chapter; therefore, the use in research and practice is limited. However, the idea of cultural marginality, since it was introduced (Choi, 2001), has been cited in various areas of nursing research and practice. The concept was used to understand experiences of Mexican American families caring for children with serious chronic conditions (Rehm, 2003) and to study stress experienced by Pakistani Ismaili Muslim girls (Khuwaja, Selwyn, Kapadia, McCurdy, & Khuwaja, 2007). The fact that

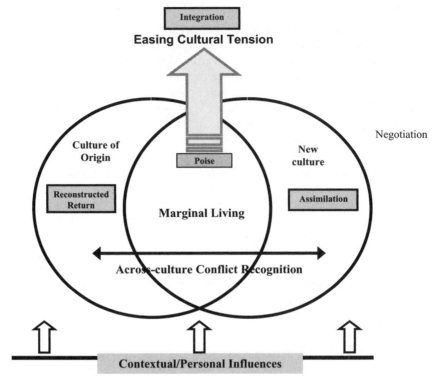

FIGURE 13.1   Cultural marginality.

researchers have used the concept of cultural marginality demonstrates the need for theory development and suggests possible applications for the theory of cultural marginality.

My research studies based on the theory of cultural marginality began with a qualitative descriptive study of Korean American adolescents and their parents. I interviewed 20 parent–child dyads to understand their perceptions about the experiences of straddling two cultures. The findings of the study revealed main sources of stress for Korean American adolescents and their parents encountered while living in between two cultures.

Another possible area of research for the theory of cultural marginality is instrument development. Researchers have developed scales to measure levels of acculturation and acculturative stress and to explain the relationships between these concepts and mental health outcomes (Hovey & King, 1997; Padilla, Alvarez, & Lindholm, 1986; Phinney, 1992; Sam & Berry, 1995; Williams & Berry, 1991), but there is no scale specifically designed to measure cultural marginality. A comprehensive instrument with items aligned according to the concepts of the theory would allow assessment of the structure of the associated concepts and of the extent to which cultural marginality influences health. Assessing the relationship between cultural marginality and mental health outcomes has significant implications for the health care of immigrants; it has particular relevance for preventive care, where nurses caring for immigrants develop approaches for recognizing those who are at risk for mental health problems.

USE OF THE THEORY IN NURSING PRACTICE

The concept of cultural marginality has been used to discuss adherence issues of Mexican clients (Barron, Hunter, Mayo, & Willoughby, 2004) and to address the gap in health care provider–client relationships and its impact on health disparities (Cupertino, n.d.). The theory can also be applied to school nurse practice to foster awareness of culturally distinct adolescent needs (Labun, 2003).

Current work in progress includes development of a mental health promotion program for Korean American adolescents and their parents based on the findings from the qualitative study. The main goal of the mental health promotion program, "Be Connected," is to promote connection between Korean American adolescents and their parents and between Korean and American cultures by modifying contextual/personal influences. Through the program, Korean American adolescents are expected to learn coping strategies, communication skills, and knowledge required to ease generational/cultural conflicts. Parents also will gain knowledge and skills needed for connected parent–child relationships. Main topics for the program will be the characteristics of adolescent development, U.S. education system, influences of culture on parent–child relationships, parenting skills, communication skills, and coping strategies. Through the program, Korean American adolescents and their parents would stay connected.

In this chapter, the theory of cultural marginality was described in the context of immigrant adolescents' experiences; however, the theory is also applicable to any immigrant who is encountering marginal living. The theory of cultural marginality can be used as a framework to explore unique experiences of diverse groups of immigrants and to provide care for them. Particularly, recognizing the influences of the contextual/personal factors has significant implications for health care providers. For instance, adjustment response patterns and health care needs among immigrants who came to this country for freedom cannot be the same as those for people who are here for educational opportunities. By recognizing these influences and modifying them when appropriate, health care providers may ease the adjustment process, promote healthy adolescent development, and elicit positive mental health outcomes. Education or health promotion programs that assess and modify personal influences such as self-esteem, coping strategies, and ethnic identities are one of the potential approaches that could be guided by the theory. Incorporation of the theory of cultural marginality into cultural competency training for health care providers could produce an evidence-based structure to enhance learning.

CONCLUSION

What is it like to be caught between cultures? How does that experience impact one's health? How can health care providers ease the experience? These questions have inspired development of the theory of cultural marginality. The goal of the theory is to highlight the complexity of living between two cultures, emphasizing the challenge to immigrant well-being. The theory elucidates essences of marginal living, across-culture conflict recognition, and striving to ease cultural tension while recognizing the fundamental importance of contextual/personal influences. Understanding of the theory concepts and the relationships among the concepts promises a framework for culturally relevant health care for immigrant people.

Regardless of the long history of immigration and the increasing number of immigrants in this country, knowledge about these populations has been limited. The theory's attention to contextual/personal influences provides wide opportunities for research and practice. To make the theory relevant to the lives of immigrant people, more research and practice tailored to their needs and sensitive to their contextual/personal influences is necessary. The theory of cultural marginality introduced in this book is a turning point of a long journey that began in doctoral study. Further reflection and the use of the theory in research and practice will contribute to the theory evolution and refinement.

REFERENCES

Anderson, T. L., & Levy, J. A. (2003). Marginality among older injectors in today's illicit drug culture: Assessing the impact of ageing. *Addiction, 98,* 761–770.

Andersson, E. P. (1995). Marginality: Concept or reality in nursing education? *Journal of Advanced Nursing, 21,* 131–136.

Barron, F., Hunter, A., Mayo, R., & Willoughby, B. (2004). Acculturation and adherence: Issues for health care providers working with clients of Mexican origin. *Journal of Transcultural Nursing, 15,* 331–337.

Bennett, J. M. (1993). Cultural marginality: Identity issues in intercultural training. In R. M. Paise (Ed.), *Education for intercultural experience* (pp. 109–135). Yarmouth, ME: Intercultural Press.

Berry, J. W. (1995). Psychology of acculturation. In N. R. Goldberger & J. B. Veroff (Eds.), *The culture and psychology reader* (pp. 457–488). New York: New York University.

Berry, J. W., & Kim, U. (1988). Acculturation and mental health. In P. R. Dasen, J. W. Berry, & N. Sartorius (Eds.), *Health and cross-cultural psychology: Toward applications* (pp. 207–236). Newbury Park: Sage.

Berry, J. W., Poortinga, Y. H., Segall, M. H., & Dasen, P. R. (1992). *Cross-cultural psychology: Research and applications.* New York: Cambridge University.

Chavez, D. V., Moran, V. R., Reid, S. L., & Lopez, M. (1997). Acculturative stress in children: A modification of the SAFE Scale. *Hispanic Journal of Behavioral Sciences, 19,* 34–44.

Choi, H. (2001). Cultural marginality: A concept analysis with implications for immigrant adolescents. *Issues in Comprehensive Pediatric Nursing, 24,* 193–206.

Choi, H., Meininger, J. C., & Roberts, R. E. (2006). Ethnic differences in adolescents' mental distress, social stress, and resources. *Adolescence, 41*(162), 263–283.

Choi, H., Stafford, L., Meininger, J. C., Roberts, R. E., & Smith, D. P. (2002). Psychometric properties of the DSM Scale for Depression (DSD) with Korean American youths. *Issues in Mental Health Nursing, 23,* 735–756.

Cupertino, A. P. (n.d.). *Provider-patient relationship: Cultural competency and literacy.* Retrieved December 20, 2006, from http://www.minorityhealthks.org/download/Cultural_COmpetence.ppt

Del Pilar, J. A., & Udasco, J. O. (2004). Marginality theory: The lack of construct validity. *Hispanic Journal of Behavioral Sciences, 26,* 3–15.

Fuertes, J. N., & Westbrook, F. D. (1996). Using the Social, Attitudinal, Familial, and Environmental (S.A.F.E.) Acculturation Stress Scale to assess the adjustment needs of Hispanic college students. *Measurement and Evaluation in Counseling and Development, 29,* 67–76.

Gil, A. G., Wagner, E. F., & Vega, W. A. (2000). Acculturation, familism, and alcohol use among Latino adolescent males: Longitudinal relations. *Journal of Community Psychology, 28,* 443–458.

Guarnaccia, P. J., & Lopez, S. (1998). The mental health and adjustment of immigrant and refugee children. *The Child Psychiatrist in the Community, 7,* 537–553.

Hall, J. M. (1999). Marginalization revisited: Critical, postmodern, and liberation perspectives. *Advances in Nursing Science, 22*(2), 88–102.

Hall, J. M., Stevens, P. E., & Meleis, A. I. (1994). Marginalization: A guiding concept for valuing diversity in nursing knowledge development. *Advances in Nursing Science, 16*(4), 23–41.

Hovey, J. D., & King, C. A. (1997). Suicidality among acculturating Mexican Americans: Current knowledge and directions for research. *Suicide and Life-Threatening Behavior, 27,* 92–103.

Hovey, J. D., & Magana, C. G. (2002). Exploring the mental health Mexican migrant farm workers in the Midwest: Psychosocial predictors of psychological distress and suggestions for prevention and treatment. *Journal of Psychology, 136,* 493–513.

Im, E. O., & Lipson, J. G. (1997). Menopausal transition of Korean immigrant women: A literature review. *Health Care for Women International, 18,* 507–520.

Keefe, S. E., & Padilla, A. M. (1987). *Chicano ethnicity.* Albuquerque: University of New Mexico Press.

Khuwaja, S. A., Selwyn, B. J., Kapadia, A., McCurdy, S., & Khuwaja, A. (2007). Pakistani Ismaili Muslim adolescent females living in the United States of America: Stresses associated with the process of adaptation to U.S. culture. *Journal of Immigrant Health, 9,* 35–42.

Labun, E. (2003). Working with a Vietnamese adolescent. *The Journal of School Nursing, 19,* 319–325.

Lazarus, R. S. (1997). Acculturation isn't everything. *Applied Psychology, 46,* 39–43.

Noh, S., & Kaspar, V. (2003). Perceived discrimination and depression: Moderating effects of coping, acculturation, and ethnic support. *American Journal of Public Health, 93,* 232–238.

Oetting, E. R., & Beauvais, F. (1990–1991). Orthogonal cultural identification theory: The cultural identification of minority adolescents. *The International Journal of the Addictions, 25,* 655–685.

Padilla, A. M., Alvarez, M., & Lindholm, K. J. (1986). Generational status and personality factors as predictors of stress in students. *Hispanic Journal of Behavioral Sciences, 8,* 275–288.

Park, R. E. (1928). Human migration and the marginal man. *The American Journal of Sociology, 33,* 881–893.

Phinney, J. S. (1992). The Multigroup Ethnic Identity Measure: A new scale for use with adolescents and youth adults from diverse groups. *Journal of Adolescent Research, 7,* 156–176.

Redfield, R., Linton, R., & Herskovits, M. J. (1936). Memorandum on the study of acculturation. *American Anthropologist, 38,* 149–152.

Rehm, R. S. (2003). Legal, financial, and ethical ambiguities for Mexican American families: Caring for children with chronic conditions. *Qualitative Health Research, 13,* 689–702.

Rogler, L. H. (1994). International migrations: A framework for directing research. *American Psychologist, 49,* 701–708.

Rudmin, F. W. (2003). Critical history of the acculturation psychology of assimilation, separation, integration, and marginalization. *Review of General Psychology, 7,* 3–37.

Sam, D. L., & Berry, J. W. (1995). Acculturative stress among young immigrants in Norway. *Scandinavian Journal of Psychology, 36,* 10–24.

Schwartz-Barcott, D., & Kim, H. S. (2000). An expansion and elaboration of the hybrid model of concept development. In B. L. Rodgers & K. A. Knafl (Eds.), *Concept development in nursing* (2nd ed., pp. 129–159). Philadelphia: WB Saunders.

Scribner, A. P. (1995). Advocating for Hispanic high school students: Research-based educational practices. *The High School Journal, 78,* 206–214.

Stonequist, E. V. (1935). The problem of the marginal man. *The American Journal of Sociology, 41,* 1–12.

Trueba, H. T. (2002). Multiple ethnic, racial, and cultural identities in action: From marginality to a new cultural capital in modern society. *Journal of Latinos and Education, 1,* 7–28.

U.S. Census Bureau (2005). 2005 American Community Survey. Retrieved December 10, 2006, from http://factfinder.census.gov/servlet/ACSSAFFFacts?_sse=on&_submenuId= factsheet_1&_ci_nbr=&qr_name=&ds_name=&reg=&_industry

Vega, W. A., Gil, A. G., & Wagner, E. (1998). Cultural adjustment and Hispanic adolescent drug use. In W. A. Vega & A. G. Gil (Eds.), *Drug use and ethnicity in early adolescence* (pp. 125–148). New York: Plenum.

Vivero, V. N., & Jenkins, S. R. (1999). Existential hazards of the multicultural individual: Defining and understanding "cultural homelessness." *Cultural Diversity and Ethnic Minority Psychology, 5,* 6–26.

Weisberger, A. (1992). Marginality and its directions. *Sociological Forum, 7,* 425–446.

Williams, C. L., & Berry, J. W. (1991). Primary prevention of acculturative stress among refugees: Application of psychological theory and practice. *American Psychologist, 46,* 632–641.

Ziller, R. C. (1973). *The social self.* New York: Pergamon.

CHAPTER 14

Theory of Caregiving Dynamics

Loretta A. Williams

Unpaid care provided by family, friends, or neighbors is a critical resource in today's health care system. The value of caregiving in the United States in 2004 was estimated to be about $306 billion (Arno, 2006). While patients are the direct beneficiaries of care, paid care providers also benefit indirectly from the care provided by unpaid caregivers. Caregivers make possible the discharge of patients from inpatient facilities and often provide the link between ambulatory care facilities and patients. Just as nurses are the health care providers who have the most contact with patients, so nurses also have the most contact with caregivers (U.S. Census Bureau, 2005). Because of the critical and frequent need to identify a caregiver for a patient and to have the patient and caregiver develop and sustain a caregiving relationship, understanding the dynamics of the caregiving relationship is especially important for nurses.

Family members, friends, or neighbors provide most of the day-to-day care for persons with health problems, who are chronically-ill, disabled, or aged (Thompson, 2004). This unpaid assistance often involves multiple tasks that may be physically, emotionally, socially, or financially demanding (Biegel, Sales, & Schulz, 1991). These caregivers are sometimes referred to as informal caregivers. The term informal is used to differentiate them from formal health care providers who receive pay for the care they provide. Informal caregivers are usually family, friends, or neighbors and are frequently key resources in the care of patients who would otherwise need institutional care (Pasacreta & McCorkle, 2000).

The dynamics of caregiving are the forces that motivate caregivers and care recipients to assume and continue the caregiving relationship.

While much caregiving inquiry has focused on the burden of caregiving, it is equally if not more important to understand the positive forces that move the caregiving relationship forward. In this middle range theory of caregiving dynamics caregiving refers to care given by family, friends, or neighbors.

PURPOSE OF THE THEORY AND HOW IT WAS DEVELOPED

The purpose of this middle range theory is to describe the positive forces that allow the caregiving relationship to change and grow. Recognition of these forces will enable nurses to identify methods for supporting the caregiving relationship. The theory began as a concept named "informal caregiving dynamics" (Williams, 2003). Informal caregiving dynamics was conceptualized as forces that stimulate and shape change in an informal caregiver–care recipient dyad.

As the concept has developed into a theory and has been presented and used, the decision was made to drop the term informal. While informal caregiving is a recognized concept in health care and social science literature, those who are unfamiliar with the term sometimes misunderstand the word informal and think that it diminishes the importance of caregiving provided by family members, friends, and neighbors.

The clinical situation that stimulated the development of this theory was the need to identify strategies to ensure reliable caregivers for patients scheduled to undergo hematopoietic stem cell transplantation (HSCT). HSCT is an intensive but potentially curative therapy for patients with life-threatening illnesses (Horowitz, Loberiza, Bredeson, Rizzo, & Nugent, 2001). In 2002, approximately 40,000 HSCTs were performed worldwide, the majority for hematological cancers (Loberiza, 2003). Over the last 15 years, caregiving by family, friends, or neighbors has become an integral and essential aspect of the bone marrow transplant process (Grimm, Zawacki, Mock, Krumm, & Frink, 2000). Patients may even be denied the treatment option of HSCT if a caregiver cannot be identified (Frey et al., 2002).

A qualitative research study was conducted based on the experiences of caregivers of patients undergoing HSCT. Forty caregivers were invited to tell their caregiving stories in a one-on-one dialogue with the researcher. Story theory (Smith & Liehr, 2003) was the theoretical foundation for the interviews. The model emerging from the study provides the structure for the middle range theory of caregiving dynamics.

CONCEPTS OF THE THEORY

The major concepts of the theory of caregiving dynamics are commitment, expectation management, and role negotiation. Self-care, new insight, and role support are related concepts, each connected to one of the major concepts. Caregiving dynamics are interacting processes of commitment, expectation management, and role negotiation supported by self-care, new insight, and role support that move a caregiving relationship along an illness trajectory.

Commitment

Commitment is enduring caregiver responsibility that inspires life changes to make the patient a priority. Commitment calls caregivers to a supportive presence whether or not they were experiencing a self-affirming loving connection with the patient (Williams, 2007). There are four dimensions of commitment. These dimensions are enduring responsibility, making the patient a priority, supportive presence, and self-affirming loving connection. *Enduring responsibility* is caregiver determination to provide care despite difficulties for however long it takes. Enduring responsibility, based on obligation, reciprocity, or love, may begin long before the illness and continue after the illness resolves; it has both the connotation of being lasting and the connotation of bearing hardship without yielding (Williams, 2007). *Making the patient a priority* is placement of patient care needs before all other needs and wants because patient well-being is the most important goal. Significant and often difficult life changes are voluntarily made in the best interest of the patient (Williams, 2007). *Supportive presence* is remaining at the patient's side with comfort, encouragement, and a positive attitude when the caregiver can do nothing else to assist the patient. The senses of the caregiver are heightened to fully understand the patient experience so that patient emotional needs and wants are accurately identified and met (Williams, 2007). *Self-affirming loving connection* is a feeling of open togetherness between the caregiver and the patient where meeting patient needs is emotionally satisfying for the caregiver (Williams, 2007).

When the caregiver and care recipient commit to the caregiving dyad, each brings with them past experiences, strengths, and weaknesses. The past histories of the caregiver and care recipient, as well as their joint history, will influence the caregiving dyad (Phillips, Brewer, & Torres de Ardon, 2001). Caregivers and care recipients may bring technical knowledge and skills (Schumacher, Stewart, & Archbold, 1998), fears about caregiving (Ferrell, Cohen, Rhiner, & Rozek, 1991), physical or emotional deficits (Cohen et al., 1993; Hadjistavropoulos, Taylor, Tuokko, &

Beattie, 1994; Ostwald, 1997), multiple other roles (Wuest, 2001), coping abilities (Folkman, 1997), previously developed support systems (Miller et al., 2001), and previous knowledge of the other member of the caregiving dyad (Phillips et al., 2001). The caregiving dyad will be influenced by these unique qualities and experiences that the caregiver and care recipient bring to the caregiving situation.

Self-Care

Self-care is a concept related to commitment. Self-care is acting to maintain health by cultivating healthy habits while letting out the feelings and frustrations of caregiving and getting away from caregiving demands when necessary. There are four dimensions of self-care. These dimensions are supportive physical environment, cultivating healthy habits, letting it out, and getting away from it. *Supportive physical environment* refers to accommodations, food, and other amenities that are comfortable and convenient for the caregiver and the patient. *Cultivating healthy habits* is taking action to maintain or improve health necessary for caregiving. The caregiver and the patient support and encourage each other to follow health-improving habits such as eating well and exercising. *Letting it out* is finding ways to express feelings and frustrations associated with caregiving. Caregivers may communicate intentionally with others to share their feelings or may disclose their thoughts and feelings through writing or other methods of expression that may not necessarily be shared with others. *Getting away from it* is finding physical or mental space to temporarily experience ordinary life separate from the demands of illness, treatment, and caregiving. Caregivers sometimes find the need to be physically away from the caregiving situation, but at other times merely leaving the situation mentally provides adequate respite. Caregivers may report feeling guilty in leaving the care recipient.

Caregivers of patients with dementia have reported using exercise to maintain their own health (Connell, 1994), while caregivers of patients with multiple sclerosis frequently seek interpersonal support to maintain their health (O'Brien, 1993). Caregivers of frail elders reported using a variety of behaviors to maintain their health, but most behaviors addressed physical health (McDonald, Fink, & Wykle, 1999). Caregivers of cancer survivors practice a high number of health maintenance activities (Bowman, Rose, & Deimling, 2005). Regardless of the population, self-care is a critical dimension of committing to a caregiving relationship over time.

Expectation Management

Expectation management is envisioning the future and yearning to return to normal. It includes taking one day at a time when the future is uncertain, gauging behavior from past experiences with the patient, and reconciling actual to anticipated treatment twists and turns (Williams, 2007). There are five dimensions of expectation management. These dimensions are envisioning tomorrow, getting back to normal, taking one day at a time, gauging behavior, and reconciling treatment twists and turns. *Envisioning tomorrow* is grappling with an ambiguous future with hope, fear, or both. Images of the future span a continuum from very certain and specific to very vague and general. Imagining a hopeful future provides caregivers with goals to strive for and a reason to endure difficulties while imagining a fearful future allows caregivers to minimize losses and prepare for future disappointments (Williams, 2007). *Getting back to normal* is seeing the light at the end of the tunnel and anticipating going back to an ordinary life of health that was lost in the demands of illness and treatment (Williams, 2007). *Taking one day at a time* is focusing in the present as a means of dealing with an uncertain future that cannot or will not be envisioned. As perspectives and priorities change with a present orientation, attempts may be made to slow down and make the most of the present rather than rushing to an uncertain future. Caregivers sometimes avoid the future because they fear what it might hold, but at other times they savor the positive aspects of the present (Williams, 2007). *Gauging behavior* is explaining, predicting, or reacting to actions or statements of the patient based on prior knowledge of and experience with the patient. Expectations developed from gauging behavior allow caregivers to react positively to even difficult patient behaviors (Williams, 2007). *Reconciling treatment twists and turns* is comparing actual to anticipated patient outcomes to confirm, explain, and eventually accept the reality of the actual outcomes (Williams, 2007).

The caregiver and care recipient naturally bring expectations to the caregiving situation. Expectations are the anticipation or looking forward to the coming or occurrence of something. Expectations consider an occurrence probable, certain, reasonable, due, necessary, or bound by duty or obligation (Merriam-Webster OnLine, 2007). Expectations may also be the strong belief that something will happen, be it the case in the future, or that someone will or should achieve something (Jewell & Abate, 2001). Realistic and congruent expectations on the part of the caregiver and care recipient improve the functioning of the caregiving dyad (Kylma, Vehviläinen-Julkunen, & Lähdevirta, 2001). Expectations may involve the behavior of the other member of the caregiving dyad, the caregiving relationship, the roles that will exist in the caregiving dyad, and the illness trajectory (Boyle et al., 2000; Speice et al., 2000). The illness trajectory is the path, progression, or line of development of the care recipient's illness (Merriam-Webster OnLine, 2007). The trajectory will be expected in the future until it occurs in the present and becomes part of the past (Padilla, Mishel, & Grant, 1992). As the trajectory becomes known, the expectation of the trajectory may need to be changed (Boyle et al., 2000). Changes in expectations are some of the transitions in caregiving (Seltzer & Li, 2000). Understanding the illness trajectory and managing to have realistic expectations is an area of caregiving dynamics where nurses and other health care professionals can make an impact (Speice et al., 2000).

New Insight

New insight is a concept related to expectation management. New insight is changing awareness through experiencing personal growth, believing that a higher power controls the situation, and recognizing positive treatment outcomes. There are three dimensions of new insight. These dimensions are experiencing personal growth, leaning on the Lord, and recognizing positive outcomes. *Experiencing personal growth* is finding unexpected benefits of new perspectives, knowledge, and skills in the caregiving experience. Caregivers gain new appreciation of the importance of relationships in their lives and develop a new confidence and sense of worth in themselves because of care they are able to provide. Experiencing personal growth often reframes the caregiving experience and allows the discovery of positive meaning in events and outcomes that may not have been anticipated or desired in the past. *Leaning on the Lord* is finding comfort in the belief that a higher power has control of the situation and will see that the final outcome will be what is best for the patient. Prayer is often used to ensure that this best outcome is achieved. Belief that a higher power has control and is acting in the best interest of the care recipient may allow acceptance of outcomes that on the surface seem negative. *Recognizing positive outcomes* is being uplifted by events pointing to improved health for the patient. These may or may not be outcomes that the caregiver originally envisioned and yet are recognized by the caregiver as part of the process of recovery.

The caregiving relationship is constantly evolving, and caregivers gain new perspectives that help them deal with caregiving challenges and consider the illness trajectory in realistic ways. These perspectives primarily assist caregivers to reframe caregiving outcomes and maintain a positive view of the caregiving situation. Caregiver perception has long been understood as one of the most important factors influencing caregiving outcomes (Zarit, Reever, & Bach-Peterson, 1980). New insights are especially helpful as the illness process moves forward, and caregivers strive to successfully manage expectations.

Role Negotiation

Role negotiation is defined as appropriate pushing by the caregiver toward patient recovery and independence after getting a handle on complex care that demands shared responsibilities. Role negotiation happens as caregivers determine action with attention to patient voice and vigilantly bridge communication between patients and the health care system. There are five dimensions of role negotiation. These dimensions are appropriate pushing, getting a handle on it, sharing responsibilities, attending to patient voice, and vigilant bridging. *Appropriate pushing* is caregiver responsibility to see that rules for recovery set by health care providers are followed. The caregiver may encourage the patient to independently follow the rules, may develop individualized, innovative methods to support the patient in following rules, or may carry out the rules if the patient is deemed unable to meet rule requirements (Williams, 2007). *Getting a handle on it* is the struggle to come to grips with the reality of and changes demanded by illness and treatment. Strategies are identified and routines organized to meet caregiving role demands (Williams, 2007). *Sharing responsibilities* is determining illness and treatment needs, identifying the appropriate person to meet each need, and accepting the division of duties. Sharing is done between the caregiver, the patient, other family, friends, and health care providers (Williams, 2007). *Attending to patient voice* is careful listening and consideration of patient perspective by the caregiver before crafting a response or deciding on a course of action. Caregivers did not always accede to patients' wishes, but they considered patients' points-of-view in relation to situations before making decisions in the patients' best interests (Williams, 2007). *Vigilant bridging* is caregiver communication with the health care system to support the best interests of the patient. Messages from the health care system are critically evaluated by the caregiver to determine if they require action or should be relayed to the patient. Caregiver knowledge and assessments of the patient are relayed to the health care system to generate action and support for the patient (Williams, 2007).

Committing on the part of the caregiver and care recipient to the caregiving relationship starts a series of ongoing negotiations to define and redefine roles in the caregiving dyad (Shyu, 2000). With negotiation, the caregiving dyad becomes a dynamic whole, where the roles of caregiver and care recipient ebb and flow reciprocally in constant adjustment to achieve a balance that is most acceptable to both the caregiver and care recipient (Schumacher, 1996). Care recipients have been found to negotiate role functions, when possible, to maintain autonomy and relieve caregivers of tasks in order to protect the caregiver and the caregiving dyad (Russell, Bunting, & Gregory, 1997; Schumacher, 1996). Likewise, some caregivers will negotiate role functions to encourage care recipient autonomy (Bunting, 2001; Wrubel, Richards, Folkman, & Acree, 2001). When the outcome of the negotiation is acceptable to the caregiver and care recipient, there is a strengthening of the caregiving dyad (Schumacher, 1996).

Role Support

Role support is a concept related to role negotiation. Role support is knowing that others care by encountering competent compassionate care, finding support for other responsibilities, and receiving helpful information. Others may also provide help in meeting financial obligations or the caregiver may discover creative ways of meeting financial obligations. There are five dimensions of role support. These dimensions are encountering competent, compassionate care; finding support for other responsibilities; knowing others care; meeting financial responsibilities; and receiving helpful information. *Encountering competent, compassionate care* is finding health care providers and workers who determine the needs of the patient and family caregiver and meet those needs in a proficient and timely way. *Finding support for other responsibilities* is accessing assistance from others in meeting responsibilities not directly related to illness and treatment caregiving. These responsibilities may be present before the need for illness caregiving. Finding support for other responsibilities involves finding others to assume roles that the caregiver relinquishes in order to provide care. *Knowing others care* is experiencing emotional support from family, friends, and acquaintances. Contact with supportive others may occur over long distances and keeps the caregiver in touch with familiar people and events. Knowing others care gives the caregiver a sense of personal value and worth. *Meeting financial obligations* is finding ways to pay for added expenses of treatment while normal income is decreased. Help may be received from family, friends, or employers, or decisions may be made to reassign financial resources to other uses. *Receiving helpful information* is gaining knowledge that is necessary and useful for performing the caregiver role. Caregivers may feel overwhelmed by some of the responsibilities they assume as part of caregiving. Being given information or knowing that information resources are accessible if needed helps with caregiving. Role support enables caregiver negotiation within the health care system to optimize care recipient movement along the illness trajectory.

There are numerous reports of resources that caregivers use to support role functions. For instance, caregivers of patients at the end of life are less stressed when they experience open communication with and find continuity of care among health care professionals (Jo, Brazil, Lohfeld, & Willison, 2007). Swanberg (2006) found that caregivers of patients with cancer were supported in the workplace by coworkers who provided help by filling in job responsibilities, contributing money to help with medical expenses, and listening when caregivers needed someone in whom to confide. Caregivers of patients with cancer use knowledge to improve their caregiving skills and decrease feelings of burden (Aranda &

Peerson, 2001; Pasacreta, Barg, Nuamah, & McCorkle, 2000; Rose, 1999; Schumacher, Beidler, Beeber, & Gambino, 2006; Soothill et al., 2001). Information also provides caregivers of patients at the end of life with a sense of power and connectedness (McGrath, 2001; Mok, Chan, Chan, & Yeung, 2002; Wilkes, White, & O'Riordan, 2000).

RELATIONSHIPS AMONG THE CONCEPTS: THE MODEL

Caregiving dynamics are interacting processes of commitment, expectation management, and role negotiation supported by self-care, new insight, and role support that move the caregiving relationship along an illness trajectory (Figure 14.1). The circles in the model represent the relationship of the caregiver and care recipient in the past, present, and future. The present relationship is most prominent, but it is continuous with the past and the future. Commitment, expectation management, and role negotiation connect the caregiver and patient and provide the force to move the caregiving relationship through time. Self-care, new insights, and role support ground the concepts of commitment, expectation management, and role negotiation, respectively. Through self-care caregivers maintain their commitment to care recipients. When physically and emotionally healthy, caregivers can continue to focus attention on the care recipients' needs. New insight comes with support for managing expectations. New understandings and ways of framing the caregiving experience help caregivers make sense of illness outcomes. Role support offers caregivers tools to successfully fulfill care demands for the care recipient. The illness trajectory overlays the caregiving relationship, moves forward through time in parallel with the relationship, and influences the relationship (Williams, 2003).

USE OF THE THEORY IN NURSING RESEARCH

The theory was initially tested and refined in a qualitative research study of 40 caregivers of patients undergoing HSCT (Williams, 2007). While the care recipients had potentially fatal malignancies, HSCT was performed with the intent to cure or provide extended remission from disease. The caregivers were asked to tell their caregiving story approximately 3 to 4 weeks after the HSCT.

Stories were collected using the story path method (Liehr & Smith, 2000) where the storyteller begins with the present, then goes to the past and finally moves to the future by talking about hopes and dreams. Data

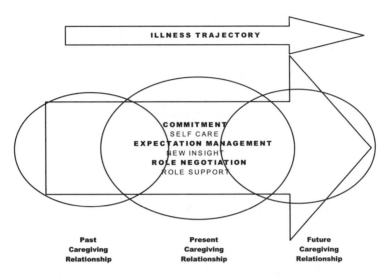

FIGURE 14.1   Caregiving dynamics.

were content analyzed using standard descriptive exploratory methods. Based on a review of literature that identified forces that motivated caregivers, expressions of commitment, expectations, and negotiation were first identified and organized into themes. The data were then searched for other forces that motivated caregivers. The caregiver stories confirmed the importance of commitment and contributed to a more precise understanding of expectation and negotiation. Expectation was renamed expectation management and negotiation was renamed role negotiation (Williams, 2007). The study concluded that (a) commitment, expectation management, and role negotiation sustain caregivers in their role; and (b) self-care, new insight, and role support were energy sources critical to caregiving dynamics.

While many of the caregivers in the study reported that they had been providing care for many months or years, possibly from the time that the patient was diagnosed with cancer, the HSCT therapy was a new experience for many caregivers and represented a chance for a possible cure. At the time these caregivers were interviewed, the care recipients were recovering from the initial effects of the HSCT. The care recipients had just come through a critical period and were doing well. The caregivers had reason to be hopeful when they told their stories and to feel that their efforts at caregiving, even if difficult at times, might contribute to a cure for the care recipient. There was concern that a theory based on the experiences of these caregivers at this stage of an illness trajectory might not apply to caregiving for patients with incurable, moribund illnesses.

A second researcher has studied caregivers of patients with primary brain tumors to determine if the theory describes their experience (Whisenant, 2006). This qualitative study of 20 caregivers used a single dialogue based on story theory (Smith & Liehr, 2003) to explore the caregiving experience. These caregivers confirmed that the six concepts in the theory were the forces that propelled their caregiving forward. No additional forces were identified. Caregivers of patients with brain tumors attached different meaning and made different use of the forces than did caregivers of patients undergoing HSCT. Caregivers of patients with brain tumors also described more negative experiences in their caregiving stories than did the caregivers of patients undergoing HSCT.

Further research is needed to test the theory in caregivers of patients at other stages in the cancer illness trajectory and in caregivers of patients with other types of illnesses. A study is currently in progress to explore the experience of caregivers of patients who develop chronic graft-versus-host disease following HSCT. While these care recipients have survived the intensity of the HSCT and are likely cured of their malignancy, they now have a chronic disease that waxes and wanes unpredictably. Caregivers of these patients may have less hope that life will ever return to normal, and they may have increased role negotiation demands as the disease waxes and wanes and the care recipients' needs change. Support from others may have declined as the immediacy of the HSCT passed. The experience of these caregivers may be different than it was during the early phase of HSCT and may be different than that of caregivers of brain tumor patients who are anticipating that the care recipient will die within months to a few years.

Because the theory considers the dyad of caregiver and care recipient, research is also needed to explore the experience of the care recipient. While research on the experience of being a caregiver is becoming more prevalent, there is little research on the experience of being a care recipient. The care recipient, as a member of the caregiving dyad, is a vital part of caregiving dynamics. It is possible that there are additional forces that move caregiving along the illness trajectory for care recipients. As further research expands understanding of the experience of caregivers and care recipients, additional modifications of the theory will be needed.

In the two studies of caregivers that have been completed, the majority of the caregivers were White. Additional research is needed to test the applicability and appropriateness of the concepts of the theory to other cultural and ethnic groups.

Intervention research based on the theory is also needed. The theory suggests interventions that could support caregivers in their roles.

Acknowledgment of the caregiver's contributions by health care professionals is an intervention that deserves further exploration. Caregivers in a variety of situations have reported feeling ignored and devalued by health care professionals (Andershed & Ternestedt, 2000; Stetz, McDonald, & Compton, 1996). How best to acknowledge caregivers and the amount of acknowledgment necessary to affect outcomes requires further exploration. Story theory (Smith & Liehr, 2003) produced an effective method of data collection among caregivers. Providing caregivers with an opportunity to tell their caregiving story to an attentive listener or to write their stories may be one method of acknowledging and memorializing their contributions.

Health maintenance and promotion is another area of intervention research suggested by the theory. Health promotion among caregivers has been studied, but most research has been descriptive (Acton, 2002; Chen, 1999; Matthews, Dunbar-Jacob, Sereika, Schulz, & McDowell, 2004; McDonald, Fink, & Wykle, 1999; O'Brien, 1993; Sisk, 2000). The caregivers of HSCT patients found exercise and eating healthy meals to be helpful in sustaining their caregiving. Interventions to encourage health promotion and make health promotion activities accessible to caregivers even when they are busy or away from home warrant further study.

USE OF THE THEORY IN NURSING PRACTICE

The first use of the middle range theory of caregiving dynamics in practice is currently in progress. The HSCT Inpatient and Outpatient Units at the University of Texas M. D. Anderson Cancer Center (Houston, TX) are using the theory to devise interventions to support caregivers.

An information book specifically for caregivers is being developed. In the past, there was a single brief chapter in the HSCT book for patients that discussed caregivers. In addition, a class for patients was conducted prior to HSCT, and caregivers were invited to attend. Three HSCT classes will now be held at various times throughout the HSCT trajectory. One class several weeks prior to the HSCT will be targeted to caregivers. A second class held immediately before the patient is admitted to the hospital for the HSCT will focus on the patient. The last class to be held immediately prior to the patient's discharge from the hospital will be divided between the patient and the caregiver. The intention of having a special book and classes for the caregiver is to acknowledge the importance of the caregiver and to strengthen the caregiver's commitment. In addition, the book and classes will provide the caregiver with helpful information that is part of role support.

Caregivers will be provided with opportunities to participate in exercise classes and will be given suggestions for healthy eating while they spend time at the hospital during the HSCT. In addition, caregivers will be provided with a variety of opportunities to express frustrations, worries, and fears associated with caregiving, such as support groups, journaling, art therapy, and an online chat community.

Other opportunities to support caregivers by providing positive forces to move caregiving forward are suggested by the theory of caregiving dynamics. Specific applications of the theory will vary among different caregiver and care recipient populations. Important considerations in deciding how best to support caregivers will include age, gender, and ethnicity of the caregiver and care recipient; the illness, treatment, and illness trajectory; and the site of caregiving. It is expected that use of the theory in practice will result in evaluation of outcomes, which serve as evidence of the usefulness of interventions suggested by the theory.

CONCLUSION

Caregiving by family members, friends, and neighbors is a crucial component of care in the current health system. While the burden of caregiving has been investigated, little attention has been paid to the forces that drive caregiving forward. The middle range theory of caregiving dynamics was developed to help understand these forces so that caregiving might be strengthened. The literature-derived model was tested, refined, and has been proposed as a middle range theory in this chapter. Further research is needed to confirm the applicability and appropriateness of the theory to care recipients, to caregivers in other situations, and to caregiving dyads of various cultural and ethnic backgrounds. Interventions suggested by the theory also need investigation. Use of the theory in practice is just beginning. As more experience is gained with the theory it will be modified to better describe the caregiving experience and to better guide nursing practice and research. Use of the theory to date has shown that it describes the caregiving situation from the perspective of the caregiver and is useful in suggesting interventions to support caregiving.

REFERENCES

Acton, G. J. (2002). Health-promoting self-care in family caregivers. *Western Journal of Nursing Research, 24,* 73–86.

Andershed, B., & Ternestedt, B. M. (2000). Being a close relative of a dying person: Development of the concepts "involvement in the light and in the dark." *Cancer Nursing, 23,* 151–159.

Aranda, S., & Peerson, A. (2001). Global exchange. Caregiving in advanced cancer: Lay decision making. *Journal of Palliative Care, 17*(4), 270–276.

Arno, P. (2006). *Economic value of family caregiving: 2004*. Retrieved March 5, 2007, from http://www.thefamilycaregiver.org/who/stats.cfm

Biegel, D., Sales, E., & Schulz, R. (1991). *Family caregiving in chronic illness: Heart disease, cancer, stroke, Alzheimer's disease, and chronic mental illness*. Newbury Park, CA: Sage.

Bowman, K. F., Rose, J. H., & Deimling, G. T. (2005). Families of long-term cancer survivors: Health maintenance advocacy and practice. *Psychooncology, 14*, 1008–1017.

Boyle, D., Blodgett, L., Gnesdiloff, S., White, J. R., Bamford, A. M., Sheridan, M., et al. (2000). Caregiver quality of life after autologous bone marrow transplantation. *Cancer Nursing, 23*, 193–203.

Bunting, S. M. (2001). Sustaining the relationship: Women's caregiving in the context of HIV disease. *Health Care for Women International, 22*, 131–148.

Chen, M. Y. (1999). The effectiveness of health promotion counseling to family caregivers. *Public Health Nursing, 16*, 125–132.

Cohen, C. A., Gold, D. P., Shulman, K. I., Wortley, J. T., McDonald, G., & Wargon, M. (1993). Factors determining the decision to institutionalize dementing individuals: A prospective study. *The Gerontologist, 33*, 714–720.

Connell, C. (1994). Impact of spouse caregiving on health behaviors and physical and mental health status. *American Journal of Alzeheimer's Care and Related Disorders and Research, 9*, 26–36.

Ferrell, B. R., Cohen, M. Z., Rhiner, M., & Rozek, A. (1991). Pain as a metaphor for illness. Part II: Family caregivers' management of pain. *Oncology Nursing Forum, 18*, 1315–1321.

Folkman, S. (1997). Positive psychological states and coping with severe stress. *Social Science and Medicine, 45*, 1207–1221.

Frey, P., Stinson, T., Siston, A., Knight, S. J., Ferdman, E., Traynor, A., et al. (2002). Lack of caregivers limits the use of outpatient hematopoietic stem cell transplant program. *Bone Marrow Transplantation, 30*, 741–748.

Grimm, P. M., Zawacki, K. L., Mock, V., Krumm, S., & Frink, B. B. (2000). Caregiver responses and needs. An ambulatory bone marrow transplant model. *Cancer Practice, 8*, 120–128.

Hadjistavropoulos, T., Taylor, S., Tuokko, H., & Beattie, B. L. (1994). Neuropsychological deficits, caregivers' perception of deficits and caregiver burden. *Journal of the American Geriatrics Society, 42*, 308–314.

Horowitz, M. M., Loberiza, F. R., Bredeson, C. N., Rizzo, J. D., & Nugent, M. L. (2001). Transplant registries: Guiding clinical decisions and improving outcomes. *Oncology, 15*, 649–659, 663–664, 666.

Jewell, E. J., & Abate, F. (Eds.). (2001). *The New Oxford American Dictionary*. New York: Oxford University Press.

Jo, S., Brazil, K., Lohfeld, L., & Willison, K. (2007). Caregiving at the end of life: Perspectives from spousal caregivers and care recipients. *Palliative and Supportive Care, 5*, 11–17.

Kylma, J., Vehviläinen-Julkunen, K., & Lähdevirta, J. (2001). Dynamically fluctuating hope, despair and hopelessness along the HIV/AIDS continuum as described by caregivers in voluntary organizations in Finland. *Issues in Mental Health Nursing, 22*, 353–377.

Liehr, P., & Smith, M. J. (2000). Using Story Theory to guide nursing practice. *International Journal of Human Caring, 4*, 13–18.

Loberiza, F., Jr. (2003). Summary slides 2003. *IBMTR/ABMTR Newsletter, 10*(1), 1, 7–10.

Matthews, J. T., Dunbar-Jacob, J., Sereika, S., Schulz, R., & McDowell, B. J. (2004). Preventive health practices: Comparison of family caregivers 50 and older. *Journal of Gerontological Nursing, 30*(2), 46–54.

McDonald, P. E., Fink, S. V., & Wykle, M. L. (1999). Self-reported health-promoting behaviors of black and white caregivers. *Western Journal of Nursing Research, 21,* 538–548.

McGrath, P. (2001). Caregivers' insights in the dying trajectory in hematology oncology. *Cancer Nursing, 24,* 413–421.

Merriam-Webster OnLine. (2007). *Merriam-Webster's Collegiate Dictionary* [Web site]. Retrieved March 5, 2007, from http://www.m-w.com/dictionary.

Miller, B., Townsend, A., Carpenter, E., Montgomery, R. V., Stull, D., & Young, R. F. (2001). Social support and caregiver distress: A replication analysis. *Journal of Gerontology Series B: Psychological Science and Social Science, 56,* S249–S256.

Mok, E., Chan, F., Chan, V., & Yeung, E. (2002). Perception of empowerment by family caregivers of patients with a terminal illness in Hong Kong. *International Journal of Palliative Nursing, 8,* 137–145.

O'Brien, M. T. (1993). Multiple sclerosis: Health-promoting behaviors of spousal caregivers. *Journal of Neuroscience Nursing, 25,* 105–112.

Ostwald, S. K. (1997). Caregiver exhaustion: Caring for the hidden patients. *Advanced Practice Nursing Quarterly, 3*(2), 29–35.

Padilla, G. V., Mishel, M. H., & Grant, M. M. (1992). Uncertainty, appraisal and quality of life. *Quality of Life Research, 1,* 155–165.

Pasacreta, J. V., Barg, F., Nuamah, I., & McCorkle, R. (2000). Participant characteristics before and 4 months after attendance at a family caregiver cancer education program. *Cancer Nursing, 23,* 295–303.

Pasacreta, J. V., & McCorkle, R. (2000). Cancer care: Impact of interventions on caregiver outcomes. *Annual Review of Nursing Research, 18,* 127–148.

Phillips, L. R., Brewer, B. B., & Torres de Ardon, E. (2001). The Elder Image Scale: A method for indexing history and emotion in family caregiving. *Journal of Nursing Measurement, 9,* 23–47.

Rose, K. E. (1999). A qualitative analysis of the information needs of informal carers of terminally ill cancer patients. *Journal of Clinical Nursing, 8,* 81–88.

Russell, C. K., Bunting, S. M., & Gregory, D. M. (1997). Protective care-receiving: The active role of care-recipients. *Journal of Advanced Nursing, 25,* 532–540.

Schumacher, K. L. (1996). Reconceptualizing family caregiving: Family-based illness care during chemotherapy. *Research in Nursing and Health, 19,* 261–271.

Schumacher, K. L., Beidler, S. M., Beeber, A. S., & Gambino, P. (2006). A transactional model of cancer family caregiving skill. *Advances in Nursing Science, 29,* 271–286.

Schumacher, K. L., Stewart, B. J., & Archbold, P. G. (1998). Conceptualization and measurement of doing family caregiving well. *Image: Journal of Nursing Scholarship, 30,* 63–69.

Seltzer, M. M., & Li, L. W. (2000). The dynamics of caregiving: Transitions during a three-year prospective study. *Gerontologist, 40,* 165–178.

Shyu, Y. I. (2000). Role tuning between caregiver and care receiver during discharge transition: An illustration of role function mode in Roy's adaptation theory. *Nursing Science Quarterly, 13,* 323–331.

Sisk, R. J. (2000). Caregiver burden and health promotion. *International Journal of Nursing Studies, 37,* 37–43.

Smith, M. J., & Liehr, P. (2003). The theory of attentively embracing story. In M. J. Smith & P. R. Liehr (Eds.), *Middle range theory for nursing* (pp. 167–187). New York: Springer Publishing.

Soothill, K., Morris, S. M., Harman, J. C., Francis, B., Thomas, C., & McIllmurray, M. B. (2001). Informal carers of cancer patients: What are their unmet psychosocial needs? *Health and Social Care in the Community, 9,* 464–475.

Speice, J., Harkness, J., Laneri, H., Frankel, R., Roter, D., Kornblith, A. B., et al. (2000). Involving family members in cancer care: Focus group considerations of patients and oncological providers. *Psycho-Oncology, 9,* 101–112.

Stetz, K. M., McDonald, J. C., & Compton, K. (1996). Needs and experiences of family caregivers during marrow transplantation. *Oncology Nursing Forum, 23,* 1422–1427.

Swanberg, J. E. (2006). Making it work: Informal caregiving, cancer, and employment. *Journal of Psychosocial Oncology, 24*(3), 1–18.

Thompson, L. (2004). *Long-term care: Support for family caregivers* [Issue Brief]. Georgetown University: Washington, DC. Retrieved March 5, 2007, from http://ltc.george town.edu/pdfs/caregivers.pdf

U.S. Census Bureau. (2005, April 29). Facts for features: Special addition: National nurses week (May 6–12) and national hospital week (May 8–14). Retrieved March 5, 2007, from http://www.census.gov/Press-Release/www/releases/archives/cb05-ffse.02.pdf

Whisenant, M. S. (2006). *Informal caregiving in patients with brain tumors: Jumping into the deep end.* Unpublished master's thesis, University of Texas–Houston School of Nursing, Houston, TX.

Wilkes, L., White, K., & O'Riordan, L. (2000). Empowerment through information: Supporting rural families of oncology patients in palliative care. *Australian Journal of Rural Health, 8,* 41–46.

Williams, L. A. (2003). Informal caregiving dynamics with a case study in blood and marrow transplantation. *Oncology Nursing Forum, 30,* 679–688.

Williams, L. A. (2007). Whatever it takes: Informal caregiving dynamics in blood and marrow transplantation. *Oncology Nursing Forum, 34,* 379–387.

Wrubel, J., Richards, T. A., Folkman, S., & Acree, M. C. (2001). Tacit definitions of informal caregiving. *Journal of Advanced Nursing, 33,* 175–181.

Wuest, J. (2001). Precarious ordering: Toward a formal theory of women's caring. *Health Care for Women International, 22,* 167–193.

Zarit, S. H., Reever, K. E., & Bach-Peterson, J. (1980). Relatives of the impaired elderly: Correlates of feelings of burden. *Gerontologist, 20,* 649–655.

CHAPTER 15

Theory of Moral Reckoning

Alvita Nathaniel

Today's health care environment, with its spiraling technology, longer life spans, power imbalance, and budget restraints, engenders an atmosphere with moral problems of ever-increasing complexity—problems for which the most basic moral beliefs about life, death, right, and wrong are challenged. An increasing number of researchers have examined nurses' responses to these types of stressors and their impact on patient care, often determining that nurses experience moral distress in many such situations. The theory of moral reckoning began with an interest in this compelling concept.

PURPOSE OF THE THEORY AND HOW IT WAS DEVELOPED

Andrew Jameton, a philosopher and ethicist, first described moral distress in nursing. When Jameton asked nurses to talk about moral dilemmas, he noticed that their stories failed to meet the definition of dilemma (Jameton, 1984, pp. 335–336). A moral dilemma forces one to choose between two undesirable, mutually exclusive alternatives—the correct choice is unclear, since all alternatives have nearly equal moral weight and none are more right or wrong than others. Relating their personal stories, nurses consistently talked to Jameton about situations in which they believed they knew the morally right actions to take, yet they felt constrained from following their convictions (Jameton, 1993). Jameton concluded that nurses were compelled to tell these stories

277

because of their profound suffering and their belief about the importance of the situations. Mentioning this concept only briefly, Jameton proposed that "moral distress arises when one knows the right thing to do, but institutional constraints make it nearly impossible to pursue the right course of action" (Jameton, 1984, p. 6). Jameton also stipulated that nurses who participate in an action that they have judged to be morally wrong experience moral distress (Jameton, 1993). Building upon Jameton's definition, Wilkinson defined moral distress as "the psychological disequilibrium and negative feeling state experienced when a person makes a moral decision but does not follow through by performing the moral behavior indicated by that decision" (Wilkinson, 1987, p. 16). In the intervening years, there has been increasing interest in moral distress. Most subsequent nursing sources rely on Jameton's or Wilkinson's definition of moral distress.

For many years, I taught a nursing ethics course and later coauthored an ethics textbook (Burkhardt & Nathaniel, 2008). The concept of moral distress caught my imagination. I wondered, for example, if we in the profession claim that nurses are autonomous professionals, why do so many nurses violate their own moral codes when faced with constraints to action? How can institutional pressure override an individual's beliefs, values, and convictions formed over a lifetime? Why do highly educated professionals view themselves as powerless in morally troubling situations? How does moral distress affect nurses, patients, and the health care system as a whole?

Even though the literature offered emotionally charged descriptions of nurses' moral distress, the knowledge was limited in four essential ways. First, there were few studies, with few informants, so even though many nurses had written about moral distress, we really knew very little about it. Second, only a handful of published studies identified moral distress in their purpose statements. In addition, most published studies were rudimentary and exploratory in nature. Third, theoretical foundations did not adequately explain moral distress. Fourth, there were gaps in the literature in terms of the impact of moral distress on nursing care and patients' health outcomes.

Awareness of these limitations prompted pursuit of understanding. I began conducting interviews with nurses who reported that they had experienced morally troubling patient care situations. My purpose was to address gaps in knowledge by seeking answers to one basic research question: What transpires in morally laden situations in which nurses experience distress? Using the inductive approach of classic grounded theory (Glaser, 1965, 1978, 1998; Glaser & Strauss, 1967), I soon recognized that more was going on in these situations than could be explained adequately by the concept of moral distress. Distinct patterns and processes emerged from the data, making it clear that nurses' experiences followed a relatively predictable pattern as each nurse made important choices before, during, and after becoming entangled in a morally significant situational bind.

As required by the classic grounded theory method, I laid aside preconceived notions, logical elaborations, and ideas gleaned from the extant literature. New concepts, processes, and tentative hypotheses began to emerge from the empirical data through careful investigation, inductive reasoning, and analysis. Early in the data-gathering phase, I noticed that nurses vividly recalled important junctures in their professional lives that included morally troubling patient care situations yet seemed to be part of a much bigger process. Extant research focusing on moral distress remained pertinent and was subsequently interwoven into the larger, more explanatory and predictive process of moral reckoning, adding depth and complexity to the resultant theory.

The theory of moral reckoning emerged through the inductive process of the classic grounded theory method. I recorded the interviews as field notes immediately after each interview. Analysis began with the first episode of data gathering and was simultaneous with other steps of the process. Using constant comparison as suggested by Glaser (1965), data were analyzed sentence by sentence as they were coded. Data were organized into concepts and further into categories. I composed conceptual-level memos as concepts became evident. As the research continued, social psychological processes began to surface. Moral reckoning emerged as the theory to which all other concepts related. Identification of moral reckoning enabled subsequent selective theoretical sampling, coding, and memoing. Theoretical sampling began when concepts seemed to require more refinement or areas needed more depth. Memos consisted of the emerging concepts and categories (highly abstract concepts). When it became clear that the indicators were saturated, I began sorting and organizing the memos.

The larger process of moral reckoning overlaps moral distress as described in the extant literature. Both moral reckoning and moral distress include a situational bind (unnamed in moral distress literature) and consequences for nurses. Because it explicates choices and actions and includes precursor conditions and long-term consequences, the substantive and more comprehensive and explanatory theory of moral reckoning effectively synthesizes, organizes, and transcends what was previously known about moral distress.

Moral reckoning captures the culmination of the process as nurses critically and emotionally reflect on motivations, choices, actions, and consequences entangled in a particularly troubling patient care situation. They are alone with their experiences; wrestling with something they have difficulty communicating. According to Strauss (1959), critical events occur in which there is a temporary gap between events and the person's understanding of them. The person is aware of this gap. Under certain social conditions, such as with moral reckoning, a person will undergo so many or such critical experiences for which conventional explanations seem inadequate that the person begins to question large segments of what was previously learned. Subsequently, there is an internal rhetorical battle. The person cannot question what was learned in the past without questioning internal purposes. If the person rejects the explanations once believed, then there will be a type of alienation—a perception of a world lost. The person may feel spiritually dispossessed as he or she embraces a set of counter explanations to recreate a world-view (Strauss, 1959).

The term *reckon* is especially suitable to describe the name of the theory. To reckon is to enumerate serially or separately; to name or mention one after another in due order; to go over or through (a series) in this manner; to recount, relate, narrate, tell; to mention; to allege; to calculate, work out, decide the nature or value of; to consider, judge, or estimate by, or as the result of calculation; to consider, think, suppose, be of opinion; to speak or discourse of something; to render or give an account (of one's conduct, etc.); and to regard in a certain light (Simpson & Weiner, 1989, pp. 335–336).

Reckoning is "the action of rendering to another an account of one's self or one's conduct; an account, statement of something" (Simpson & Weiner, 1989, p. 336).

CONCEPTS OF THE THEORY

Concepts in the middle range theory of moral reckoning include ease, situational binds, resolution, and reflection. The named concepts of the theory are processes that comprise the stages of moral reckoning. The second concept situational bind is an event that interrupts the stage of ease.

Ease

Ease is a state of naturalness, a sense of comfort. Ease assumes a certain measure of freedom from constraint, worry, hardship, and agitation. Ease also denotes readiness and skillfulness. Nurses who experience ease are comfortable. They have technical skills and feel rewarded to practice within the boundaries of self, profession, and institution. They know their patients and witness their suffering, making the implicit promise that they have skill and knowledge to relieve suffering. These nurses are competent and confident. They know what others expect of them and experience a sense of flow and at-homeness. When at ease, nurses have high standards and are proud of their technical abilities and skill at communicating with patients and others. As long as the work of nursing fulfills the nurse and the nurse experiences a sense of comfort with the integration of core beliefs and professional and institutional norms, then ease continues.

Situational Binds

Situational binds are serious and complex conflicts within individuals and tacit or overt conflicts between nurses and others—all having moral overtones. The concept *situational bind* was discussed by Strauss (1959), who theorized that when situational binds occur the person questions his or her central purpose, asking to what, for what, or to whom he or she is committed. The person experiences turmoil and inner dialogue that leads to a decision.

Situational binds lead to life turning points. These incidents transform identity and force a person to recognize that "I am not the same as I was, as I used to be" (Strauss, 1959, p. 93). Critical incidents lead to "surprise, shock, chagrin, anxiety, tension, bafflement, self-questioning—and also the need to try out the new self, to explore and validate the new and often exciting or fearful conceptions" (Strauss, 1959, p. 93). Situational binds lead to decisions that ultimately change people's lives.

Resolution

Resolution is a move to set things right, to resolve the turmoil and to relieve the tension. Resolution occurs when a person terminates the intolerable condition by finding a solution to the problem, deciding on a course of action, and bringing a situation to a conclusion. The person might make a declaration or carry out a plan. Resolution tends to disentangle one from a situational bind.

Reflection

Reflection is contemplating, pondering, and thinking about past events. Having made and acted upon a decision, a person reflects as he or she reckons past behavior and actions. The person carefully considers the events and generates opinions. Reflection raises questions about previous judgments, particular acts, and the essential self. Reflection may extend over a lifetime.

RELATIONSHIPS AMONG THE CONCEPTS: THE MODEL

Moral reckoning consists of a three-stage process as nurses reflect on motivations, choices, actions, and consequences of a morally troubling patient care situation (Nathaniel, 2004, 2006). The relationship among the stages is depicted in Figure 15.1. In the middle range theory of moral reckoning the stage of ease is disrupted by a situational bind and then followed by the processes of resolution and reflection.

The Stage of Ease

After the initial novice phase, nurses experience a stage of ease in which they enjoy a sense of satisfaction and at-homeness in the workplace. They feel comfortable with their knowledge and skills. Properties central to the stage of ease include becoming, professionalizing, institutionalizing, and working. There is a fragile balance among the properties during the stage of ease such that each property is related to the other, creating a feeling of comfort.

Becoming. As Strauss once wrote, "The human experience of time is one of process: the present is always a becoming" (Strauss, 1959, p. 31). Through the process of becoming every person evolves a set of core beliefs and values, which are a product of lifelong learning about what is important and how to behave in society. Core beliefs evolve through experience, from the testimony of authority, and from the modeling of parents, teachers, ministers, peers, and others. Integration and consistency of core values produce moral integrity (Beauchamp & Childress,

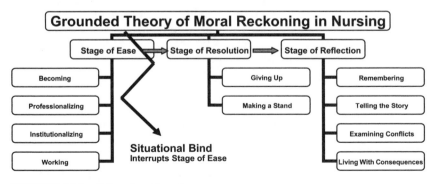

FIGURE 15.1   Moral reckoning.

Reprinted from: Nathaniel, A. K. (2006). Moral reckoning in nursing. *Western Journal of Nursing Research, 28*(4), 419–438.

2001). Through the lifelong process of becoming, nurses develop core beliefs and values.

Professionalizing. The process of becoming a nurse includes inculcation of certain cultural norms learned in nursing school and early practice. Professional norms are conceptual ideals that contribute to the nurse's idea of what a good nurse should be or do. Explicitly, nurses learn that they have unique relationships with patients and are responsible to keep promises, which are sometimes implicit in the relationship. Penticuff identified moral goals that are part of nursing's common perspective, such as "the protection and enhancement of human dignity, the alleviation of vulnerability, the promotion of growth and health, and the enhancement of coping and comfort in the face of hardship" (Penticuff, 1997, p. 51). Likewise, nurses honor the common professional norms of knowing patients as persons, listening to their needs and preferences, supporting their everyday choices through advocacy, and maintaining their dignity (Doutrich, Wros, & Izumi, 2001).

Professionalizing is supported by the theoretical work of Strauss (1959) and Glaser (1998). Strauss suggested that to become a member of a group, a person must invest in the goals of the group. Investment in a group occurs through the transmission of ideas and signifies shared meanings. Insofar as the person thinks of himself or herself as an integral part of the group, he or she embraces its goals. The person, then, has dual commitment to the group and to self. Strauss also suggested that a person may be so heavily identified with the group that "he is no longer quite himself" (Strauss, 1959, p. 37). Validation by the group is so important that the person reinterprets activity and meaning. Thus, as can be seen in moral reckoning, the person's core values may be either supported or challenged by the values of the group as the person becomes professionalized. Similarly, Glaser (1998) proposed that personal identities may merge with properties of a profession so that members find it difficult to break through the boundaries (Glaser, 1998). In this situation, the unit identity becomes the person's self-image. Professional norms sometimes lead nurses to act according to role-set behavior, governed by blind adherence to professional norms and by their perception of the expectations of others.

Institutionalizing. The third property rests on the premise that the nurse works in an institutional setting with both implicit and explicit institutional norms. This is corroborated by the studies of Liaschenko (1995) and Ehrenreich and Ehrenreich (1990), who propose that institutionalized medicine is a complex interconnected tangle of practice patterns, cultural beliefs, and values in which the practice of nursing takes place. Institutional health care delivery norms constitute basic social structural processes within which the practice of nursing takes place. Explicit institutional norms include completing a job according to institutional standards and respecting lines of authority. Implicit institutional norms include such concepts as assuring that the business makes a profit, following orders, and handling crises without making waves.

Working. The work of nursing is varied, challenging, and rewarding. Nurses attend to the most personal and private needs and learn much about patients' hopes, fears, and desires (Penticuff, 1997). They get to know patients who stay on their unit for extended periods or return many times. Doing the work of nursing includes knowing patients intimately, witnessing their suffering, accepting the responsibility to care, desiring to do the work well, and knowing what to do.

Situational Binds

Sometimes, troubling events occur that challenge the integration of core beliefs, professional norms, and institutional norms. When this happens, nurses find themselves in *situational binds* that force them into a critical juncture in their professional lives (Nathaniel, 2004, 2006).

A situational bind terminates the stage of ease and throws the nurse into turmoil when core beliefs and other claims conflict. Three types of situational binds include conflicts between core values and professional or institutional norms, moral disagreement among decision makers in the face of power imbalance, and workplace deficiencies that cause real or potential harm to patients (Nathaniel, 2004, 2006). These binds produce dramatic consequences for nurses when they must choose one value or belief over another—forcing a turning point in their professional lives.

Situational binds in nursing involve an intricate interweaving of many factors including professional relationships, divergent values, workplace demands, and other implications with moral overtones. Situational binds vary in their complexity, context, and particulars but are similar in terms of their immediate and long-term effects. When situational binds occur, nurses must make critical decisions—choosing one value or belief over another. Specific types of binds include conflict between the nurse's core beliefs and professional or institutional norms, power imbalance complicated by differences in beliefs and values, conflicting loyalty, and serious workplace deficiencies (Nathaniel, 2004, 2006). Types of cases most frequently mentioned in the extant literature included causing needless suffering by prolonging the life of dying patients or performing unnecessary tests and treatments, especially on terminal patients; lying to patients; incompetent or inadequate treatment by a physician; and coercing consent from poorly informed patients (Bamford, 1995; Bassett, 1995; Corley, 1995; Rodney, 1988; Wilkinson, 1987).

The disruption of ease that nurses experience during situational binds results from a number of dynamic internal and external tensions (Nathaniel, 2004, 2006). For example, the ability to act on moral decisions may be constrained by socialization to follow orders, self-doubt, lack of courage, and conflicting loyalty. Penticuff (1997) also found that nurses struggle with conflicting loyalties to patients, nursing peers, physicians, and institutions. Asymmetrical power relationships and powerlessness often lead to situational binds. Nurses may have insight into the problem at hand yet believe they cannot participate in the decision-making process. They sense a moral responsibility, want the best outcome for patients, know what is needed, and yet believe they are powerless to get it done. In some instances, nurses experience distress when they know the professional and institutional norms, are aware of their own core beliefs, and yet are unable to uphold them because of workplace deficiencies. Workplace deficiencies include such factors as chronic staff shortage, unreasonable institutional expectations, and equipment inadequacy (Nathaniel, 2004, 2006). Situational binds force nurses to make difficult decisions in the midst of crises characterized by intolerable internal conflict. Something must be done to rectify the situation: one must make a choice.

In the midst of the situational bind or soon after, nurses experience consequences such as profound emotions, reactive behaviors, and physical manifestations. Nurses may experience feelings of guilt, anger, powerlessness, conflict, depression, outrage, betrayal, and devastation. Physical manifestations such as lightheadedness, crying, sleeplessness, and vomiting may also occur.

During the time of or after situational binds, nursing care is affected—sometimes negatively and sometimes positively. Some nurses are unable to care for the patient or to even return to the unit after a troubling incident. Some nurses make up for what they consider to be wrongdoing by giving more compassionate care—even to the point of sacrificing personal time. For others, care improves in the long term because of lessons learned in the process.

The Stage of Resolution

Situational binds constitute crises of intolerable internal conflict. The nurse seeks to resolve the problem and set things right. This signifies the beginning of the stage of resolution. This stage often alters professional trajectory. There are two properties of the stage of resolution: making a stand and giving up. These properties are not mutually exclusive. In fact, a nurse might give up, reconsider, and make a stand.

Making a Stand. In the midst of a situational bind, some nurses choose to make a stand. Making a stand takes a variety forms—all of which include professional risk. Nurses may even make a stand by stepping beyond the proscribed boundaries of the profession to do what, to them, seems to be the morally correct action. Nurses may make a stand by refusing to follow physicians' orders, initiating negotiations, breaking the rules, whistle blowing, and so forth. Making a stand is rarely successful in the short term. Not a single informant in Liaschenko's (1995) study reported an instance where treatment was stopped on his/her testimony. Nevertheless, making a stand may occasionally improve the overall situation in the long term.

Giving Up. Sometimes nurses resolve a morally troubling situation by giving up. Giving up may overlap with making a stand in some instances. Nurses often give up because they recognize the futility of making an overt stand. They are simply not willing to sacrifice for no purpose. They may give up to protect themselves or to seek a way or find a place where they can better integrate core beliefs, professional norms, and institutional norms. Giving up includes participating (with regret) in an activity they consider to be morally wrong or leaving the unit, the institution, or the profession altogether. Sometimes nurses seem to give up in the short term but move toward more advanced or autonomous roles or toward leadership positions—all of which prepare them to make a stand in the future.

The Stage of Reflection

During the stage of reflection the nurse thoughtfully examines beliefs, values, and actions. Properties of the stage of reflection include remembering, telling the story, examining conflicts, and living with the consequences. During this stage, which may last a lifetime, nurses reflect on the moral problem and their response. Nurses recall vivid mental pictures and evoked emotions such as feelings of guilt and self-blame, lingering sadness, anger, and anxiety. Moral reckoning continues over time as nurses remember, tell the story, examine conflicts, and live with the consequences.

Remembering. One of the more intriguing properties of moral reckoning is the manner in which nurses remember critical events. After particularly troubling situations, nurses retain vivid mental pictures, which tend to evoke emotions many years later. Nurses remember sensual particulars of the incident—the sights, sounds, and smells. Even after many years, the images are seared into their minds. Remembering evokes emotions including feelings of guilt and self-blame, lingering sadness, anger, and anxiety. Lingering emotional effects may be profound for many.

Strauss (1959) proposed that a remembered act is never finished. As a person recalls the act, he or she selectively reconstructs it, remembering certain aspects and dropping others. The person reassesses acts many times, seeking new perspectives or new facts. Thus, learning leads to revision of concepts that, in turn, leads to reorganization of behavior. Strauss further proposed that the process of continual learning and revision results in a new identity. This sort of ambiguity raises challenges and the discovery of new values through which transformation takes place.

Telling the Story. Nurses want to tell the story to sympathetic others. They may tell a friend or family member immediately after an incident occurs or meet with other nurses to discuss the event. Nurses rely upon others to hear the story and to understand it from their perspective. A listening, non-judgmental person allows the nurse to tell the story as he or she attempts to seek meaning and to reckon belief and action. Nurses continue the process over time—telling and re-telling the story as they try to make sense of it. Smith and Liehr (2003) address story-gathering in the chapter (11) describing Story Theory. They say that engaging in dialogue about unique human experience catalyzes the beginning of a process of personal change. Through following the story path as recollected, one begins a process of discovery, self-revelation, and reckoning. As the story unfolds, the person attempts to understand the meaning of experiences and gain new perspectives and wisdom. The person goes into the depths of the story to find unique meanings and reconstruct a story that has a beginning, middle, and end. Consistent with the theory of moral reckoning, Smith and Liehr propose that as the person tells the story, he or she gains a full-dimensional, reflective awareness of bodily experiences, thoughts, feelings, emotions, and values. Patterns are discerned, made explicit, and named. Telling the story relieves pain and creates possibilities for human development.

Examining Conflicts. As nurses tell their stories, they begin to examine conflicts in the troubling situation. They examine their values and ask themselves questions about what actually happened, who was to blame, and how they can avoid similar situations in the future. As they thoughtfully examine the conflicts, some intellectualize their participation, some set limits, and some gain strength to make a stand and accept the consequences in future situations.

Nurses continue to struggle with conflicts between personal values and professional ideals. They want to be able to identify themselves as good nurses. Similarly, Kelly (1998) reported that some nurses have a painful awareness of the discrepancy between who they aspired to be and what they have become. These nurses suffered the loss of their own professional self-concept, their vision of the kind of nurses they wanted to be, and their image of nursing as they believed it was.

As nurses think about their roles in what they consider past moral wrongdoing, some set limits or make pronouncements about their future actions. Some identify a point beyond which they will not again be willing to go. Others vow to step outside their boundaries to help a patient in the future, fully aware and willing to accept the consequences of their future actions. Thus, the nurse's ethical practice evolves through the iterative process of experience and reflection.

Living With the Consequences. Nurses live with the consequences of morally troubling situations for a prolonged period of time. Consequences other than those already mentioned include fracturing professional relationships and changing one's life trajectory. Following a situational bind in which the nurse believes another person committed moral wrongdoing, he or she may be unable to work collaboratively with that person or others who were unsupportive. They lose faith in the person's integrity or lose respect for them as practitioners. Since they are no longer comfortable in the original workplace and have fractured professional relationships, many nurses change their work setting and often their life trajectory following a situational bind. They may change employers or specialties and they are likely to seek further education, many times intending to correct the type of moral wrongs they experienced in the past.

USE OF THE THEORY IN NURSING RESEARCH

The theory calls for programs of research that will further explore and more fully develop the concepts, begin to identify causes, and make comparisons and predictions. Vigorous theoretical sampling is needed to (a) allow a more thorough and useful understanding of the concepts of ease, situational bind, resolution, and reflection and different ways that nurses might progress through them, (b) provide a better understanding of core values as they intersect with professional and institutional norms, and (c) modify the theory to include different levels of nursing practice.

In addition, nursing ethics research is needed to shed light on what nurses understand about nursing ethics, the depth of this understanding, how the understanding of nursing ethics factors into everyday decision making, and what kind of learning leads to empowered, patient-centered, ethical decision making. Further qualitative and quantitative research is needed to determine the characteristics of nurses who experience moral distress and moral reckoning versus those who do not and the quality of patient care provided by each group. Correlational research is needed to identify nurses who leave the bedside and those who stay, particularly in relation to whether or not they have experienced situational binds. In the face of the nursing shortage, this has implications for nurse recruiting and retention. If caring and sensitive nurses leave the bedside, it is important for research to identify strategies to retain them.

Research on moral reckoning should not be limited to the profession of nursing. Investigators have an opportunity to use the theory with a wide variety of populations. For instance, people who live through disasters such as September 11, 2001, or Hurricane Katrina may experience moral reckoning. Significant losses, such as the death of a child or the loss of a family-sustaining job, create a context for moral reckoning. In addition, the obvious use of the theory with other disciplines deserves consideration, particularly as related to nursing practice and patient outcomes.

USE OF THE THEORY IN NURSING PRACTICE

Implications for Nursing Ethics Development

Moral reckoning points to a chasm between the ethical practice of nurses and formal ethics theory. This may indicate what MacIntyre (1988) terms an "epistemological crisis" in nursing: a crisis that occurs when events bring into question ideals and convictions of a tradition and when previous methods of inquiry, conceptualization, and principles fall into question. MacIntyre suggests that an epistemological crisis can be resolved successfully through innovations that meet three requirements: (1) new concepts and new theory must furnish a systematic and rational solution to a previously unmanageable problem; (2) innovations must explain what it was that made the tradition ineffective, and; (3) the new tradition must carry out tasks in a way that exhibits some fundamental continuity of new conceptual and theoretical structures with the tradition's shared beliefs (MacIntyre, 1988). Such ethics will allow for consideration of the uniqueness and particularity of patient situations, while acknowledging diverse moral perspectives. As MacIntyre (1988) suggests, nurses should come to understand rival perspectives as different, yet comprising complementary understandings of reality.

Implications for Nursing Educators

The middle range theory of moral reckoning brings several implications for nursing education. Recommendations include strengthening nursing ethics education, teaching strategies to improve nurses' empowerment, and helping students learn effective ways to establish intra- and interprofessional relationships. Nurse educators teach students to be ethically self-aware and provide opportunities for them to learn about normative ethics. Educators can closely examine implicit messages transmitted to students, particularly traditions of the discipline that inhibit meaningful dialogue and sustain conflict and power imbalance. In this manner, they help students learn strategies and language that prepare them to enter into ethical dialogue with other professionals, and to prepare students for the realities of practice.

Specifically, the middle range theory of moral reckoning uncovers a basic social process seldom considered before nurses come to the workplace. Nurse educators help to prepare novice nurses through curricula that include recognition of the conditions of the stage of ease—becoming, professionalizing, and institutionalizing. To help prepare students for the real world, educators can facilitate dialogue that uncovers sources of conflict between core beliefs, professional traditions, and institutional expectations. They can acknowledge the unique relationship between nurses and patients, recognizing special elements of the relationship such as knowing intimately and witnessing suffering.

Nurse educators can also prepare students for situational binds related to asymmetrical power relationships, loyalty conflicts, and workplace deficiencies. When students practice dealing with these problems in simulated educational circumstances, they may find better ways to deal with situational binds before encountering them in the workplace. Educators might also prepare students for the stage of resolution and the properties of giving up and making a stand in order to be better prepared to follow integrity-preserving courses of action.

Implications for Practicing Nurses

Avoiding situational binds and searching for integrity-saving compromise in morally troubling situations may help practicing nurses engaged in morally troubling situations. A structured discussion of the process of moral reckoning may lead to an increase of satisfaction with nursing care. In these discussion groups nurses can purposely examine core values and their relationship to professional and institutional norms.

CONCLUSION

This middle range theory of moral reckoning encompasses moral distress yet reaches further—identifying a life event experienced through disruption of ease as one confronts a situational bind demanding resolution and reflection. The concepts of the theory—ease, situational bind, resolution, and reflection—name the stages of the basic social process of moral reckoning. The theory has been developed in the context of the discipline of nursing, but its use in other contexts promises meaningful guidance and ongoing development.

REFERENCES

Bamford, P. (1995). *Moral distress: An inability to care.* Unpublished dissertation, Adelphi University, Garden City, NY.

Bassett, C. C. (1995). Critical care nurses: Ethical dilemmas: A phenomenological perspective. *Care of the Critically Ill, 11*(4), 166–168.

Beauchamp, T. L., & Childress, J. F. (2001). *Principles of biomedical ethics* (5th ed.). New York: Oxford University Press.

Burkhardt, M. A., & Nathaniel, A. K. (2008). *Ethics & issues in contemporary nursing* (3rd ed.). New York: Delmar.

Corley, M. C. (1995). Moral distress of critical care nurses. *American Journal of Critical Care, 4*(4), 280–285.

Doutrich, D., Wros, P., & Izumi, S. (2001). Relief of suffering and regard for personhood: Nurses' ethical concerns in Japan and the USA. *Nursing Ethics, 8*(5), 448–458.

Ehrenreich, B., & Ehrenreich, J. (1990). The system behind the chaos. In N. F. McKenzie (Ed.), *The crisis in health care: Ethical issues* (pp. 50–69). New York: Meridian.

Glaser, B. G. (1965). The constant comparative method of qualitative analysis. *Social Problems, 12,* 10.

Glaser, B. G. (1978). *Theoretical sensitivity: Advances in the methodology of grounded theory.* Mill Valley, CA: Sociology Press.

Glaser, B. G. (1998). *Doing grounded theory: Issues and discussion.* Mill Valley, CA: Sociology Press.

Glaser, B. G., & Strauss, A. L. (1967). *The discovery of grounded theory: Strategies for qualitative research.* Chicago: Aldine.

Jameton, A. (1984). *Nursing practice: The ethical issues.* Englewood Cliffs, NJ: Prentice-Hall.

Jameton, A. (1993). Dilemmas of moral distress: Moral responsibility and nursing practice. *Clinical Issues in Perinatal and Women's Health Nursing, 4*(4), 542–551.

Kelly, B. (1998). Preserving moral integrity: A follow-up study with new graduate nurses. *Journal of Advanced Nursing, 28*(5), 1134–1145.

Liaschenko, J. (1995). Artificial personhood: Nursing ethics in a medical world. *Nursing Ethics, 2*(3), 185–196.

MacIntyre, A. C. (1988). *Whose justice? Which rationality?* Notre Dame, IN: University of Notre Dame Press.

Nathaniel, A. K. (2004). A grounded theory of moral reckoning in nursing. *Grounded Theory Review, 4*(1), 43–58.

Nathaniel, A. K. (2006). Moral reckoning in nursing. *Western Journal of Nursing Research, 28*(4), 419–438; discussion 439–448.

Penticuff, J. H. (1987). Neonatal nursing ethics: Toward a consensus. *Neonatal Network, 5*(6), 7–16.

Penticuff, J. H. (1997). Nursing perspectives in bioethics. In K. Hoshino (Ed.), *Japanese and western bioethics* (pp. 49–60). The Dordrecht: Khower Academic Publishers.

Rodney, P. (1988). Moral distress in critical care nursing. *Canadian Critical Care Nursing Journal, 5*(2), 9–11.

Simpson, J. A., & Weiner, E. S. C. (1989). *The Oxford English dictionary, Vol. XIII* (2nd ed.). New York: Oxford University Press.

Smith, M. J., & Liehr, P. (2003). The theory of attentively embracing story. In M. J. Smith & P. Liehr (Eds.), *Middle range theory for nursing* (pp. 167–187). New York: Springer Publishing.

Strauss, A. L. (1959). *Mirrors and masks: The search for identity.* Glencoe, IL: Free Press.

Wilkinson, J. M. (1987). Moral distress in nursing practice: Experience and effect. *Nursing Forum, 23*(1), 16–29.

CHAPTER 16

Evaluation of Middle Range Theories for the Discipline of Nursing

Marlaine C. Smith

Theories are patterned ideas that provide a coherent way of viewing complex phenomena. Middle range theories have a more limited view of circumscribed phenomena than do grand theories. However, because nursing is a professional discipline, all of the theories within it should be evaluated from a perspective that considers the salient elements of the discipline in the evaluation. While there are many sets of criteria for evaluating nursing conceptual models and grand theories (Chinn & Kramer, 2004; Fawcett, 2004; Fitzpatrick & Whall, 2004; Parse, 1987; Stevens, 1998), few focus particularly on theories at the middle range. In addition, there has been little guidance for beginning nursing scholars on the purpose and the process of critical analysis and evaluation of theories. A common course assignment on the evaluation of nursing theory becomes a pedantic exercise, ending in a rather cynical view of theory development. One is reminded of the aphorism, when our only tool is a hammer, all we see are nails. In other words, the tool of critical evaluation taught to students is often weighted toward finding the faults, errors, and inconsistencies within the theoretic structures. It is no wonder that there is evidence of some devaluation of nursing theory and a reticence to engage in its development.

The atheoretical measurement of outcomes of practice, while a worthy endeavor, has eclipsed the compelling need to create systems of thought with potential to describe and explain the nature of phenomena of concern to nursing science. The nursing scholars who contribute to the development of theory for the discipline, including those who are featured in this text, are innovative pioneers who courageously offer their ideas for the advancement of the discipline and the betterment of health care. It is important, then, to balance the identification of theoretic weaknesses with the aspects of appreciation, recognition, and affirmation of their strengths. The purposes of this chapter are to provide tools for a balanced and reasoned evaluation of middle range theory for the discipline of nursing. Describing the purposes of theory evaluation, articulating a set of criteria to guide evaluation of middle range theory, and elaborating a process for conducting this evaluation organize the chapter.

THE PURPOSE OF THEORY EVALUATION: TOWARD A POSTMODERN VIEW

Evaluation is one of the most popular indoor sports of the organizations in which we live. Because these organizations are accountable to various stakeholders, evaluation is used as a measure of assurance and accountability. The meaning of evaluation carries an onerous tone because of baggage that is often attached to it. Students receive grades that reflect evaluation of achievement in a course. A score or category is received when one is evaluated for job performance. Often this evaluation is attached to some reward. The memory of the evaluation of papers, projects, and practice may be more often marked by the red ink of what was done wrong than by what was achieved or done well.

The common, modern definition of evaluation is a process of determining or fixing the value, worth, or significance of something. This definition reflects the anxieties that are experienced surrounding evaluation, connoting the determination of a static and absolute outcome of worth or value. A postmodern meaning of evaluation is quite different. It reflects the presence of subjectivity and contextuality, the diversity of opinions from a community, and, ultimately, the tentative nature of any outcome. It becomes an informed and flawed opinion rendered at a particular moment in time by a person with inherent biases and values. This opinion, which one hopes is not arbitrary or capricious, is based on some sound, reasonable measures or criteria that can be applied consistently. However, it is important to note that the criteria and the evaluator's application of them are value-laden. In this way, they should be viewed not as absolute judgments of worth but as one honest examination by a member of a community.

The evaluation of theory, then, is a process of coming to an opinion about its worth or value. Kaplan (1964), in his discussion of the validation of theory, states that its purpose is to examine a theory's value or worth for advancement by the scientific community. When evaluating nursing theory we ask questions about its worthiness to be used as a guide for inquiry and practice and to be taught to students. Theory, by its definition in any paradigm of science, is a creative constellation of ideas, offered as a possible explanation or description of an observed or experienced phenomenon. In the process of evaluation one is not determining the truth of the theory but its value for further exploration within the scientific community. History affirms the tentative nature of theory evaluation. Theories that were judged by the scientific community as valid were often later abandoned. Ptolemaic theory on the geocentric nature of the planetary system was abandoned later for the Copernican theory that the Earth and the planets revolved around the sun.

Many revolutionary ideas of our time were evaluated initially as worthless. Rogers's (1970) conceptual system, describing the integral nature of human–environment energy fields, was an object of ridicule in the early 1970s. Thirty years later, its correspondence to burgeoning contemporary thought is stunning.

Members of a disciplinary community bear the responsibility to participate in authentic dialogue around ideas within the field of study. The purpose of evaluation of theory in this context is to share in the evolution of the discipline through reflection and comment on the ideas offered up within the community. The greater value of evaluating theory is to participate as individuals in the community's structuring of ideas. While the theory is given to the community, the community re-forms it through critique, testing, and application. The life of any theory is determined by the scientific community's engagement with it. Evaluation of theory is essential to the life of the theory, leading to its extension, revision, and refinement. Based on the preceding discussion, it is important that the evaluator stay true to the purpose of evaluation of theory. The stance of the one evaluating theory from a postmodern perspective is characterized by intellectual empathy, curiosity, honesty, and responsibility. The empathic stance is the attempt to understand the perspective of the theorist and is defined by Paul (1993) as "to imaginatively put oneself in the place of others in order to understand them" (p. 261). Here, the evaluator listens carefully to the point of view. Listening is being aware of one's own biases but trying to put them aside to thoughtfully consider others' ideas, even if the evaluator does not share them. The stance of empathy requires an appreciation of others' points of view and a seeking out of the origin and context of those points of view. Curiosity is the second characteristic of the critical stance. Here, the evaluator raises questions in the process of studying the theory that are born from a quest to understand. The evaluator plays with the theory in different circumstances and imagines ways of testing or understanding it more deeply. The evaluator engages fully in trying to understand and acquire a range of sources on the theory and its application. The third stance is one of honesty. The evaluator trusts individual inner wisdom and recognizes the need to honor that wisdom in sharing the evaluation. Knowing personal biases and limitations, the evaluator is still willing to share reflections on the theory. One of the major hurdles in learning to evaluate theory is to rely on one's own opinions rather than jumping on the bandwagon of others who are considered wiser or more learned. From the postmodern perspective each evaluation should stand on its own, one voice among many diverse ones in the community. It may be difficult to publish negative comments, but it is important to remember that these may be the needed stimuli to make important clarifications or changes in the theory. Finally, the evaluator must be a responsible steward of the discipline. As a member of the scientific community, the evaluator has an obligation to care about the nature of evolution of nursing knowledge. That responsibility entails a thoughtful and scholarly response to the critique, applying the criteria fairly and drawing conclusions that can be useful in the revision or extension of the theory as others use it. Once a theory is published it no longer belongs to the theorist. The voice of the theorist becomes one of many in the community using the theory to guide processes of knowledge development and practice.

In summary, the purpose of a postmodern approach to the evaluation of middle range theory in nursing is to come to a decision about the merits and limitations of the theory for nursing science. The evaluator approaches the evaluation from a stance of empathy, curiosity, honesty, and responsibility. Evaluation of theory is acknowledged as necessary to the evolution of the theory in the context of the scientific community.

THE ORIGIN OF EVALUATIVE FRAMEWORKS

Theories are the language of science. "Science is the process of systematically seeking an understanding of phenomena through creating some unifying or organizing frameworks about the nature of those phenomena. In addition, science involves the evaluation of these frameworks for their credibility and empirical honesty" (Smith, 1994, p. 50). The organizing or unifying frameworks of science are theories. Rigorous and systematic standards of inquiry govern the development and testing of theories. Theories are evaluated for their credibility and empirical honesty by judging them against established standards.

The nature of science, and, therefore, of the theories of science, have undergone change. Philosophies of science have evolved from a sole reliance on the assumptions of logical–positivist views toward expanding philosophies of the post-positivist or postmodern era (Smith, 1998). For example, the traditional or empirical–analytic view of science defines theories as sets of interrelated propositions that describe, explain, or predict the nature of phenomena (Kerlinger, 1986). In the human science view, encompassing phenomenology, hermeneutics, critical, and poststructural perspectives, the purpose of theory is to create an understanding of phenomena through description and interpretation. Therefore, the structural rules, which apply to traditional science, do not apply to human science. For this reason, the frameworks used to evaluate theories must be inclusive enough to encompass these differences.

Kaplan's (1964) perspective on the "validation" of theories is open enough to encompass a diversity of theoretic forms. He emphasizes that the evaluation of any theory is not a matter of pronouncement of its truth. "At any given moment a particular theory will be accepted by some scientists, for some of their purposes, and not by other scientists, or not for other contexts of possible application" (p. 311).

The evaluation of theory involves the exercise of good judgment in determining a relative and tentative truth, and is by its nature normative in that the community ultimately determines the outcome. "The validation of a theory is not the act of granting an imprimatur but the act of deciding that the theory is worth being published, taught, and above all, applied—worth being acted on in contexts of inquiry or of other action" (Kaplan, 1964, p. 312). Kaplan identifies three major philosophical conceptions or norms of truth that can be exercised in the process of evaluating theory: correspondence or semantical norms, coherence or syntactical norms, and pragmatics or functional norms.

The norm of correspondence refers to the substantive meaning of the theory. Through application of this norm, one judges the degree to which the theory fits the facts. While facts are in themselves understood through a theoretic lens, Kaplan argues that this does not necessarily present a tautology. Any theory must in some way pass the test of common sense. While he acknowledges that significant discoveries have flown in the face of common sense, these discoveries in some way could be explained through their relationship to accepted knowledge or some convergence of evidence that supported the plausibility of the theory. Through the norm of correspondence one evaluates the extent to which the theory fits comfortably within the nexus of existing knowledge.

The norm of coherence relates to the integrity of the theory's structure. Kaplan describes the experience of the "click of relation, when widely different and separate phenomena suddenly fall into a pattern of relatedness, when they click into position" (p. 314).

This experience of truth or wholeness occurs when all the fragments of the theory come together to form an integrated whole. Simplicity is the most widely applied norm of coherence. Descriptive simplicity is the quality of expressing the complex ideas of the theory parsimoniously. Inductive simplicity refers to the phenomenon being described by the theory. The theory must encompass a manageable number of ideas; too many will overwhelm the capacity of the theory to serve its purpose to provide a framework for understanding. Kaplan warns that a theory can be too simple in that it goes too far in reducing the complexities. Theories should introduce the degree of complexity necessary for clear understanding, nothing more. He quotes Whitehead's axiom: "Seek simplicity and distrust it" (p. 318). Another norm of coherence is esthetics, that is, the beauty perceived upon the contemplation of the theory. The beauty of the theory involves some sense of symmetry and balance, but Kaplan warns, "Beauty is not truth" (p. 319). The process of developing theory is creative, and that creativity is expressed in a product that possesses an aesthetic quality.

The final norm is pragmatics and refers to the effectiveness or functional capability of the theory. In a professional discipline, the norm of pragmatics instructs us to consider the degree to which the theory can guide practice and research to advance the goals of the discipline. On the other hand, Kaplan states that the theory is not judged by the extent to which it makes some external difference alone; he acknowledges that other factors might interfere with or enhance the success of application. The theory is also judged by what it can do for science, "how it guides and stimulates the ongoing process of scientific inquiry" (pp. 319–320). So the degree to which the theory has spawned research questions is relevant. "The value of the theory lies not only in the answers it gives but also in the new questions it raises" (p. 320).

A theory is validated when it is put to good use in the application of concerns to the discipline. The evaluative framework for middle range theories is based on these norms. Criteria will be clustered into the following three categories: substantive foundation, structural integrity, and functional adequacy.

An abundance of evaluative frameworks for nursing theories have evolved over the past several decades (Chinn & Kramer, 2004; Fawcett, 2004; Fitzpatrick & Whall, 2004; Parse, 1987; Stevens, 1998). Some of these frameworks are applicable to middle range theories while others are not. Liehr and Smith (1999) summarized the literature about the nature of middle range theories. They concluded that middle range theories are identified by their scope, level of abstraction, and proximity to empirical findings. Scope refers to the breadth of phenomena addressed by the theory. Compared to conceptual models and grand theories, middle range theories offer constellations of ideas or concepts about more circumscribed phenomena of concern to the discipline. In this way they are intermediate in scope, focusing on a limited number of concepts focused on a limited aspect of reality (Liehr & Smith, 1999). Level of abstraction locates middle range theories between the abstract level of conceptual models and grand theories and situation-specific theories. The language of middle range theory describes concepts and relationships between them more concretely. Finally, middle range theories are more proximal to empirical findings than are conceptual models and grand theories. They are developed through an analysis of empirical findings or at a level of immediate testability. These three qualities of middle range theories should be represented in the evaluative frameworks for them.

The following criteria (Table 16.1) have been developed from Kaplan's norms for validating theories and are informed by the essential qualities of middle range theories to create an evaluative framework specific to theories of the middle range.

Substantive Foundation

Substantive foundation is the first category of criteria for the evaluation of middle range theory in nursing. This category includes criteria based

TABLE 16.1   Framework for the Evaluation of Middle Range Theories

Substantive Foundations

1. The theory is within the focus of the discipline of nursing.
2. The assumptions are specified and are congruent with the focus.
3. The theory provides a substantive description, explanation, or interpretation of a named phenomenon at the middle range level of discourse.
4. The origins are rooted in practice and research experience.

Structural Integrity

1. The concepts are clearly defined.
2. The concepts within the theory are at the middle range level of abstraction.
3. There are no more concepts than needed to explain the phenomenon.
4. The concepts and relationships among them are logically represented with a model.

Functional Adequacy

1. The theory can be applied to a variety of practice environments and client groups.
2. Empirical indicators have been identified for concepts of the theory.
3. There are published examples of use of the theory in practice.
4. There are published examples of research related to the theory.
5. The theory has evolved through scholarly inquiry.

on Kaplan's norm of correspondence and leads to questions about the meaning or semantic elements of the theory. A middle range theory in nursing contributes to the knowledge of the discipline of nursing and is developed from assumptions that are clearly specified. The theory provides knowledge that is at the middle range level of abstraction. There are four major criteria related to substantive meaning: (1) the theory is within the focus of the discipline of nursing, (2) the assumptions are specified and are congruent with the focus of the discipline of nursing, (3) the theory provides a substantive description, explanation, or interpretation of a named phenomenon at the middle range level of discourse, and (4) the origins are rooted in practice and research experience. Each of these criteria and the questions that guide the application of the criteria in evaluating the theory will be discussed. The first criterion emphasizes that a middle range theory in nursing is judged by its location in and contribution to the discipline of nursing. The question, "What makes a middle range theory in nursing a *nursing* theory?" is interesting to consider. Some (Fawcett, 2004; Parse, 1987) assert that nursing theories are only those identified as the conceptual models and grand theories developed by nurses in the 1960s through the 1980s. From this perspective, legitimate middle range theories in nursing are those deduced from or inductively developed within existing conceptual models and grand theories of nursing. This is problematic in that it fixates theory development in what has been considered legitimate in the past. It is important to leave space for the possibility of emergent conceptual models or grand constructions that may be articulated as sets of foundational assumptions upon which middle range theories are constructed. The evaluator should expect that a middle range theory in nursing contributes to knowledge about human–environment health relationships, caring in the human health experience, and/or health and healing processes (Fawcett, 2004; Newman, Sime, & Corcoran-Perry, 1991; Smith, 1994). It should be possible to locate the theory within a paradigmatic perspective endorsed by nursing, such as the particulate–deterministic, interactive–integrative, unitary–transformative schema (Newman et al., 1991), the totality or simultaneity paradigm (Parse, 1987), or the reaction, reciprocal interaction, or simultaneous worldview (Fawcett, 2004).

The second criterion regarding the specification of assumptions in the category of substantive foundations is that the origins and ontological foundations of the theory are specified. The developer of the middle range theory holds philosophical assumptions that are either explicitly stated or implied by the meaning of the theory. Fawcett (2004) argues that the belief that middle range theory is developed outside the context of a conceptual frame of reference is absurd. She emphasizes the contextual nature of theory building. The assumptions of a middle range theory identify the context for theory building and should be identifiable. A stronger middle range theory would explicate the assumptions.

The ideas of parent theories or models should be clearly identified in the explication of the meaning of the theory. The developers should cite primary sources from any parent theories that may be accessed for greater depth in understanding. While some middle range theories will not be explicitly derived from nursing conceptual models, parent ideas that shaped theory development would be clearly described.

Finally, the meaning of the theory should be consistent with its foundational assumptions. This consistency is essential. If Rogers's Science of Unitary Human Beings (SUHB) forms the assumptions of a middle range theory, the meaning of the concepts within the theory should not violate these assumptions. One would not use the language of adaptive responses in a theory purportedly derived from the SUHB. If the assumptions are not derived from an existing conceptual model/grand theory, the synthesized assumptions provide a frame of reference for this analysis. Without this, one is left to analyze inferred foundations and how the middle range theory corresponds to their meaning.

The third criterion related to substantive meaning states that the middle range theory provides substantive knowledge about a named circumscribed phenomenon of concern to nursing. Liehr and Smith (1999) contend that a middle range theory is known by the way it is named and that it should be "named in the context of the disciplinary perspective and at the appropriate level of discourse" (p. 86). Middle range theory is defined by its focus on providing knowledge about a specific phenomenon of concern to nursing. The theory should offer a substantive description, explanation, or interpretation of this particular phenomenon that leads to a new understanding or different way of considering the phenomenon. It is incumbent on the developer of the theory to provide adequate explanation substantiated by logical reasoning and reference to existing knowledge sources that lead to a full understanding of the meaning of the concepts and their relationships to each other.

Finally, the theory should capture the complexities of the phenomenon that it addresses. A theory is a map of some aspect of reality; like a map it cannot capture the landscape. However, to the extent possible the theory should approximate the fullest range of conceptual relationships that it addresses.

The fourth criterion deals with the rooting of the origins of the theory in practice and research experience. Middle range theory grows out of the research and practice experiences of nurses, who articulate a set of concepts to describe and explain a phenomenon that they have observed in their work. The evaluator will seek out the practice and research roots of the theory. It may be that one set of roots (practice or research) is sturdier than the other. This assessment may indicate a next direction for further application of the theory. Well-developed middle range theory will have documented development related to both practice and research.

Structural Integrity

A middle range theory is a framework that organizes ideas. Like any framework, it has a structure. The structure provides strength, balance, and the aesthetic qualities that ensure its integrity. Structural integrity is the category that was derived from Kaplan's (1964) norm of coherence. There are four criteria for evaluation of the structural integrity of middle range theories: (1) the concepts are clearly defined, (2) the concepts of the theory are at the middle range level of abstraction, (3) there are no more concepts than are needed to explain the phenomenon, and (4) the concepts and relationships among them are logically represented with a model. The four criteria for structural integrity and their application are discussed below.

The first criterion is that the ideas and the relationships among them are clearly presented within the theory. Concepts are the names given to the abstract ideas that constitute the theory. The relationships among the ideas are developed into statements or propositions. In any middle range theory, the concepts within it should be clearly defined. Any neologisms (newly coined terms) should be adequately defined. The relationship statements, whether called propositions or not, should articulate the relationships among the central ideas or concepts within the theory. Concepts, even within the context of middle range theory, are abstractions, and, as such, it takes some willingness to understand them. However, the definitions should lead to this understanding and provide precise meaning.

The second criterion related to structural integrity is that the ideas of the theory are at the middle range level of abstraction. All concepts should be on the ladder of abstraction at a similar level. For example, health may be considered a concept at the metaparadigm level; adaptation, at the level of grand theory; and anxiety, at the level of the middle range. Mixing these as concepts within one theory would be an example of concepts at differing levels of abstraction. Similarly, the concepts in the theory should consistently be presented at the middle range level, more concrete and circumscribed than concepts at a higher level of abstraction. The deductive or inductive processes of theory development should be transparent in the presentation of the theory. Movement up the ladder of abstraction to paradigms or down the ladder to empirical indicators should be logical, reasoned, and clear.

The third criterion is that there should be no more concepts than necessary to describe the theory as named. The theory should be organized and presented parsimoniously. That means that the ideas should be synthesized and communicated in the simplest, most elegant way possible. Extraneous concepts or unclear differentiation of concepts creates complexity that confuses rather than clarifies.

The fourth or final criterion is that the ideas of the theory are integrated to create an understanding of the whole phenomenon, which is presented in a model. This criterion leads to consideration of the internal consistency, balance, and aesthetics of the theory. The concepts and statements of the theory should be logically ordered so that they lead to an appreciation and apprehension of the theory meaning. The relationships among the ideas can be represented in a schema, a model, or a list of logically ordered statements. In any case, it is the responsibility of the developer to make these relationships accessible. All ideas (concepts and related statements) in the theory should have semantic congruence, that is, the meanings should not be contradictory. Middle range theories are creative products of science. As such, there should be balance and harmony in the way they are presented.

Functional Adequacy

For a professional discipline, functional adequacy is arguably the acid test of a middle range theory. Middle range theories are closely tied to research and practice. They may be generated from research findings or deduced from larger models to form a set of testable hypotheses. They may have been developed in relation to a practice dilemma, and they can be used to create practice guidelines. Middle range theories build nursing knowledge and are valuable in and of themselves for this contribution. There are five criteria for functional adequacy of middle range theories: (1) the theory can be applied to a variety of practice environments and client groups, (2) empirical indicators have been identified for concepts of the theory, (3) there are published examples of use of the theory in practice, (4) there are published examples of research related to the theory, and (5) the theory has evolved through scholarly inquiry. Each of these criteria will be described below.

The first criterion of functional adequacy is that the theory is able to provide guidance for a variety of practice populations and environments. One would expect literature that documents use of the theory with more than one population and in more than one setting. Because the theory is middle range rather than situation specific, this generality criterion is important and limited to the central phenomenon of the theory.

The second criterion is that there are empirical indicators identified for the concepts of the theory. Empirical adequacy is an essential aspect of middle range theory. Empirics are meant to go beyond empiricism and include perceptions, symbolic meanings, self-reports, observable behavior, biological indicators, and personal stories (Ford-Gilboe, Campbell, & Berman, 1995; Reed, 1995). Researchers working with the middle range theory may have selected empirical indicators for measurement of theoretical constructs or they may have developed the middle range theory from descriptions and stories. Both of these examples support the theory's empirical adequacy. Empirical adequacy is an indication of the maturity of the theory.

The third criterion is that there are published examples of how the theory has been used in practice. This criterion offers evidence to support that the theory makes a difference in the lives of people. Published reports of the theory should demonstrate that use of the theory enhances well-being and quality of life. When the middle range theory is taken to practice there are expectations about emergent outcomes. These outcomes may be identified and tested by those conducting evaluation studies on theory-guided practice.

The fourth criterion is that there are published examples of research related to the theory. This criterion is a strong indicator of functional adequacy. The research findings can be examined for the level of support of the theory. In addition, middle range theories may generate hypotheses or research questions. Any refinements to the theory based on research findings should be examined; this indicates that the theory is open enough to change through the incorporation of further testing or development of ideas. In the process of evaluating this criterion, it is important to examine the evolution of the theory over time through inquiry and reflection.

The fifth criterion is that the theory has evolved through scholarly inquiry. Theories should evoke thinking, raise questions, invite dialogue, and urge us toward further exploration. This engaging quality of the theory is a hallmark of its potential for advancing the discipline. In order for the theory to grow, a community of scholars must engage with it in practice and research. Middle range theories build the discipline of nursing through expanding knowledge related to specific phenomena. The speculations offered by the theory push the boundaries of what is currently known and will invite continuing systematic inquiry. In this way the theory evolves and contributes to the development of nursing science and art.

APPLYING THE FRAMEWORK TO THE
EVALUATION OF MIDDLE RANGE THEORIES

The evaluation of middle range theory involves preparation, judgment, and justification. In the preparation phase those evaluating the theory should spend time understanding the theory as fully as possible through dwelling with it. Dwelling with is investing time in reading and reflecting on the theory. The elements of the critical stance—empathy, curiosity, honesty, and responsibility, as articulated earlier in this chapter—are applied during preparation. It is important to gather a variety of sources on and about the theory, including primary sources written by the author of the theory, research reports, critiques, and practice papers. Reading the theory repeatedly to understand the ideas is the first step. In this process of beginning analysis, it is important to identify the central ideas and the structure of the theory. Middle range theories are developed from parent theories, empirical findings, or practice insights. Depth in understanding a theory may require going to the source documents that were critical to its development. Critical evaluation requires attending to questions and reactions to the theory that surface during the reading. It is important to record these questions and reactions. The next step in preparation is studying the practice and research reports related to the theory. Note how the theory was tested or extended through research. Examine how the theory has been applied in practice and any outcome studies that relate to the application of practice approaches or models based on the theory. Written critiques by others will provide another source of information. Because they may interfere with or unduly influence one's own evaluation, it is preferable to read those critiques or evaluations after one's own is completed.

The judgment phase is the heart of the evaluative process. In this phase the evaluator reads and reflects on the criteria in the evaluative framework. The evaluator trusts self as the instrument of judgment, one who has seriously and rigorously engaged in studying the theory. The evaluator reflects on and refers to the notes and responses created during the analysis process. The criteria in the evaluative framework are a guide toward making decisions about the meaning, structure, and practice and research applications. The strengths and the weaknesses of the theory should receive equal weight in the judgment phase. Both of these elements of the evaluation can contribute to the development of the theory. In the justification phase the evaluator supports judgments with explicit reasons for the decisions and with examples that illustrate points. In this phase the evaluator can refer to other written critiques that may support or refute judgments about the theory. The evaluation is written in a narration structured by the criteria in the framework. Each criterion is addressed through weaving judgments and support of those judgments. A balanced evaluation identifies both the strengths and limitations of the theory and suggests specific recommendations for clarification, extension, or revision.

The goal of this chapter was to explicate the purpose, structure, and process of evaluating middle range theories. Middle range theories are at the frontier of nursing science. The development of substantive knowledge through middle range theories promises movement toward disciplinary maturity. These theories will direct and spawn new inquiry and will stimulate the development of nursing practice approaches to enhance health and well-being. The evaluation of nursing theory is an essential activity within the scientific community. It leads to the advancement, refinement, and extension of substantive knowledge in the discipline. It is a critical skill of any scholar and is honed through practice and mentoring.

REFERENCES

Chinn, P. L., & Kramer, M. K. (2004). *Integrated knowledge development in nursing.* St. Louis: Mosby.

Fawcett, J. (2004). *Analysis and evaluation of contemporary nursing knowledge.* Philadelphia: F. A. Davis.

Fitzpatrick, J. J., & Whall, A. L. (2004). *Conceptual models of nursing.* Stamford, CT: Appleton & Lange.

Ford-Gilboe, M., Campbell, J., & Berman, H. (1995). Stories and numbers: Coexistence without compromise. *Advances in Nursing Science, 18,* 14–26.

Kaplan, A. (1964). *The conduct of inquiry.* San Francisco: Chandler.

Kerlinger, F. N. (1986). *Foundations of behavioral research* (3rd ed.). New York: Holt, Rinehart & Winston.

Liehr, P., & Smith, M. J. (1999). Middle range theory: Spinning research and practice to create knowledge for the new millennium. *Advances in Nursing Science, 21*(4), 81–91.

Newman, M. A., Sime, A. M., & Corcoran-Perry, S. A. (1991). Focus of the discipline of nursing. *Advances in Nursing Science, 14*(1), 1–6.

Parse, R. R. (1987). *Nursing science: Major paradigms, theories, and critiques.* Philadelphia: W. B. Saunders.

Paul, R. (1993). *Critical thinking: How to prepare students for a rapidly changing world.* Santa Rosa, CA: Foundation for Critical Thinking.

Reed, P. (1995). Treatise on nursing knowledge development for the 21st century: Beyond postmodernism. *Advances in Nursing Science, 17,* 70–84.

Rogers, M. E. (1970). *An introduction to the theoretical basis of nursing.* Philadelphia: F. A. Davis.

Smith, M. C. (1994). Arriving at a philosophy of nursing: Discovering? Constructing? Evolving? In J. Kikuchi & H. Simmons (Eds.), *Developing a philosophy of nursing* (pp. 43–60). Thousand Oaks, CA: Sage.

Smith, M. C. (1998). Knowledge building for the health sciences in the twenty-first century. *Journal of Sport and Exercise Psychology, 20,* S128–S144.

Stevens, B. (1998). *Nursing theory: Analysis, application, evaluation.* Boston: Little, Brown.

Appendix

MIDDLE RANGE THEORIES: 1988–2007

TABLE A.1

Year	Full Citation (APA)	Name of Theory
1988	Mishel, M. H. (1988). Uncertainty in illness. *Image: Journal of Nursing Scholarship, 20*(4), 225–231.	Uncertainty in illness
1990	Mishel, M. H. (1990). Reconceptualization of the uncertainty in illness theory. *Image: Journal of Nursing Scholarship, 22*(4), 256–262.	
1989	Thompson, J. E., Oakley, D., Burke, M., Jay, S., & Conklin, M. (1989). Theory building in nurse-midwifery: The care process. *Journal of Nurse-Midwifery, 34*(3), 120–130.	Nurse midwifery care
1990	Kinney, C. K. (1990). Facilitating growth and development: A paradigm case for modeling and role-modeling. *Issues in Mental Health Nursing, 11,* 375–395.	Facilitating growth and development

(Continued)

307

TABLE A.1 *(Continued)*

Year	Full Citation (APA)	Name of Theory
1991	Reed, P. G. (1991). Toward a nursing theory of self-transcendence: Deductive reformulation using developmental theories. *Advances in Nursing Science, 13*(4), 64–77.	Self-transcendence
1991	Burke, S. O., Kauffmann, E., Costello, E. A., & Dillon, M. C. (1991). Hazardous secrets and reluctantly taking charge: Parenting a child with repeated hospitalizations. *Image: Journal of Nursing Scholarship, 23*(1), 39–45.	Hazardous secrets and reluctantly taking charge
1991	Thomas, S. P. (1991). Toward a new conceptualization of women's anger. *Issues in Mental Health Nursing, 12,* 31–49.	Women's anger
1991	Swanson, K. M. (1991). Empirical development of a middle range theory of caring. *Nursing Research, 40*(3), 161–166.	Caring
1994	Powell-Cope, G. M. (1994). Family caregivers of people with AIDS: Negotiating partnerships with professional health care providers. *Nursing Research, 43*(6), 324–330.	Negotiating partnership
1995	Lenz, E. R., Suppe, F., Gift, A. G., Pugh, L. C., & Milligan, R. A. (1995). Collaborative development of middle-range nursing theories: Toward a theory of unpleasant symptoms. *Advances in Nursing Science, 17*(3), 1–13.	Unpleasant symptoms
1997	Lenz, E. R., Pugh, L. C., Milligan, R. A., Gift, A., & Suppe, F. (1997). The middle-range theory of unpleasant symptoms: An update. *Advances in Nursing Science, 19*(3), 14–27.	Unpleasant symptoms
1995	Jezewski, M. A. (1995). Evolution of a grounded theory: Conflict resolution through culture brokering. *Advances in Nursing Science, 17*(3), 14–30.	Cultural brokering

TABLE A.1 *(Continued)*

Year	Full Citation (APA)	Name of Theory
1995	Tollett, J. H., & Thomas, S. P. (1995). A theory-based nursing intervention to instill hope in homeless veterans. *Advances in Nursing Science, 18*(2), 76–90.	Homelessness-hopelessness
1996	Good, M., & Moore, S. M. (1996). Clinical practice guidelines as a new source of middle-range theory: Focus on acute pain. *Nursing Outlook, 44*(2), 74–79.	Balance between analgesia and side effects
1998	Good, M. (1998). A middle-range theory of acute pain management: Use in research. *Nursing Outlook, 46*(3), 120–124.	Acute pain management
1997	Auvil-Novak, S. E. (1997). A middle-range theory of chronotherapeutic intervention for postsurgical pain. *Nursing Research, 46*(2), 66–70.	Chronotherapeutic intervention for postsurgical pain
1997	Olson, J., & Hanchett, E. (1997). Nurse-expressed empathy, patient outcomes, and development of a middle-range theory. *Image: Journal of Nursing Scholarship, 29*(1), 71–76.	Nurse-expressed empathy and patient distress
1997	Brooks, E. M., & Thomas, S. (1997). The perception and judgment of senior baccalaureate student nurses in clinical decision making. *Advances in Nursing Science, 19*(3), 50–69.	Intrapersonal perceptual awareness
1997	Polk, L. V. (1997). Toward a middle-range theory of resilience. *Advances in Nursing Science, 19*(3), 1–13.	Resilience
1997	Gerdner, L. (1997). An individualized music intervention for agitation. *Journal of the American Psychiatric Nurses Association, 3*(6), 177–184.	Individualized music intervention for agitation
1997	Acton, G. J. (1997). Affiliated-individuation as a mediator of stress and burden in caregivers of adults with dementia. *Journal of Holistic Nursing, 15*(4), 336–357.	Affiliated individuation as mediator of stress

(Continued)

TABLE A.1 *(Continued)*

Year	Full Citation (APA)	Name of Theory
1998	Eakes, G. G., Burke, M. L., & Hainsworth, M. A. (1998). Middle-range theory of chronic sorrow. *Image: Journal of Nursing Scholarship, 30*(2), 179–184.	Chronic sorrow
1998	Huth, M. M., & Moore, S. M. (1998). Prescriptive theory of acute pain management in infants and children. *Journal of the Society of Pediatric Nurses, 3*(1), 23–32.	Acute pain management in infants and children
1998	Levesque, L., Ricard, N., Ducharme, F., Duquette, A., & Bonin, J. (1998). Empirical verification of a theoretical model derived from the Roy Adaptation Model: Findings from five studies. *Nursing Science Quarterly, 11*(1), 31–39.	Psychological adaptation
1998	Ruland, C. M., & Moore, S. M. (1998). Theory construction based on standards of care: A proposed theory of the peaceful end of life. *Nursing Outlook, 46*(4), 169–175.	Peaceful end of life
1998	Kearney, M. H. (1998). Truthful self-nurturing: A grounded formal theory of women's addiction recovery. *Qualitative Health Research, 8*(4), 495–512.	Truthful self-nurturing
1998	Burns, C. M. (1998). A retroductive theoretical model of the pathway to chemical dependency in nurses. *Archives of Psychiatric Nursing, 21*(1), 59–65.	Pathway to chemical dependency in nurses
1999	Jirovec, M. M., Jenkins, J., Isenberg, M., & Baiardi, J. (1999). Urine control theory derived from Roy's conceptual framework. *Nursing Science Quarterly, 12*(3), 251–255.	Urine control theory
1999	Smith, A. A., & Friedemann, M. (1999). Perceived family dynamics of persons with chronic pain. *Journal of Advanced Nursing, 30*(3), 543–551.	Family dynamics of persons with chronic pain

TABLE A.1 *(Continued)*

Year	Full Citation (APA)	Name of Theory
1999	Smith, M. J., & Liehr, P. (1999). Attentively embracing story: A middle-range theory with practice and research implications. *Scholarly Inquiry for Nursing Practice: An International Journal, 13*(3), 187–204.	Attentively embracing story
2000	Doornbos, M. M. (2000). King's systems frameworks and family health: The derivation and testing of a theory. *The Journal of Theory Construction & Testing, 4*(1), 20–26.	Family health
2000	Meleis, A. I., Sawyer, L. M., Im, E., Messias, D. K. H., & Schumacher, K. (2000). Experiencing transitions: An emerging middle-range theory. *Advances in Nursing Science, 23*(1), 12–28.	Experiencing transitions
2000	August-Brady, M. (2000). Prevention as intervention. *Journal of Advanced Nursing, 31*(6), 1304–1308.	Prevention as intervention
2000	Leenerts, M. H., & Magilvy, J. (2000). Investing in self-care: A midrange theory of self-care grounded in the lived experience of low-income HIV-positive white women. *Advances in Nursing Science, 22*(3), 58–75.	Self-care
2000	Sanford, R. C. (2000). Caring through relation and dialogue: A nursing perspective for patient education. *Advances in Nursing Science, 22*(3), 1–15.	Caring through relation and dialogue for patient education
2001	Wuest, J. (2001). Precarious ordering: Toward a formal theory of women's caring. *Health Care for Women International, 22*, 167–193.	Precarious ordering: Theory of women's caring
2001	Kolcaba, K. (2001). Evolution of the mid range theory of comfort for outcomes research. *Nursing Outlook, 49*(2), 86–92.	Comfort

(Continued)

TABLE A.1 *(Continued)*

Year	Full Citation (APA)	Name of Theory
2001	Hills, R. G. S., & Hanchett, E. (2001). Human change and individuation in pivotal life situations: Development and testing the theory of enlightenments. *Visions, 9*(1), 6–19.	Enlightenment
2001	Engebretson, J., & Littleton, L. Y. (2001). Cultural negotiation: A constructivist-based model for nursing practice. *Nursing Outlook, 49*(5), 223–230.	Cultural negotiation
2001	Woods, S. J., & Isenberg, M. A. (2001). Adaptation as a mediator of intimate abuse and traumatic stress in battered women. *Nursing Science Quarterly, 14*(3), 215–221.	Adaptation as a mediator of intimate abuse and traumatic stress in battered women
2002	Barnes, S., & Adair, B. (2002). The cognition-sensitive approach to dementia: Parallels with the science of unitary human beings. *Journal of Psychosocial Nursing and Mental Health Services, 40*(11), 30–37.	The cognition-sensitive approach to dementia
2002	Smith, C. E., Pace, K., Kochinda, C., Kleinbeck, S. V. M., Koehler, J., & Popkess-Vawter, S. (2002). Caregiving effectiveness model evolution to a midrange theory of home care: A process for critique and replication. *Advances in Nursing Science, 25*(1), 50–64.	Caregiving effectiveness
2002	Roux, G., Dingley, C. E., & Bush, H. A. (2002). Inner strength in women: metasynthesis of qualitative findings in theory development. *Journal of Theory Construction and Testing, 6*(1), 86–93.	Inner strength in women
2002	Whittemore, R., & Roy, C. (2002). Adapting to diabetes mellitus: A theory synthesis. *Nursing Science Quarterly, 15*(4), 311–317.	Adapting to diabetes mellitus

TABLE A.1 *(Continued)*

Year	Full Citation (APA)	Name of Theory
2003	Lawson, L. (2003). Becoming a success story: How boys who have molested children talk about treatment. *Journal of Psychiatric and Mental Health Nursing, 10,* 259–268.	Becoming a success story
2003	Tsai, P. (2003). A middle-range theory of caregiver stress. *Nursing Science Quarterly, 16*(2), 137–145.	Caregiver stress
2003	Tsai, P., Tak, S., Moore, C., & Palencia, I. (2003). Testing a theory of chronic pain. *Journal of Advanced Nursing, 43*(2), 158–169.	Chronic pain
2003	Dorsey, C. J., & Murdaugh, C. L. (2003). The theory of self-care management for vulnerable populations. *The Journal of Theory Construction & Testing, 7*(2), 43–49.	Self-care management for vulnerable populations
2004	Walton, J., & Sullivan, N. (2004). Men of prayer: Spirituality of men with prostate cancer. *Journal of Holistic Nursing, 22*(2), 133–151.	Spirituality
2004	Dunn, K. S. (2004). Toward a middle-range theory of adaptation to chronic pain. *Nursing Science Quarterly, 17*(1), 78–84.	Adaptation to chronic pain
2005	Dunn, K. S. (2005). Testing a middle-range theoretical model of adaptation to chronic pain. *Nursing Science Quarterly, 18*(2), 146–156.	Adaptation to chronic pain
2004	Mefford, L. C. (2004). A theory of health promotion for preterm infants based on Levine's Conservation Model of Nursing. *Nursing Science Quarterly, 17*(3), 260–266.	Health promotion for preterm infants
2006	Register, M. E., & Herman, J. (2006). A middle range theory for generative quality of life for the elderly. *Advances in Nursing Science, 29*(4), 340–350.	Generative quality of life for the elderly

(Continued)

TABLE A.1 *(Continued)*

Year	Full Citation (APA)	Name of Theory
2006	Peters, R. M. (2006). The relationship to racism, chronic stress emotions, and blood pressure. *Journal of Nursing Scholarship, 38*(3), 234–240.	Chronic stress emotions
2006	Johnson, M. E., & Delaney, K. R. (2006). Keeping the unit safe: A grounded theory study. *Journal of the American Psychiatric Nurses Association, 12*(1), 13–21.	Violence prevention
2007	Bu, X., & Jezewski, M. A. (2007). Developing a mid-range theory of patient advocacy through concept analysis. *Journal of Advanced Nursing, 57*(1), 101–110.	Patient advocacy
2007	Penrod, J., Yu, F., Kolanowski, A., Fick, D. M., Loeb, S. J. & Hupcey, J. E. (2007). Reframing person-centered nursing care for persons with dementia. *Research and Theory for Nursing Practice: An International Journal, 21*(1), 57–72.	Need driven dementia—compromised behavior

Index

Middle Range Theory Development Using King's Conceptual System

Christina Leibold Sieloff, PhD, RN, CNA
Maureen A. Frey, RN, PhD, Editors

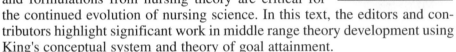

"This book...provides a fresh look at the development and testing of nursing knowledge and includes new middle-range theories from refereed publications as well as master's theses and doctoral dissertations."

—Doody's Book Review Service

Continuing development and testing of propositions and formulations from nursing theory are critical for the continued evolution of nursing science. In this text, the editors and contributors highlight significant work in middle range theory development using King's conceptual system and theory of goal attainment.

Explored in the three sections of this volume are:

- An overview of the foundations on which middle range theories are built from within King's conceptual system, including a chapter by Dr. King

- Presentation of a variety of middle range theories applied to individuals, groups and families, and organizations—from children to the elderly

- Examination of post-middle range theory development and challenges for further nursing research and education

Each chapter has a consistent format and includes a wide range of perspectives and geographical locations, allowing readers to compare knowledge-building efforts across international lines.

2007 · 336pp · 978-0-8261-0238-6 · Softcover

11 West 42nd Street, New York, NY 10036-8002 • Fax: 212-941-7842
Order Toll-Free: 877-687-7476 • Order Online: www.springerpub.com